PRAISE FOR

The Patient Will See You Now

"Eric Topol has written a must-read manifesto for patients who feel helpless. Filled with knowledge and engaging stories, this book shows how you can harness technology to be the master of your medical care—or at least, a better partner for your doctor. I want Dr. Topol for my doctor."

—ELISABETH ROSENTHAL, M.D., *The New York Times*

"It's your blood, your DNA, and your money; shouldn't the images, records, and data belong to you, too? Dr. Topol's deeply researched, powerfully presented arguments will ruffle feathers in the medical establishment—but he maintains that the new era of smartphones, apps, and tiny sensors is putting the patient in charge for the first time. And he's right."

—DAVID POGUE, FOUNDER OF YAHOO TECH
AND HOST OF PBS' "NOVA"

"Dr. Eric Topol is uniquely positioned to map out a new era of democratized medicine—a time when each individual will not only have immediate access to all of their own medical data, but even generate much of it and play a principal role in their healthcare."

—SANJAY GUPTA, M.D.,
CHIEF MEDICAL CORRESPONDENT FOR CNN

"We are seeing a sea-change in medicine, a time when the old paradigms no longer apply. As a physician and a scientist, Eric Topol has been both contributor and commentator to this revolution and therefore, one of the few people who can weave together and explain the stunning advances in seemingly unrelated fields. His personal voice, his ability to explain the most complex developments in science in a simple and engaging manner, and the clarity of his vision of the future make this compelling reading. I couldn't put this book down and I learned so much. It has changed my perspective of what is to come."

—ABRAHAM VERGHESE, AUTHOR OF *Cutting for Stone*

"Topol expertly builds upon his earlier path-finding work and explores how smartphone adoption, big data, new digital monitors of medically relevant information streams, ubiquitous computing, and larger networks are all combining to revolutionize health care far beyond what most now expect—with the exciting promise of lower costs and higher quality simultaneously. Coming from a world-class physician with a unique perspective on the rapidly changing nature of medicine, Topol's prescription for patient empowerment is a must read."

—AL GORE,
FORMER VICE PRESIDENT OF THE UNITED STATES

"The most extraordinary time for health care lies ahead. Dr. Topol presents a highly innovative vision and model for how, in an era of big data for each individual, medicine can be democratized."

—MITT ROMNEY, FORMER GOVERNOR OF MASSACHUSETTS

"Dr. Eric Topol is a pioneer of the medicine of the future and the future is now! Read this book and empower yourself for total well-being." —DEEPAK CHOPRA

"I have experienced Dr. Topol's healing touch as my personal physician after a 99% heart blockage, in his capacity as cardiology advisor to *Men's Health* magazine's 12 million readers, and as the visionary author of *The Creative Destruction of Medicine*. With *The Patient Will See You Now*, he's extending his healing powers where they'll do the most good: to the patients themselves. Book an appointment to read it now, and you'll save yourself a lot of copays later."

—PETER MOORE, EDITOR OF *Men's Health* MAGAZINE

"Eric Topol's book focuses us on the most important development in health care today: putting the patient at the center of everything. This is the pathway to the most effective and efficient innovation, development and reform of health care practices, products and policies globally."

—ALEX GORSKY, CEO OF JOHNSON & JOHNSON

"Dr. Topol clearly captures the challenges and major disruptions occurring in medicine today. A revolution in healthcare is finally happening—one that will not only improve outcomes, but the individual patient's experience. This is a book that everyone needs to read. The practice and future of medicine are indeed being turned upside down."

—JOHN E. KELLY III, DIRECTOR OF RESEARCH AT IBM

"Dr. Eric Topol has the vision for how smartphones will play a central part in health care in the coming years. Consumers will take on a powerful new role in medicine of the future—*The Patient Will See You Now* reveals to us how that will occur."

—JK SHIN, PRESIDENT AND CEO OF SAMSUNG ELECTRONICS

"In *The Patient Will See You Now*, Dr. Eric Topol has helped to define a new era in healthcare when the role of the patient has evolved, empowered by the rapid adoption of digital health technologies. We fully agree with Dr. Topol's vision of the future of healthcare becoming increasingly seamless and giving consumers access to care—where, when, and at the value point they want." —GREG WASSON, CEO OF WALGREENS

"Eric Topol understands better than anybody else the growing battle between technology- and information-empowered patients on one side, and the incumbent medical establishment on the other. He also understands who should win it. Read this book and you'll join him in fighting the good fight."
—ANDREW MCAFEE, AUTHOR OF *The Second Machine Age*

"In this extraordinary book, Topol has, in effect, provided us with a prescription for the future of medicine. He outlines the challenges of the current practice of medicine, and gives us a powerful vision of what can be changed—and how. Topol writes about the future more effectively than any physician or scientist that I know. If you want to know about what medicine looks like today, you should read this book. But if you want to know what medicine will look like tomorrow, then you must absolutely read this book."
—SIDDHARTA MUHKERJEE, M.D., AUTHOR OF
The Emperor of All Maladies: A Biography of Cancer

The Patient Will See You Now

ALSO BY ERIC TOPOL

The Creative Destruction of Medicine

THE PATIENT WILL SEE YOU NOW

The Future of Medicine Is in Your Hands

ERIC TOPOL

BASIC BOOKS
New York

Library of Congress Cataloging-in-Publication Data
  Topol, Eric J., 1954-
  The patient will see you now : the future of medicine is in your hands / Eric Topol.
    pages cm
  Includes bibliographical references and index.
  ISBN 978-0-465-05474-9 (hardback)—ISBN 978-0-465-04054-4 (ebook) 1. Medicine—Data processing—Social aspects. 2. Medical informatics—Social aspects. 3. Medical care—Forecasting. 4. Physician and patient. I. Title.
  R858.T657 2015
  610.285—dc23
                                                                    2014035830

10 9 8 7 6 5 4 3 2 1

For Susan, Sarah, Evan, Antonio and Julian . . .
without them these pages would be empty.

TABLE OF CONTENTS

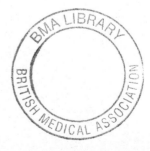

Readiness for a Revolution

Chapter 1

Medicine Turned Upside Down

"Every patient is an expert in their own chosen field, namely themselves and their own life."
—EMMA HILL, EDITOR, *The Lancet*[1]

"Health care will be less frustrating when the power shifts from sellers to buyers, and when the patients are more in charge."
DAVID CUTLER, PROFESSOR OF APPLIED ECONOMICS, HARVARD UNIVERSITY[2]

"It is no exaggeration to say that billions of people will soon have a printing press, reference library, school, and computer all at their fingertips."
—ERIK BRYNJOLFSSON AND ANDREW MCAFEE, *The Second Machine Age*[3]

"Every aspect of Western mechanical culture was shaped by print technology, but the modern age is the age of the electric media . . . electronic media constitutes a break boundary between fragmented Gutenberg man and integral man."
—MARSHALL MCLUHAN, 1966[4]

Way back in 1996, the *Seinfeld* TV show told the story of the "difficult" patient.[5] Elaine Benes, played by Julia Louis-Dreyfus, developed a skin rash, but doctors kept refusing to see her. The problem was that her doctor had called her "difficult" after an appointment four years earlier, when she had not wanted to change into a gown to get a mole examined. She wanted to have her chart delete this discredit, but the doctors wouldn't cooperate. Instead, they labeled her "very difficult." So she worked with Kramer, who posed as Dr. Van Nostrand, to try to steal her chart. That backfired. She never got her diagnosis or chart, and even Kramer was written up in a medical record for impersonating a doctor. The segment is hilarious and at the same time sobering, since it's a slice of medical life (see https://www .youtube.com/watch?v=ZJ2msARQsKU).

Now let's fast-forward to two decades later. Doctors are still labeling patients as difficult.[6,7] Patients are typically unable to see, let alone keep or contribute to *their* office visit notes about *their* condition and *their* body that *they* paid for. Frequently they have to consult multiple doctors for the same condition. It may take weeks to get an appointment. The time with a doctor is quite limited, typically less than ten minutes, and much of that is without eye contact because the doctor is pecking away at a keyboard.[8]

But a new model of medicine is taking hold, one that is democratized— not difficult, but easy. If Elaine wanted to have her skin rash assessed today, all she would have to do is take a picture of it with a smartphone and download an app to process it. Within minutes, a validated computer algorithm, which is more accurate than most doctors, would deliver by text a diagnosis of her skin rash. The text would include specific next steps, perhaps treatment with a topical ointment or a visit to dermatologist for further assessment. Elaine could even download apps to see the ratings of nearby dermatologists, how expensive a visit would be, and even if the doctors themselves were difficult to deal with. When seen by a doctor, she could demand a copy of her office visit notes and also request to review and edit them (especially if she is mislabeled).[9] Most likely, however, she wouldn't have to see any doctor. She'd have immediate access at any moment in time, at any location, to a diagnosis of her medical condition. She would not only avoid the delay, inconvenience, and unnecessary expense, but she wouldn't even have to find someone to steal her chart.

The difference between these two scenarios represents the essence of a new era of medicine. It is powered by unplugged digitization, with the smartphone as the hub. We have seen this model already adopted in retail, travel, dining, entertainment, banking, and virtually every other industry.[10] It's all on demand and instantaneously executed. This has moved far beyond just having a prosthetic brain for a search or a built-in navigation GPS. In almost any endeavor, getting things done in a flash has become the norm, except in medicine. But that is now inevitable.

Getting first-rate health care will always be quite different from ordering something from Amazon. We're talking about the most precious part of life—one's health—not buying a book. But the common thread is the power of information and individualization. We are embarking on a time when each individual will have all their own medical data and the computing power to process it in the context of their own world. There will be comprehensive medical information about a person that is eminently accessible, analyzable, and transferable. This will set up a tectonic (or "tech-tonic") power shift, putting the individual at center stage. No longer will MD stand for medical deity. What have been dubbed the six most powerful words of the English language—"The doctor will see you now"[8]—will no longer be true. Indeed you will still be seeing doctors, but the relationship will be radically altered.

The doctor will see you now via your smartphone screen without an hour of waiting, at any time, day or night.[8] It might not be your primary care doctor, but it will be likely be a reputable physician who is conducting part of his or her practice through secure video consults. And those consults will involve doing parts of the standard physical examination remotely. More importantly, they will incorporate sharing your data—the full gamut from sensors, images, labs, and genomic sequence, well beyond an electronic medical record. We're talking about lots of terabytes of data about you, which will someday accumulate, from the womb to tomb, in your personal cloud, stored and ready for ferreting out the signals from the noise, even to prevent an illness before it happens.

The Power Shift

More is at play than just your "little" big data. Let's drill down on the term *democratization,* meaning "to make something available to all people." Until now, the flow of medical data has been to the doctor. If a patient was fortunate enough, *their* data, such as results of lab tests or scans, might arrive in the mail. More likely, but still rare, would be for the bottom line (like "everything is normal") to be relayed via a phone call, often via a nurse or office assistant. The really lucky patient (with a less than 1 out of 10 chance in the United States) might even get an e-mail with attachments that include all their data.

But the world is changing now. Patients are generating their own data on their own devices. Already any individual can take unlimited blood pressures or blood glucose measurements, or even do an electrocardiogram (ECG) via their smartphone. The data are immediately analyzed, graphed, displayed on the screen, updated with new measurements, stored and, at the discretion of the individual, shared. The first time I had an ECG e-mailed to me by a patient with the subject line "I'm in atrial fib, now what do I do?," I knew the world had changed. The patient's phone hadn't just recorded the data—it had interpreted it! A smart algorithm was now trumping one of my skills as a cardiologist. Putting this power in everyone's pocket could preempt an emergency room visit or an urgent clinic appointment. In our unplugged world full of mobile devices, a diagnosis could now be made anywhere, anytime, by anybody. Or by a machine.

Three other experiences over the past couple of years, attending to airplane passengers in distress, have reinforced my sense that medicine has already transformed. The first passenger turned patient was having chest discomfort and sweating; I was able to confirm with a mobile phone electrocardiogram that he was indeed having a heart attack, which led to an emergency landing. Had the smartphone sensor and app been available, a flight attendant or any other passenger could have done the same thing. Were there any ambiguity, the ECG could have been wirelessly sent from the plane to medical personnel on the ground to help make the call. A young woman having a panic attack with difficulty breathing and a very rapid pulse was the second passenger I met up with. The ECG showed atrial fibrillation, with a heart rate of 140, and upon questioning her it was pretty clear she had an overactive thyroid, which was later confirmed. An amalgam of verbal reassurance and handholding was all that was needed. More recently, a man lost consciousness in his seat soon after takeoff. In this case I performed a smartphone physical exam in the air, with an ECG, blood pressure measurement, a sensor for blood oxygen concentration, and high-resolution ultrasound imaging of the heart, which collectively revealed the passenger was stable, had likely suffered a transient very slow heart rhythm, and that the flight was fine to go on. None of these passengers required a doctor on the plane to make their diagnosis. Although the

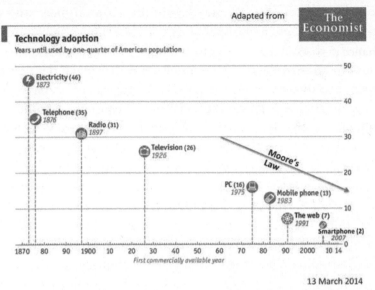

Technology adoption
Years until used by one-quarter of American population

Adapted from **The Economist**

- Electricity (46) 1873 — 50
- Telephone (35) 1876 — 40
- Radio (31) 1897
- Television (26) 1926 — 30
- Moore's Law — 20
- PC (16) 1975
- Mobile phone (13) 1983 — 10
- The web (7) 1991
- Smartphone (2) 2007 — 0

1870 80 90 1900 10 20 30 40 50 60 70 80 90 2000 10 14

First commercially available year

13 March 2014

FIGURE 1.1: When the technology was introduced and the number of years (in parentheses, y-axis) for each to be used by 25 percent of Americans. Source: Adapted from "Happy Birthday World Wide Web," *The Economist* (2014): http://www.economist.com/blogs/graphicdetail/2014/03/daily-chart-7.

flight crew had asked if there were doctors on board, all that was needed were the tools to collect the data.

These tools aren't just for the heart. The sensors now extend to virtually any physiologic metric (such as brain waves, eye pressure, lung function, and mood). Anyone can do multiple parts of their own physical examination, including all vital signs, skin, eyes, ears, throat, heart, and lungs. And just about any routine lab test will soon be available to be assayed via one's smartphone.

To truly qualify as democratized this has to be capable of spreading among common people, not just the elite or affluent. This is possible. It turns out that smartphones are the most rapidly adopted technology in the history of man. While it took thirteen years for 1 out of 4 Americans to use cell phones, it took only two years for them to use smartphones (Figure 1.1). Indeed, 1 out of 4 people worldwide now use smartphones.[11] But we've still got the challenge of more than 7.25 billion people on the planet and only approximately 2 billion with smartphones.[11] It's not just about having phones, of course: they need to connect to broadband Internet. And this is coming, too. Internet.org and other initiatives are working to provide free Internet services to people worldwide.[12]

Fortunately, we've got Moore's law in play. We can now stuff over 2 billion transistors into a smartphone, which has exponentially dropped the costs of the technology needed to make democratized, digital medicine available to all. Almost all of the innovations that make the smartphone the hub of medicine's future are amazingly frugal. For example, the cost of manufacturing the ECG sensors is about fifty cents. Beyond the cost of writing code and developing it, software is free. Smartphones are in the midst of becoming remarkably cheap—projected to cost less than $35, perhaps without all the bells and whistles, but with the key features of an expensive phone intact.[13-15] So anywhere there is a mobile signal, such as in the remote hinterlands of Timbuktu, there is the ability to do all these medical things: capture real-time biosensor metrics, perform various components of the physical exam, and run a bunch of lab tests. That's a good start for spreading a new medical model for all people. It may just mean that the best way to cut the ever-increasing costs of health care around the world will be to provide cheap smartphones with Internet service to those who otherwise could not afford to buy them.

The Rise of Smart Patients

Patients are intrinsically remarkably smart—they know their own bodies and the context of their lives—and no one has a bigger interest in their own health. That doesn't mean, however, that they do all (or any of) the right things to stay healthy, but when things do go wrong, they are pretty darn good at detecting a problem.[6,16-18] But we've learned that, in general, doctors don't like smart patients. In fact, a recent study of physician attitudes found that: "patients who have in-depth knowledge of their condition encounter problems when their expertise is seen as inappropriate in standard healthcare interactions."[6]

Those attitudes won't be enough to hold back a whole new generation of even smarter patients and hopefully more supportive and smarter doctors. Indeed, they're already all around us (Figure 1.2). First, consider Jeanette Erdmann, a research colleague of mine who lives in Germany and published her own very personal case report "Forty-five Years to Diagnosis."[19] At age four she realized she was much slower climbing stairs compared with all the other kids. Her condition precipitously declined when she was working on her PhD thesis, to the point where she was put on a ventilator at night for the rest of her life. But it wasn't until age forty-five when she "consulted Google" and put in her illness descriptors (muscular dystrophy, hip dislocation, and keloid scarring) that she came up with a rare condition, with less than three hundred cases worldwide, known as Ulrich muscular dystrophy (UMD). A genomic scientist, she had her exome sequenced to confirm that she had the specific mutation that is the known root cause of UMD.

Second, consider Elena Simon, who at age twelve developed a rare type of liver cancer (fibrolamellar hepatocellular carcinoma, FL-HCC).[20–24] There are no known drug treatments for FL-HCC, and its biologic basis was, at the time, unknown. FL-HCC affects approximately two hundred young people every year, and not infrequently proves to be fatal. Fortunately for Elena, surgery to remove the carcinoma proved successful. For a high school science project four years after she was diagnosed, Elena worked with her surgeon and researchers at Rockefeller University to sequence her tumor specimen along with those from fourteen other patients. This led to finding a gene mutation that was present in each and every patient, but not in controls with other types of cancer. That is, they found the cancer's cause, likely the first step in finding an effective treatment. This led Elena not only to publish their findings in the prestigious journal *Science* in 2014, but also to develop a website to connect all the individuals affected by FL-HCC around the world.

Lastly, consider Grace Wilsey, who had another rare disease manifest when she was a baby. Dubbed "kids who don't cry,"[25,26a] the disease is in fact far more complicated and leads to loss of muscle tone, seizures, development delays, and liver damage. Her father, along with another father of a child with the same condition, was able to find via social media eight other families with similarly affected children and, by genetic sequencing, to identify a mutation in the NGLY1 gene that was the root cause of the condition.[26b] Multiple potential treatments have been identified as a result, and these are currently undergoing testing. Wilsey's father and one other father published an editorial in a biomedical journal calling attention to the capabilities of parents, social media, and "individuals outside the box" to change medicine, and calling for researchers and physicians not to ignore them.[26a] The lead author of the NGLY1 report, Gregory Enns, said, "This represents a complete change in the way we're going about clinical medicine."[27] As David Cutler wrote in *MIT Technology Review*, "the single most unused person in health care" is the patient.[2] That's a call for democratization.

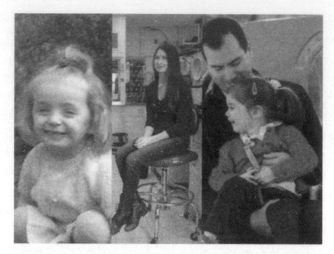

FIGURE 1.2: Three individuals with rare diseases and a molecular diagnosis: Jeanette Erdmann (left), Elena Simon (middle), and Grace Wilsey with her father Matt Wilsey (right).

I don't cite these three individuals just because they deserve recognition. Although they all had rare or undiagnosed conditions that were deciphered via sequencing, yielding a precise molecular diagnosis, there's another important common thread—connectivity.[24] This is seen by Jeanette's use of an Internet search engine, Elena's ability to bring a substantial number of individuals with FL-HCC together, and Matt Wilsey's (along with other parents') use of social media to nail down the root cause of his kid's condition. That we are indeed electronically hyperconnected to one another and to machines is yet another critical feature of the new democratic model of medicine.

Hyperconnected?

If there's any question as to whether electronic connectivity between people has taken hold, just consider that Facebook—dating only from 2004— now has 1.3 billion registrants, roughly equal to the population of China, the largest country in the world, and still growing. That represents more than 1 of every 6 people on the planet.

The importance of online health communities, exemplified by PatientsLikeMe, cannot be underestimated. When patients with like conditions can connect with and learn from each other, without the constraints of

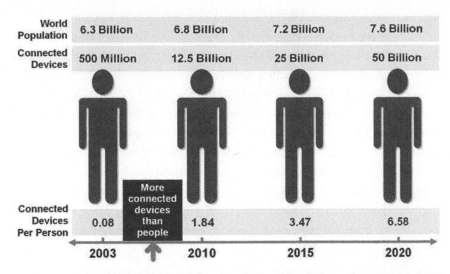

World Population	6.3 Billion	6.8 Billion	7.2 Billion	7.6 Billion
Connected Devices	500 Million	12.5 Billion	25 Billion	50 Billion

Connected Devices Per Person	0.08	More connected devices than people	1.84	3.47	6.58

| 2003 | 2010 | 2015 | 2020 |

FIGURE 1.3: The rise in connected devices on the Internet of Things from 2003 to 2020, projected. Source: D. Evans, "The Internet of Things: How the Next Evolution of the Internet is Changing Everything," Cisco Internet Business Solutions Group, April 2011, http://www.cisco.com/web/about/ac79/docs/innov/IoT_IBSG_0411FINAL.pdf. Courtesy of Cisco Systems, Inc. Unauthorized use not permitted. August 1, 2014.

time or place as they would have with a doctor's visit, yet another critical dimension of democratized medicine is discernible.

The marked connectivity is taken further when one considers the Internet of Things (IoT). That is the unbridled growth of not only people but also devices that are wirelessly connected via the Internet. The projections range from twenty-eight to fifty billion connected devices by 2020,[28] and the implications are profound. This doesn't just refer to Nest thermometers or connected cars—the bulk of the growth is actually expected to come from sensors, particularly wearable ones that track medical data. As shown in Figure 1.3, the average person is projected to have between six and seven connected devices by 2020. This represents a quadrupling of connected devices in the span of a decade with only 10 percent of growth of the population during that time. The impressive growth of our connectivity—between both people and machines—represents a formidable technologic force that makes medicine's democratization more likely and more powerful.

These connected medical devices—I call them the IoMT (Internet of Medical Things)—enable sharing not just with a physician or nurse, but with anyone: family members, such as an elderly individual with her care-giver daughter, or peers, such as a network of friends to set up a managed competition ("coopetition") for best physiologic metrics. And of course sharing could be with machines and algorithms to provide data processing and automated feedback to the individual.

All of these movements of self-generated data by smart, hyperconnected patients represent a serious challenge to medical paternalism. The traditional power structure is top-down. In the book *Doctor in the House,* Richard Gordon (a physician) wrote, "doctors consider themselves the most evolved of the human species."[18] The boss has been the doctor, who has long been portrayed, as "doctor knows best." While the doctor may indeed have the most knowledge, that doesn't mean he or she knows best. In the new model, the information is no longer flowing from the top. Data and information are not knowledge, of course, and for the latter, the doctor will continue to be its purveyor. Moreover, the intimacy at the heart of the best doctor-patient relationship—where a patient can reveal their secrets and worst fears, or experience the physician's touch to promote confidence and healing—cannot be compromised and should never be lost.

Still, the relationship is changing and must change. If we liken the new model to the business world, the patient becomes the chief operating officer (COO)—a notable promotion from nobody to senior management. The COO monitors *all* the operations of the body. He is fully in charge, including of the team in information technology (IT), getting all the relevant data accurately and rapidly analyzed and reported back directly to him. The IT group in this company is really into data visualization and makes graphics for the COO that a small child on the street could understand. The graphic tools make him look brilliant. The COO has periodic and ad hoc reporting to the chief executive officer (CEO), the doctor. The doctor likes being the CEO but is really into delegating responsibility. She's got many irons in the fire and really doesn't want to be bothered by the COO unless it's particularly important. But when that occurs, the CEO is ready to plug in and offer guidance and all her experience, knowledge, and wisdom to deal with a problem. Beyond that, the CEO is a kind and compassionate manager, exceptionally good at both communication and multitasking. The CEO is really into IT, too, realizing that both her performance and the company's are greatly enhanced when everyone can make full use of computer resources.

How We Get There

In the *The Creative Destruction of Medicine*,[29] I delved into how medicine would become digitized, how we had a new capability of digitizing human beings. But that is a far cry from medicine becoming democratized. As Wael Ghonim wrote in *Revolution 2.0*, "the power of the people is greater than the people in power."[30] While his book was about the Egypt part of the Arab Spring, enabled by smartphones and social media, the assertion now clearly pertains to medicine, too. When each individual owns and takes part in generating their entire set of medical data and information, including records, notes, labs, images, omics, sensors; when they have complete assurance of privacy and security, such that their identity will not be revealed and their data will not be sold or misused; when individuals become fully respected by their doctors and on an equal footing; when the individual now unabashedly asks the right questions, drives the process, and makes the choices; when individuals have full access to the cloud, supercomputing, and telemedicine, and there is total transparency for data on doctors and hospitals with respect to outcomes, costs, and ratings; when it is for all ordinary people, anywhere in the world. When all that is true, we're not just talking medical empowerment. We're talking medical emancipation.

We'll be taking a deep dive into democratization in this book. It's divided into three sections. First, we'll look at medical paternalism parallels from Gutenberg, *the* historic precedent for change, to explore the new attitudes we all need if, like one leading public figure, we can ever take charge of our medical care. Second, we'll look at the challenges and opportunities of dealing with our newly acquired data and information. We'll go through what it will mean to have our own information system, our labs and scans, records and medications, cost and interactions with our doctor. Third, the full impact of these titanic changes will be probed, including the need for hospitals in the future, sharing medical data openly on a massive scale while finding the right balance of privacy and security, and the ability to preempt illness, to flatten the Earth, and to medically emancipate each of us.

In 1450, less than 8 percent of the population in Europe knew how to read, and reading was only for the elite. Johannes Gutenberg liberated the printed word, not to mention the human mind and the common man. No longer was reading only for the elite, such as the high priests. By making books and all forms of printed materials available to ordinary people, the world was democratized in an unprecedented fashion. Knowledge was disseminated widely like never before. Movable type enabled the culture to change far more than at any other time in human history.

Marshall McLuhan, "the metaphysician of media," was asked in 1969 about Gutenberg and why he thought practically every aspect of modern life is a direct consequence of the printing press.[4] He said that, first, the mechanization of book printing was the blueprint of all mechanization to follow. Typography became the first uniformly repeatable commodity, and led to Henry Ford, the first assembly line, and the first mass production. Furthermore, it led to widespread literacy, which shaped not only production and marketing procedures but all other areas of life, from education to city planning, as well as industrialism itself. Now—in 1969—he saw another shift as radically concluding:

> Every aspect of Western mechanical culture was shaped by print technology, but the modern age is the age of the electric media, which forge environments and cultures antithetical to the mechanical consumer society derived from print. Print tore man out of his traditional cultural matrix while showing him how to pile individual upon individual into a massive agglomeration of national and industrial power, and the typographic trance of the West has endured until today, when the electronic media are at last demesmerizing us.[4]

If Marshall McLuhan were alive today, he might think we are at a similar break boundary in medicine. But instead of the Gutenberg press, it's the smartphone. The percentage of people who have and understand their own medical data is in the single digits, but there's the new potential for information parity and equality and, as a result, emerging authority for you to be the decision maker. But the paternalistic tendency in medicine is strong. Let us now turn to where it comes from and what we can do about it.

Chapter 2

Eminence-Based Medicine

THE LONG HISTORY OF PATERNALISM

"The era of paternalistic medicine, where the doctor knew best and the patient felt lucky to have him, has ended."
—MICHAEL SPECTER, *New Yorker*, 2013[1a]

"This refusal to come to terms with our own decay is, finally, no more realistic than blind faith in fellow mortals ordained as doctors."
—HOLLY BRUBACH, *New York Times*, 2014[1b]

Meet Kim Goodsell, one of the most interesting patients I have seen in recent years. High-spirited, athletic, a lover of the outdoors, and remarkably energetic, she competed as a world-ranked Ironman triathlete in her twenties and thirties (Figure 2.1).[2–5a] But in stark contrast to her physical appearance is her medical history. Sixteen years ago she collapsed from a heart arrhythmia and was resuscitated. She had an extensive workup that suggested she suffered from a very rare heart condition known as arrhythmogenic right ventricular dysplasia (ARVD). The incidence of this condition is 1 in 10,000, and it usually presents in adolescence, not at age forty, which

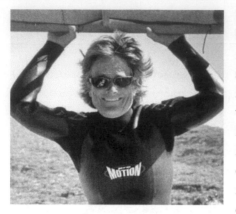

FIGURE 2.1: Kim Goodsell.

Kim was at the time of her first brush with sudden death. ARVD results from infiltration of fatty, and subsequently fibrous, tissue into the heart muscle, particularly the right ventricle, and it is typically inherited as a so-called autosomal dominant trait, meaning it appears in every generation. Although Kim never had any family history of sudden death or serious heart rhythm abnormalities, her physicians nevertheless treated her according to a diagnosis for ARVD: she had an internal defibrillator implanted in her heart that would sense any further episodes of serious ventricular arrhythmias and would deliver an internal shock to restore her heart rhythm to normal.

Unfortunately, Kim has had many breakthrough, recurrent episodes of ventricular tachycardia, and her defibrillator has shocked her several times over the past decade. This is even more traumatic than you might imagine, as she has been fully alert each time the shock has been delivered. It feels like a two-by-four piece of lumber whacked across her chest—incredibly scary, painful, and emotionally disruptive. Despite that, Kim continued to lead an exceptionally dynamic lifestyle, taking bike trips that could run hundreds of miles.

Then things got worse for Kim, when five years ago she started developing muscle weakness and many new neurologic symptoms. She couldn't hold a utensil to eat. Her gait became extremely unsteady and walking was difficult. She had severe pins and needles sensations in her legs and atrophy of muscles in her calves. This prompted her to go to the Mayo Clinic, which led to her being diagnosed with a rare disease: Charcot-Marie-Tooth (CMT), Type 2.

The incidence of CMT (of any subtype) in the general population is approximately 1 in 2,500 people, and, like ARVD, it usually presents early in adulthood and is an inherited condition. Just as Kim had no relatives showing signs of ARVD, however, she had no relatives with CMT or other neurologic disorders. This led Kim to wonder why she had developed two rare diseases. If you do the math, and multiply 1/10,000 by 1/2,500, you get 0.00000004. That is not just 1 in a million but considerably lower—a

4 in 10,000,000 chance. This is far less than the chance of being hit by an asteroid. When Kim asked her doctors how she could have both, she was told she just had very bad luck.

Kim didn't believe in "just bad luck," so, without any medical background, she began a two-year search to find out the root cause of her conditions. She spent countless hours reading every article she could find on the Internet, including the most technical and esoteric papers. With no formal science background outside of college biology, she taught herself a lot about genetics. She became facile in looking up particular genes and molecular pathways that were showing up in the articles that she reviewed. Ultimately, she found a rare mutation of a gene called LMNA that tied her problems with her heart and nervous system together. She went back to Mayo Clinic and requested to have sequencing of her DNA for this particular gene, and indeed she carried the mutation. Knowing the mutation and the biologic pathway involved led her to change her diet, and that has alleviated some of her neurologic symptoms.

This is a remarkable case of an individual making her own root-cause diagnosis of a very complex combination of rare genetic diseases.[5h] A few years ago this could not have been accomplished. Only in recent times has there been enough knowledge of the human genome sequence and mutations to be potentially useful for cracking such a case. Although it required access to all the scientific literature and genetic databases, the real driver was Kim. No one could possibly have been more vested in learning about her conditions, or more likely to reject the authoritative word from her doctors that there was no unifying diagnosis. Moreover, it is increasingly common nowadays for patients to question the information or challenge directives from their doctors. In fact, from the beginning of the medical profession there is evidence of extreme paternalism. And in many ways that tradition has carried on to the present. Medicine will be unable to move forward if consumers continue to be suppressed and treated as second-class citizens. Since paternalism is such a critical force that is holding us back, understanding its roots may ultimately help us overturn it.

From Root Cause to the Root of Doctor Knows Best

Going way back to 2600 BC, Imhotep, the most important figure in ancient Egyptian medicine, is considered to be the earliest physician. He was also a high priest.[6]

The ancient Greek physician Hippocrates, regarded as the "father of medicine," made lasting contributions to the understanding of many diseases and the critical need for professionalism in medicine.[7] He is credited for understanding that diseases were not due to a supernatural force but rather were based on natural circumstances. He originated the word *cancer* (*karkinos,* from the Greek word for "crab") and described many superficial tumor types (there was no going into the body in that era), such as those of the breast, skin, tongue, and jaw. On cancer, he wrote that it is "best left untreated, since patients live longer that way." Known for keeping his fingernails at a precise length, Hippocrates espoused the need for physicians to be well groomed, kind to their patients, and to maintain the highest integrity. But if he was the father of medicine, he was also the father of medical paternalism:[8–11] he made no secret of how he viewed the relationship between doctor and patient, writing that physicians should conceal "most things from the patient" including "the patient's future or present condition."[12] Hippocrates felt strongly that medical formulas were to be kept secret from patients and that knowledge had to be compartmentalized to physicians.

In the famous Hippocratic Oath, the archetype code of professional ethics, he wrote "to give a share of precepts and oral instruction and all the other learning to my sons and to the sons of him who has instructed me and to pupils who have signed the covenant and have taken an oath according to the medical law, but to no one else."[13] As summarized by Kurtz in his essay "The Law of Informed Consent," "The Hippocratic Oath is deadly silent on communication between doctor and patient relevant to the patient's treatment."[12] It has been harshly criticized by Robert Veatch in *Patient, Heal Thyself* as the "paternalistic Hippocratic patient-benefitting principle"[8] that, by not supporting honesty toward patients, therefore violates their rights. A review in the *New Republic* of Veatch's book took the oath critique a step further: "The words of the Oath, revered and recited to the present day, clearly provide a warrant for paternalism—though such an attitude was already encouraged, as it still is, by the simple fact that the healer has always been possessed of a body of knowledge and skills unavailable to his patient."[14] Medical students still recite a version of this oath today.[15]

The term "silence" comes up frequently when reviewing the historic physician-patient relationship. The title of Jay Katz's influential book *The*

Silent World of Doctor and Patient conveys the paternalism reflected by un-informed patients having no involvement in decision-making.[9] Katz points out how in *Decorum*, Hippocrates emphasizes concealment, arguing that: "the silence that has pervaded [the doctor-patient relationship], also bears testimony to physicians' inattention to their patients' right and need to make their own decisions," and that "the emphasis on patients' incapacities to apprehend the mysteries of medicine, and therefore, to share the burdens of decision with their doctors" is responsible for Hippocrates ignoring any need for disclosure or a patient's consent.[16]

Hippocrates, although he taught physicians to patronize their patients, saw clearly the limits of their powers. He even wrote that "the gods are the real physicians."[17] Nevertheless, he believed that a patient would think his physician was the worst doctor in the world "if he does not promise to cure what is curable and to cure what is incurable."[16] Plato likewise thought it was fine to employ "lies for good and noble purposes" when physicians were treating patients.[18] Veatch, in *Patient, Heal Thyself*, addressed a physician's duty to tell the truth (or not).[8] He wrote: "For many centuries of paternalistic medicine, the professional Hippocratic physician ethics commanded the physician to assess whether disclosure would benefit or hurt the patient. If the disclosure was thought not to be helpful, it was the clinician's duty to withhold—to use a euphemism, to use jargon, or to just plain lie."[19]

The model established by Hippocrates was only strengthened in the centuries that followed. Katz summed up the medieval doctor–patient relationship as: patients must honor doctors since they have received their authority from God; patients must have faith in their doctors; and patients must promise obedience.[9] To back this up, Katz provides many extraordinary examples from physician writings, such as this from the late eighth century, "Honor the physician of necessity for the Most High created him. And do not hesitate to take what potions he gives you."[17] In the ninth century, an Arab physician wrote: "Then he who blames the art of medicine blames the acts of Allah, the exalted Creator."[17] Also in the ninth century, from a Jewish physician, "Reassure the patient and declare his safety even though you may not be certain of it, for by this you will strengthen his Nature."[20] This same physician, Isaac Israeli, also encouraged his colleagues to refuse to work with difficult patients: "Should the patient not submit to your discipline, and should his servants and members of his household not be diligent in following your command quickly, nor honor you as is proper, do not persevere in the treatment."[20] Sounds too much like today! On medicine in the eleventh century, Daremburg wrote: "On departing the physician promises the patient he shall recover; to those who are about the sickbed, however, he must affirm that the patient is very ill; if the patient recovers the physician's reputation will be enhanced, should he die the physician can state that the outcome was predicted."[16] A French surgeon in the fourteenth century agreed with his forbearers: "The surgeon . . . should promise that if the patient can endure his illness and will obey the surgeon for a short time he will soon be cured and will escape all of the dangers which have been pointed out to him; thus the cure can be brought about more easily and more quickly. If the patient is defiant, seldom will the result be successful."[21]

It seems that only by the sixteenth and seventeenth centuries—some two thousand years after Hippocrates—were there physicians, such as Samuel de Sorbière, John Gregory, and later Thomas Percival, who started to acknowledge patients might or should have a voice in their care. This does not mean the attitude was common, however. Dr. Benjamin Rush, who is regarded as both a founding father of the United States and the father of American psychiatry, wrote that doctors should "avoid sacrificing too much to the taste of (their) patients. . . . Yield to them in matters of little consequence, but maintain an inflexible authority over them in matters essential to life."[12] This was during the so-called "Age of Enlightenment."[22] Interestingly, Rush was known for his extreme use of bloodletting, which is not exactly helpful to patients except in very rare circumstances. Imagine then, as a patient, raising any objections to bloodletting as a treatment for dysentery or cancer and having a paternalist like Rush ignore them.

Cumulatively what has been called the Age of Paternalism lasted for thousands of years.[23] The crux of this long era was captured by Mark Siegler in the *Archives of Internal Medicine:* "This model of medicine—the 'doctor knows best' model—was premised on trust in the physician's technical skills and moral stature, was buttressed by an attribution of magical powers to the healer, and was characterized by patient dependency and physician control."[23] Many will argue we are still hanging on to that era today.

With so much of modern medicine having its roots from the ancient Greeks, it is not surprising that the symbol of the profession had its origin at that time. The caduceus, as the symbol is called, is easily recognizable,

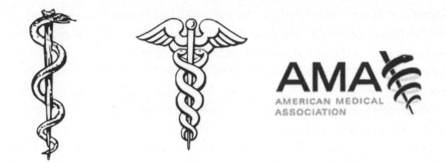

FIGURE 2.2: Evolution of the caduceus symbol in medicine and its adoption by the American Medical Association. Sources: (left and middle) "Caduceus," Wikipedia, accessed August 13, 2014, http://en.wikipedia.org/wiki/Caduceus; and (right) "History of AMA Ethics," American Medical Association, accessed August 13, 2014, http://www.ama-assn.org/ama.

but its meaning is elusive and has engendered controversy.[24] The original symbol was actually a single snake entwined around the upright staff of Aesculapius, the Greek God of medicine and son of Apollo. In the Age of Faith, God anointed Aesculapian physicians and many have therefore contemplated the caduceus as a representation of the godly nature of medical care. Later, the single snake was given a partner entwined around the staff and wings to represent Hermes, the Olympian god and patron of commerce. In the mid-1800s, this version of the caduceus started to appear in US Army hospitals and eventually was used to create the symbol of the US Military Medical Corps. The American Medical Association (AMA) has adopted the original Rod of Aesculapius as its symbol. That may be especially apropos, given the symbol's original suggestion of a godlike nature of physicians, and the tradition of paternalism that the AMA, along with many physicians, inherited from the ancient world.

The American Medical Association

The American Medical Asssociation was founded in 1847, and for more than 160 years since, says its website, the AMA's *Code of Medical Ethics* has been the "authoritative ethics guide for practicing physicians."[25] Authoritative it has been.

The AMA is the largest professional organization of physicians in the United States, with over 215,000 members in 2010, but a third of this membership consists of medical students and residents who are not yet in medical practice. So although the AMA has more than 100,000 practicing physicians in its ranks, it represents only 15 percent of practicing physicians in the country.[26] This reflects substantial attrition from the 1950s when the AMA had roughly 75 percent of American physicians as members. Despite representing only a minority of physicians in the United States, the AMA has immense lobbying power with the government and a history of exerting this force on health care policy, such as with the Affordable Care Act, the origins of Medicare, and the influence of health maintenance organizations.

In the interest of full disclosure, back in 2012, I had a bit of a flap with the AMA after the *Wall Street Journal* published an interview with me on innovation in medicine, which contained the following:

> *WSJ: What are roadblocks for moving to this new world?*
>
> DR. TOPOL: But what has really gotten me stirred up is the issue of whether patients should have access to their own health data. The AMA [American Medical Association] was lobbying the government that consumers should not have access directly to their DNA data; that it has to be mediated through a doctor. The AMA did a survey of 10,000 doctors, and 90% said they have no comfort using genomics in their clinical practice. So how could they be the ultimate mediator by which the public gets access to their DNA data? That really speaks to medical paternalism.[27]

The AMA was upset that I was calling out the organization on its paternalistic efforts to prevent individuals from obtaining their own DNA results without having to go through a physician, and shortly after that interview was published, I received a call from Dr. James Madera, the CEO and executive vice president of the AMA, who wanted to discuss this issue. He started out the phone call with the line, "Eric, we're not your father's AMA." But it was only on researching the history of paternalism in medicine did I realize the deep roots of this problem with the AMA. This wasn't just your father's AMA; it was your great-great-grandfather's AMA.

The original 1847 *Code of Ethics* is telling.[28]

Here are some of the salient passages in order of appearance, with a few key words highlighted, from the Introduction and the Code:

1. As it is the duty of a physician to advise, so he has a right to be attentively and respectfully listened to.
2. It is a delicate and **noble task** . . . to prevent disease and to prolong life; and thus to increase the productive industry and, without assuming the office of moral and religious teaching, to add to the civilization of an entire people.
3. Impressed with the **nobleness of their vocation,** as trustees of science and almoners of benevolence and charity, physicians should use unceasing vigilance to prevent the introduction into their body of those who have not been prepared by a suitably preparatory moral and intellectual training.
4. The most learned men and best judges of human nature.
5. A physician should not only be ever ready to obey the calls of the sick, but his mind ought also to be **imbued with the greatness of his mission.**
6. They (physicians) should . . . unite tenderness with firmness, and **condescension with authority,** as to inspire the minds of their patients with gratitude, respect and confidence.
7. A physician should not be forward to make gloomy prognostications, because they savor of empiricism, by magnifying importance of his services in the treatment or cure of the disease.
8. The life of a sick person can be shortened not only by the acts, but also the words or the manner of a physician.
9. Medicine, confessedly the most difficult and intricate of the sciences, the world ought not to suppose that knowledge is intuitive.
10. A patient should never weary his physician with a tedious detail of events or matters not appertaining to his disease.
11. The **obedience of a patient to the prescriptions of his physician** should be prompt and implicit. He should never permit his own crude opinions as to their fitness, to influence his attention to them.
12. A patient should never send for a consulting physician without the express consent of his own medical attendant.
13. Patients should always, when practicable, send for their physicians in the morning, before his usual hour of going out, for, by being early aware of the visits he has to pay during the day, the physician is able to apportion his time in such a manner as to prevent an interference of engagements. Patients should also avoid calling on their medical adviser unnecessarily during the hours devoted to meals or sleep. They should always be in readiness to receive the visits of their physician, as the detention of a few minutes is often serious inconvenience to him.

14. A patient should, after his recovery, entertain a just and enduring sense of the value of the services rendered to him by his physician, for these are of such a character, that no mere pecuniary acknowledgment can repay or cancel them.

15. There is no profession, from the members of which **greater purity of character,** and a **higher standard of moral excellence** are required than the medical; and to **attain such eminence,** is a duty every physician owes alike to his profession, and to his patients.

16. There is no profession, by the members of which eleemosynary services are more liberally dispensed, than the medical.

17. The benefits accruing to the public and indirectly from the active and un-wearied beneficence of the profession, are so numerous and important, that physicians are justly entitled to the utmost consideration and respect from the community.

Much of the language conveys the sense of a self-congratulatory orgy; nobility, authoritative command, and eminence are pervasive. The AMA has revised this document several times, but the original *Code of Ethics* has set a lasting tone.

The first revision did not occur until more than fifty years later, in 1903. The *Principles of Medical Ethics* included only a slight change in the statement on the readiness of physicians for calls of the sick.[29] Instead of "imbued with the greatness of his mission" (#5 above) there was a downgrade to "should be mindful of the high character of their mission and of the responsibilities they must incur in the discharge of momentous duties."[30] On gloomy prognostications (#7 above), there was an interesting kicker clause added: "This notice, however, is at times so peculiarly alarming when given by the physician, that its deliverance may often be preferably assigned to another person of good judgment."[29] In the revision, the doctor's powers were augmented as it was pointed out "life may be lengthened" by the words or manner of the physician (compared with only shortened, #8 above). An important statement about communication to the patient was added: "A solemn duty is to avoid all utterances and actions having a tendency to discourage and depress the patient."

It is striking that the first mention of informed consent by the AMA did not occur until the 1957 revision,[31] where it was stated that "a surgeon is obligated to disclose all facts relevant to the need and the performance of the operation," and "that an experimenter is obligated, when using new drugs and procedures, to obtain voluntary consent of the person."[31] It is indeed hard to imagine it took from the origin of medicine until 1957 to formalize the concept of informed consent and the right of the patient. Nevertheless, it did.

Later AMA revisions and documents on ethical affairs in the 1980s included two statements that give considerable authority to physicians based on their judgment. On informed consent, the AMA

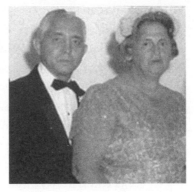

FIGURE 2.3: My maternal grandparents.

contended that physicians should be entitled "to treat without consents when the physician believes the consent would be 'medically contraindicated,'" and maintained that "disclosure need not be made when risk disclosure poses such a serious psychological threat of detriment to the patient as to be 'medically contraindicated.'"[32] Of note is the progressive shortening of the AMA codes and policies: in 1847, it was 5,600 words; in 1903, 4,000; in 1912, 3,000; in 1957, 500; and by 1980, reduced to 250.[28,29,31,32] While the words were markedly reduced overall, there were never any added to raise awareness that patients need a voice.

My maternal grandparents, Miriam and Herman Lepp, experienced as good examples of this medical paternalism as any. Both healthy into their early sixties, within a six-month period in 1965–1966, they were each diagnosed with a bowel obstruction. They each underwent surgery to decompress the bowel obstruction, but later this recurred along with severe jaundice. That they had the same symptoms, at nearly the same time, the same treatment, and the same rapid deterioration could have made one think this was an infectious disease. It wasn't, but they never knew: through the entire saga, the doctors never disclosed to either patient that they had widely metastatic colon cancer, nor that this was unequivocally a terminal condition. Shockingly, neither Miriam nor Herman was ever told they had cancer, because in the 1960s doctors rarely, if ever, used the "C" word. In fact, a study published in *Journal of the AMA* in 1961 reported that 88 percent of physicians had a policy of not telling their patients they had a diagnosis of cancer.[33] It was a long-lasting habit; in *The Emperor of All Maladies,* Siddhartha Mukherjee wrote about a cancer ward at the National Institutes of Health in 1973, where the staff still actively avoided mentioning *cancer* to their patients.[34] Of course, not saying *cancer* couldn't hide the dire reality of the situation. In visiting my grandparents on multiple occasions, in the hospital and for the short time they were able to get back to their home (a trailer in a trailer park), it was readily apparent, even to a young boy, that they were terminally ill. But the doctors were only willing to tell them that there was an obstruction, a "mass," and that the abdominal surgery that each underwent was "successful" for relieving the obstruction and removing the mass. To this day I am in disbelief that this was the ordinary practice for physicians at any point in time.

Signs of Persistent Paternalism

The contrast between the story of Kim Goodsell, making her own complex molecular diagnosis, and the Lepps, who were not even told of their diagnosis, despite it being a common disease and easily identified, is striking. But in the case of Goodsell, the doctors could have made the LMNA mutation diagnosis had they had the interest and time to pursue extensive searching of the medical and genetic literature. In the era when the Lepps presented, *cancer* was taboo as a term, and there was no easy way for a patient to access medical information. They would have been pressed to even get a doctor to answer a question. We have indeed made progress. Now it would be unacceptable for a doctor to withhold the diagnosis from a patient, so long as it was certain, and no matter whether it was cancer or any other condition. Now anyone can Google search well beyond symptoms, as Kim Goodsell did, and get to extensive databases of publicly available information. Still, however, the majority of biomedical publications are inaccessible without a subscription, and purchase of a single article is ridiculously expensive (often $30–$50). We'll come back to this issue and the need for open access later, but at least for now an abstract, or summary, of each article is usually available.

There is a common thread about Goodsell and the Lepps that is fundamental—information asymmetry. Doctors have all the data, information, and knowledge. Patients can remain passive or ignorant of their medical information, or, if they choose to be active, they typically have to call repeatedly or beg to get their data, such as the results of laboratory tests or a scan.

Before it can change, we have to deal with some entrenched clinical terms and practices that exemplify the problem. The first is *doctor's orders.*[35] As a third-year medical student doing my first clinical rotation, I distinctly remember being instructed about writing orders in the hospital chart of a patient I was following. They had to be countersigned by a licensed physician, which usually meant the intern or resident on the team. But the idea that I would write an order for a patient to receive a medication, lab test, scan, transfusion, or undergo some procedure seemed to exude some magical power, like "Open Sesame." My handwritten lines in the chart (once appropriately countersigned) would be picked up in the chain of command by the nurse or ward clerk, and then get executed. What a sense of authority this conveyed to a medical student seeing patients for the first time, and already ordering what was going to be done to or for them. It was plain to see how a doctor could easily be seduced by this sense of supremacy, and how authoritarian tendencies might be self-perpetuating. With the simple stroke of a pen, a whole staff of people was at my beck and call, not to mention the patient.

The term *doctor's orders* has to go. It conveys the problem. Going forward, the doctor should never order anything. Any medications, lab test, scan, procedure, or operation needs to be fully discussed, making the decision to act a shared one. Even though it is every patient's right to fully participate in any diagnostic or treatment component of his or her care, we don't practice shared decisions yet. And we won't so long as patients are subject to doctor's orders—and even as long as they are patients.[36] The term originally meant "one who suffers," derived from the Greek verb *pashkein,* "to suffer." As a noun it is defined as "a person receiving or registered to receive medical treatment," which implies a particularly passive role. Interestingly, as an adjective, the definition of patient is "able to accept or tolerate delays, problems, or suffering without becoming annoyed or anxious." How fitting this is, given that the waiting time on average to see a doctor for an office visit in the United States is over sixty minutes. It is not easy to think of what we should call a patient; many other terms, such as *consumer, customer,* or *client* do not capture any clinical sense of the interaction but instead seem to signify a business relationship. While it may be difficult to come up with a better term, whatever it is it ought to convey an individual who is an active participant in his or her care, who commands the same level of respect as the doctor, and who is privy to any and all data and medical information that is about that person. One phrase and acronym that comes to mind is *individual, active participant (IAP)*.

In contradistinction to the IAP profile, we still are well aware of a general physician lack of due respect for patients today. That also extends from the doctor to other health care professionals on the team caring for patients. Lucian Leape is a pediatric surgeon who has dedicated his career to promoting patient safety and especially in the past decade to "rooting out disrespect."[37, 38] At a major medical meeting in late 2013 of seven thousand critical care nurses, he asked the audience "how many had witnessed or suffered abusive behavior in their workplace during the past three months." The majority of attendees raised their hands.[37] Leape considers disrespect for patients as not just waiting, or having them fill out the same, innumerable clipboard forms each time they have a doctor's visit, but also not giving them full communication about their condition, or when there is a mistake, not being truthful. As Leape recently wrote, "the time has come for health care organizations to do something about this invidious problem and cultivate a culture of respect." This brings home the saying and mantra for the future—"Nothing about me without me"—which should and will undeniably apply to individuals when they assume the role of IAPs.[38]

But, this simply doesn't happen today. A compelling example is when a doctor orders a medical imaging test for a patient. Many of these scans involve ionizing radiation, such as computerized axial tomography (CAT scans), positron emission tomography (PET scans), nuclear tests (single photon emission computer tomography, SPECT, such as thallium or sestamibi imaging for heart disease), angiograms, and X-rays.[39] When such tests are ordered, the amount of radiation that the patient is going to be exposed to is never discussed, despite the fact that the amount of radiation can be readily quantified or certainly estimated using the units of millisieverts (mSv). The dose of radiation for a stress test with nuclear imaging, of which there are more than nine million performed each year in the United States alone, is about 40 mSv, which is the equivalent of two thousand chest X-rays.[40] I have not yet met a patient who was told this information before or after undergoing a nuclear heart scan. However, this information is especially important, given the overuse of medical imaging in the United States and the known association that ionized radiation has with the risk of inducing cancer, on a cumulative basis, many years after exposure.[41] In 2011, there were over eighty-five million computerized tomography (CT) scans and nineteen million nuclear imaging tests performed in the United States.[42] How many of these millions of patients do you think had their radiation dose measured or discussed with them before the scan was performed? The first sign of light came in 2013, when Intermountain Healthcare, a highly regarded health care system in Salt Lake City, introduced a program to systematically inform patients about the radiation exposure they would receive if they choose to undergo a medical scan.[43]

That brings us to informed consent. Most physicians seek consent the same way that a software company does when you download an update or a smartphone app: by presenting you with an extremely long legal document and asking you to press "I agree." There must be someone out there who has read all the terms of the new operating system or app download, but I have yet to meet that person. Have you ever tapped "I decline?" And so it goes for informed consent. For participation in a clinical research protocol or for undergoing a major medical procedure, patients are typically given a document (not infrequently six to eight pages, single-spaced) to read and sign. Although doctors call this "informed consent," it is at best quasi- or pseudo-informed, since most individuals don't read the materials, or if they try to they often find they are not understandable. And there's the compulsory aspect to this story. Let's say you are scheduled to have an operation with a surgeon, whom you have thoroughly researched, and before going into the operating room you are given a consent form to sign. In the form it stipulates that you waive all rights to sue the doctor for any untoward result of the surgery. Whether or not this form is legally enforceable, do you refrain from signing and have the operation cancelled? This is not informed consent—it should be called "coercive consent," as the patient is left with little viable or practical alternative. It's just like the software upgrade download, but regarding a much more serious matter. Today's patients may be better informed than their ancient Greek counterparts, but there is a ways to go before we have people who are fully informed, engaged, and enthusiastic about moving forward.

Similar problems arise when it is time to leave medical care. If you've ever been hospitalized, you are likely familiar with the infamous hospital discharge order. In *Patient, Heal Thyself,* Veatch, a pharmacist and ethicist, describes the tone of such documents as "language more fitting for the military or a prison."[44] He's right: the orders have no regard for the autonomy of a person in a hospital's care. The policy at most hospitals is that a patient cannot leave until the doctor has signed the discharge order. So after many sleepless nights, the day has finally come to get out of the hospital (which has often come to seem like jail), and the family arrives early in the morning ready to go. The intravenous line is taken out and all the belongings of the patient are packed up. A wheelchair is brought to the room, since patients are not allowed to walk out of the hospital. And then you sit and wait and sit and wait. Many times it will take several hours before the doctor gives the discharge order and you get a piece of paper that summarizes the discharge instructions, including medications. This highly frustrating end-of-the-hospital-stay experience reeks of disrespect for the patient, and is yet another flagrant example of not-so-benevolent paternalism.

Of course, a patient is not a prisoner; an interesting choice for the patient in this situation, or at any point during the stay in the hospital or even the emergency room when things are not proceeding in an acceptable manner: signing out against medical advice, which entails signing a sheet of paper acknowledging that one is defying the doctor and health care team and accepting all liability. Since this action is considered absolute insubordination, it is rare that patients and their family members ever elect to sign out on their own. Regarding the hospital discharge order and signing out of a hospital, Veatch aptly points out: "No other professional, to my knowledge, would claim the authority to discharge or release a client. None would require the client to sign a release form to leave against the professional's advice."[44]

A recent experience I had with a patient family member helps bring home the issues. When my ninety-two-year-old mother-in-law was being evaluated for low blood pressure, some lab work indicated she had a very low blood sodium level, so she was hospitalized. I was unfortunately out of town when this occurred, but questioned whether it was a laboratory error since she had no symptoms, and had a long history of very labile blood pressure, at times especially high and difficult to control, and occasionally quite low. Nonetheless, she was checked into the hospital. Her blood sodium level was checked again. It was low, but not at a threshold that would require hospitalization (if she hadn't already been there) or aggressive treatment with a high sodium intravenous infusion. Nevertheless, she did indeed have an intravenous line put in and got the treatment to boost up her sodium level. That was day 1. On day 2, her doctors had written an order for her to receive a dose of subcutaneous heparin, a blood thinner, because of the concern that an elderly woman lying in bed in the hospital was at risk for developing a blood clot. My wife was visiting her mother in the hospital at that moment and on the phone with me. She told me that the nurses were getting ready to give her the injection. "No, don't let them give her the heparin injection," I told her, as I quickly remembered that my mother-in-law had been taking Eliquis, a potent blood thinner, to reduce her risk of stroke because of her underlying chronic atrial fibrillation arrhythmia. Giving her a second blood thinner could have killed her. Fortunately the mistaken procedure was aborted. To lessen the chances of subsequent medical errors, I suggested to my wife that she have her mother sign out of the hospital (against medical advice, of course). But my wife and her parents, acknowledging that they may have just dodged a bullet, were too intimidated by the doctors and staff to take on that act of defiance. Later in the day the resident doctor apologized for the mistake (an apology for a mistake is a highly unusual occurrence in medicine)—for not having realized that Eliquis, a newly released medication, was a blood thinner. On day 3, it was time for hospital discharge. My wife was instructed to come at 8 AM to pick up her mother. But, the doctors wanted to check another sodium level, which was not even drawn until 10 AM. It was just before 2 PM by the time the hospital discharge order was signed and the discharge instructions given. This episode, and so many more like it, reminds me of the comedian Rodney Dangerfield's classic line, "I don't get no respect." Patients still today do not get the respect they deserve.

The last major source of persistent paternalism comes from the guidelines physicians get to guide their actions. In medicine, professional guidelines are particularly important because they define the standard of care, the prevailing practice for assessing cases of malpractice. Guidelines in medicine are issued by professional organizations, and are often couched with the proviso that they are not intended to be dictatorial, and that the individual patient merits consideration. That usually doesn't matter in the courtroom, however, so physicians seeking to avoid lawsuits often follow the guidelines to the letter.[45] Paradoxically, it has been pointed out that "patients can face grave risks when doctors stick to the rules too much."[46]

The guidelines on statins issued in November 2013 by the American Heart Association and American College of Cardiology (AHA/ACC) are an excellent example of the problem with guidelines.[47-50] Nearly ten years previously there were guidelines on use of statins to achieve specific target goals of the LDL (bad) cholesterol in the blood. For patients with exist-ing heart disease (namely a prior heart attack, stent, bypass operation, or angina), the target was less than 70 mg/dl. For individuals who had not manifested heart disease, but who had risk factors such as high blood pres-sure or diabetes, the target was less than 100 mg/dl. Use of statins for this latter group is termed "primary prevention," because it is intended to pre-vent heart attacks or blockages of the coronary arteries from occurring in the first place. The statin guidelines from 2004 led to almost forty million Americans taking statins by 2012—1 of every 4 individuals over the age of forty-five. Part of this can be attributed to wide-scale TV commercials and newspaper and magazine advertisements, sponsored by the manufac-turers of statins, asking the consumer, "Do you know your LDL?" Doctors around the country were evaluated by "quality metrics" as to whether their patients had reached target LDL levels. But in 2013, the new guidelines eliminated these target numbers. The panel of experts pointed out that there was no scientific basis for the target numbers in the first place—they had never been prospectively validated by rigorous, randomized clinical tri-als. Instead, the panel provided a risk calculator that asks data on age, sex, race, total cholesterol and HDL ("good") cholesterol, cigarette smoking, diabetes, and blood pressure. If, according to the calculator, one's risk for developing heart disease was at least 7.5 percent over ten years, then use of a statin is advised.

There are many problems with this risk calculator. First, if you are a male sixty-two years or older or a female seventy-two years old or older (and of European ancestry), without ANY risk factors for heart disease, a statin is indicated. Right, just your age alone would qualify you to take a statin daily for the rest of your life. Second, the data indicating benefit for statins in primary prevention are marginal: the largest trial, which treated patients with atorvastatin (Lipitor), showed only a 2 percent reduction in heart at-tacks or other serious heart problems. Or taken the other way, 98 per 100 only had a better LDL lab test but no improvement in outcomes (reduced heart attack or death). Third, there are clear-cut risks of statins beyond the relatively common muscle inflammation, which is usually transient and limited when the drug is discontinued. Statins, particularly potent ones, induce diabetes in at least 1 of 200 individuals treated. That reduces the overall benefit of statins by 25 percent, right off the bat. Fourth, the risk calculator ignores family history, arguably the most important risk factor, as it reflects genetic predisposition and is especially noteworthy for families with precocious heart disease (for men, precocious usually means before age forty-five). The three clinical trials from which the 7.5 percent risk threshold risk was derived grossly overestimated the risk of heart disease or stroke, and the 7.5 percent threshold was never prospectively assessed by following a large cohort of patients over a long period of time—it was just imputed from reviewing clinical trial data. That doesn't equate to finding a magical threshold above or below which benefit to a class of drugs is established or certain. Fifth, the number of Americans who would be projected to fulfill the new guideline would potentially double the number of statin users to 80 million. Of note, the cost of treating patients with a lipid abnormality that shows up in a lab test, but without any evidence of heart disease, increased from $9.9 billion in 2000 to $38 billion in 2010.[51] This is the highest growth rate (14.4 percent) of expenditures for any of the top ten medical conditions, and the only one driven not by the incidence of a disease or actual symptoms, but only by a single lab value. Finally, and particularly germane, the AHA/ACC guidelines were not released to the public for comment before handed down. Unlike the US Preventive Services Task Force, which releases a draft for public comment before finalizing any guidelines, the statin guidelines were held secretly by the AHA/ACC until they were released. When the chairman of the guidelines committee, Dr. Neil Stone, was asked why there was no opportunity for public comment, he responded, "I can't answer that. In retrospect that sounds fine. We will probably do that the next time."[52]

This embodies the "tyranny of experts" and what has been referred to as "eminence-based" rather than "evidence-based" medicine. Why consult with the public, even though this drug class accounts for the most commonly prescribed medication in use today, and you are potentially raising the number of people with statin prescription from 1 of every 4 to 1 of every 2 adults? The very fact that *statin* is a common word, well known and widely used by the public, makes it clear that the public should have been engaged on the topic. On the general topic of guidelines, Veatch wrote: "If doctors cannot know what is best, they cannot write guidelines or protocols that tell how to do what is best for patients."[53] Unfortunately, the new cholesterol guidelines came across as the equivalent of Moses handing down the Ten Commandments, with this one entitled "Thou Shall Use Statins." In response, the *New York Times* Sunday cartoonist, Brian

McFadden, featured a frame captioned "Check Your Pulse. If You Have One, You Should Be Taking Statin Drugs."[54] Guidelines are not just another dimension of population, mass medicine instead of an individualized approach; in their present form, as reflected by the AHA/ACC example, they are authoritarian and disrespectful. Table 2.1 presents eight guidelines for routine testing or diagnoses that have been in place for many decades but have recently been seriously questioned or overturned.[48–50,55–63] This includes the routine use of pelvic examinations, annual physicals, mammography, indirect methods of screening for fetal chromosome abnormalities, the use of PSA testing and Pap smears, how mental disorders should be diagnosed and classified, as well as LDL targets. The place for medical guidelines in the future seems uncertain, unless the recommendations that are provided are unequivocal, based on well-established facts that the public is fully engaged in and buys into, and are not considered the standard of medical practice but rather only a rough guide to help in the real objective—providing guidance on precise care and treatment for an individual.

The Knowledge Chasm

From the era of Hippocrates to the *Code of Ethics* of the AMA to the modern issuance of guidelines, doctors have largely controlled the flow of medical information. Katz called this the "Medical Monopoly"—the historical belief that physicians, and not patients, should control all aspects of medical practice.[64] While Katz, writing thirty years ago, characterized this as a silence,[9] I see it more as a profound gap in information. At the individual level, it might be that the data originates from the patient via a lab test or a scan, but without the doctor, the patient is likely to find the results hard to come by. This may be because a physician is trying to "protect" the patient by not disclosing adverse, anxiety-provoking information. Historically, this took the form of not telling patients they had cancer, as illustrated by my grandparents' experience, among other things. In the context of informed consent, the doctor does really know all the complications that might occur, what his track record is in performing the procedure or operation, or what the risks of participation in a clinical trial might impose. The patient should not be "protected" from this information. But no matter how much information the patient gets on a consent form, the patient will never be privy to the same information that is harbored in the

Routine Test or Guideline	When Introduced	When It Should Be Discontinued
Pap Smear	1940s	2014
PSA	1987	2013
Mammography	1967	2014
Standard Prenatal Aneuploidy Screening	1970s	2014
Diagnostic and Statistical Manual of Mental Disorders	1952	2013
LDL Cholesterol Targets	1988/2004	2013
Annual Checkup	1920s	2013
Pelvic Exam	1940s	2014

TABLE 2.1: Guidelines for Routine Testing or Diagnosis That Have Been Seriously Questioned or Overturned.[46–49,54–62]

doctor's mind and experience. And no matter how much one searches the Web, that's general information about the population, not the individual; further, the quality of that information is not assured.

Although we can close the information gap, the knowledge gap is much tougher. Without question, doctors and health care professionals are extensively trained and have acquired substantial knowledge. Doctors who practice general internal medicine have had dedicated preparation through four years of medical school and three years of residency; specialists have yet another two to five additional years. Individuals without medical backgrounds, notwithstanding unlimited searching on the Internet, are not going to ever come close to the knowledge level of physicians. Their determination and power, even with today's inherent obstacles, is not to be underestimated, as illuminated by Kim Goodsell's experience, but the knowledge gap will remain. Nevertheless, data and information will ultimately be accessible evenly by all people. But it will take the end of paternalism for patients to seamlessly access the knowledge base of physicians.

That will be forthcoming as we move away from the paternalistic model to one of partnership, from autocratic to far more autonomous. For this to occur, it will require not only a change in culture within the medical community, but also new technology to drive it from the outside, like the printing press did several hundred years ago.

Chapter 3

A Precedent for Momentous Change

"*Changed the whole face and state of the world.*"
— Sir Francis Bacon, 1620

"*History bears witness to the cataclysmic effect on society of inventions of new media for the transmission of information among persons.*"
— N. St. John, 1967[1]

"*Man the food-gatherer reappears incongruously as information-gatherer.*"
— Marshall McLuhan, 1962[2]

In late 2013, the most expensive book ever sold in the world—*Bay Psalm Book*—went for $14.2 million.[3,4] The book was one of eleven surviving copies of the 1,700 originally printed. They were the first books printed in British North America. The purchaser was David Rubenstein, an American financier and billionaire who had also bought the Magna Carta, a manuscript from 1215, back in 2007 for $21.3 million. The Codex Leicester, a seventy-two-page manuscript handwritten by Leonardo da Vinci around 1508, sold for a higher amount than the most expensive printed book—for $30.8 million to Bill Gates.[4]

Hand-scribed or a printed book—why so expensive? Certainly a one-of-a-kind handwritten book hits the supply and demand mismatch, but the printed book was literally mass-produced. What makes it valuable is its status as an early product of the invention with the greatest impact in history.

It was 1440 when Johannes Gutenberg, after incubating a secret for a decade, came to Mainz, Germany, and launched the era of typography. His invention relied on three components: the type, the individual letters, made of metal (just the thing a goldsmith like Gutenberg would know how to make); the oil-based ink with the right viscosity to stick to the type; and the modified screw press (derived from a device that made wine in Germany), which brought the paper or parchment in contact with the type. His first book off this press became known as the Gutenberg Bible.

The most in-depth account of the impact of this invention took fifteen years for Elizabeth Eisenstein to pull together in her classic two-volume book *The Printing Press as an Agent of Change.*[5] She briefly summarized the transformation: "A new method for duplicating handwriting—an *ars artificaliter scribendi*—was developed and first utilized five centuries ago. It brought about the most radical transformation in the conditions of intellectual life in the history of western civilization. . . . Its effects were sooner or later felt in every department of human life."[6] This was indeed a turning point in civilization like no other—we can consider it as a world before printing press (BPP) and after printing press (APP). BPP was a scribal culture, with manuscripts that were remarkably expensive: about a florin, or roughly $200 today, per five pages, or on average about $20,000 per book.[7] The cost of the same book APP would be approximately $70, about three hundred times less. It would take three individuals a lifetime to hand-scribe three hundred manuscripts; by 1470, three men could print three hundred books in three months. Within fifty years APP, there were more books made than previously in the history of mankind.[8] By 1500, an estimated one thousand printing presses had spread throughout Europe and had produced millions of books.

The error rate BPP was quite high, due to relying on a scribe, and manuscripts suffered from erosion, corruption, and loss of content. In contrast, APP led to permanent, reliable, perfect copies, but if the original contained an error, this went into mass production. Perhaps the most notable example of this showed up a couple of centuries later in the Wicked Bible of 1631,[9] which mistakenly recited the Seventh Commandment as "Thou shall commit adultery."

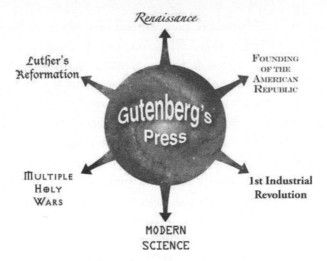

FIGURE 3.1: The impact of Gutenberg's press.

The immediate contrast was from "the age of the ear" to the "age of the eye," since only the highly affluent, nobility, and priests had access to manuscripts BPP and could read—that comprised only 8 percent of Europeans. Otherwise, the common man was left only to listen to readings. Fairly quickly APP, the public became literate as book printing in terms of soaring numbers and plummeting cost exponentially enhanced access.

As Eisenstein asserted, this was a revolution in communication, an explosion of knowledge, which "changed relationships between men of learning as well as between systems of ideas."[1] The flow of information had drastically and irrevocably changed. Stanley Morison, in *The Learned Press as an Institution,* put it this way: "The cumulative effect of the continuing revolution wrought in every aspect of human thought and activity by the invention associated with the city of Mainz is too immense ever to be fully describable. Its consequences to religion, politics and industry are too vast for assessment by available historians and bibliographers or by any assemblage of scholars to be foreseen at present."[10]

In the conventional retrospective view of the era, we can see a series of tectonic changes in the world summarized in Figure 3.1. This is the usual way the printing press's impact is assessed, by leading to the Reformation, the first religious movement that had the aid of printing, more than ten religious wars, the Renaissance, and so on. That is to say, were it not for Gutenberg's invention, each of the subsequent six major epochs of civilization would not have been possible. Although Eisenstein stopped short of claiming that the first industrial revolution was an outgrowth of the printing press, many others have claimed this. Marshall McLuhan, in *The Gutenberg Galaxy,* wrote: "The invention of typography confirmed and extended the new visual stress of applied knowledge, providing the first uniformly repeatable commodity, the first assembly-line, and the first mass-production."[11] More recently, Nate Silver, in *The Signal and the Noise,* asserted that the industrial revolution of 1775 was sparked by the printing press, whereby the economic growth rate that was stagnant at 0.1 percent per year then grew faster than the growth rate of the population.[12]

But I prefer to principally assess the Gutenberg transformative effects by the specific attributes that they induced or cultivated instead of as a precursor for subsequent momentous periods in history. The rationale for this, in my view, is that the communications revolution that began in 1440 is about to repeat itself 575 years later. Table 3.1 summarizes the predominant attributes affected by Gutenberg's press and compares them to the smartphone, or what some term as the "phablet" (a combination of smartphone and tablet). At first glance you will note a check mark in every box. But here I'll explain why the parallels can be seen as striking.

Without question, APP was associated with an explosion of knowledge and too much information. So too is our era. Back in the fifteenth century, as Nate Silver summed up, "the amount of information was increasing much more rapidly than our understanding of what to do with it, or our ability to differentiate the useful information from the mistruths."[13] Here in the twenty-first century, we call that "big data," with more data generated in the past two years than in the history of humankind. And an ever-increasing proportion of that is derived from and is passing through mobile devices. In *The Shallows,* Nicholas Carr recounts the lines from a play in 1612: "so many books—so much confusion! All around us is an ocean of print. And most of it covered in froth."[14] Today we're at about three quintillion bytes of data generated a day; our digital universe is expected to increase fifty-fold in the current decade (2010–2020) from less than one thousand exabytes to greater than forty thousand. Just as the sudden availability of what was previously a rare commodity—a book—was perceived by many as a supernatural intervention in the late 1400s, the prototypic smartphone's inventor, Steve Jobs, has been equated to Jesus, the Book of Job, and God.[15]

Innovation accelerated APP. All forms of learning were revolutionized. Minds were liberated, bent, and reshaped. There was a remarkable sharing of ideas that set up newfound cross-fertilization, which Eisenstein labeled

Attribute	Gutenberg's Press	Smartphone
Explosion of Knowledge	✔	✔
Spur Innovation	✔	✔
Promote Individualism	✔	✔
Promote Revolution, Wars	✔	✔
Basis of Social Networks	✔	✔
Reduce Interpersonal Interaction	✔	✔
Spread Ideas/Creativity	✔	✔
Promote Do-It-Yourself	✔	✔
Flatten the Earth	✔	✔
Marked Reduction of Cost	✔	✔
Archive	✔	✔
Relieve Boredom	✔	✔

TABLE 3.1: Comparison of Key Attributes Between the Printing Press and Smartphones.

"combinatorial intellectual activity,"[16] with books inspiring exponentially increased creativity. While there were innovations BPP, there was no certain or easy way of documenting them. But APP, between 1469 and 1474 in Venice, a printer started operating and the first law related to patenting was written. Gutenberg's press led to "explicit recognition of individual innovation and by the staking of claims to inventions, discoveries, and creations."[17] Nowadays, we have worldwide app developers for mobile devices; tens of thousands of young millennials have largely been the code-writers for several million smartphone and tablet apps—none of which existed prior to 2007! Books initially led to idea exchange in a world population of only about four hundred million people; today the vast majority of seven billion people on the planet has a cellphone and communicates with one another incessantly.

At the root of innovation and idea exchange APP was the cultivation of the individual, who was now engaged in a solo activity instead of being part of a listening group. Noted by McLuhan, "The portability of the book, like that of the easel-painting, added much to the cult of individualism."[18] With private reading, Eisenstein concluded there was "awakening of personality with a new spirit of independence and a new claim to shape

one's own life."[1] The permanence of print and its wide distribution motivated ambition, recognition, and personal achievement. BPP there was
little room for widely circulating an individual's identity without recording
of personal histories or being able to publicize their names or faces.

Just as Gutenberg's press aroused individuality, so has the smartphone.
"Selfie" was named word of the year for 2013, referring to the remarkably
common practice of using one's smartphone to take a picture of oneself and
posting it onto a social networking website such as Facebook or Twitter.
Besides serving as the repository for so much personal data—texts, e-mails,
pictures, videos—the smartphone is the conduit for self-expression, the
primary outlet for posts on social media. Sherry Turkle, in *Alone Together,*
made the case for this technology forming the basis of one's identity: "The
self shaped in a world of rapid response measures success by calls made, e-
mails answered, texts replied to, contacts reached. The self is calibrated on
the basis of what technology proposes."[19] Each of us has a distinct online,
virtual identity, largely developed via our smartphone connectivity, which
may or may not correlate with our physical identity.

Social Networks

Social networking was alive and well in the fifteenth century, thanks to
the rising popularity of books. The communal gathering places consisted
of reading rooms, coffeehouses, and bookshops.[20] The coffeehouses weren't
just for drinking coffee, but were used to discuss the latest books, pam-
phlets, and new-sheets. By the seventeenth century, many of the coffeehouses were specialized for particular topics such as science, literature, or
politics. A coffeehouse argument accounted for Isaac Newton's canonical
book *Principia Mathematica,* published in 1687, which laid the foundation
for classical mechanics, the laws of motion and gravity, and much more.[21]
We'll come back to Newton shortly. Later in the 1700s, the preeminent
economist Adam Smith actually wrote *The Wealth of Nations* in a coffeehouse, after having repeatedly circulated drafts for input among the
regulars there. Beyond this physical confluence and interaction based on
printed materials, Eisenstein pointed out: "That identical images, maps
and diagrams could be viewed simultaneously by scattered readers consti-
tuted a kind of communications revolution in itself."[22] In parallel, we have
seen a social media revolution the likes of which no one could have anticipated. With well over 1.3 billion Facebook registrants, and five hundred

million Twitter users, the vast majority makes their posts, tweets, and likes via mobile devices. In the United States, over 80 percent use a smartphone or tablet to access these social media.[23] For every minute on the Internet, there are over two million Facebook likes, over seventy hours of YouTube video uploaded, three hundred thousand tweets, two hundred thousand Instagram and one hundred thousand Snapchat photos shared, and tens of thousands of interactions on LinkedIn, Pinterest, tumblr, flickr, and countless other social media networks.[3] While not all of this connectivity is occurring via smartphones and tablets, it is quickly and asymptotically approaching that endpoint.

But connecting people can also create wars and revolutions. As a result of the printing press, there were more than eleven religious wars, beginning with the Spanish Inquisition in 1480 and carrying on for two centuries through German, French, Irish, Scottish, and English civil wars. Here books and printed materials propelled the bloodiest era of human history, with millions of people dying in European battlefields "as mankind came to believe it could predict its fate and choose its destiny."[24]

The likeness of the impact on stimulating unrest and revolutions in the era of smartphones is fairly striking. It's remarkably easy and instantaneous to share ideas, emotions, speeches, pictures, and videos with a large number of people. To agitate people, this multimedia, rich graphic capability builds considerably on the clout of books. A 2013 cover of *The Economist* depicted the smartphone as the contemporary icon of protest.[25] But without mobile devices and the social networks that they have in turn proliferated, this augmented power to protest or revolt would not exist. The modern smartphone propagated uprisings and revolutions that continue around the world,[26] beyond the Middle East, in places such as the Ukraine and Bulgaria.

Just as books and smartphones have brought people together for protests and social networks, they clearly have both also contributed to reduced interpersonal interaction. Of the products of Gutenberg's press, the move to reading individually resulted in "the replacement of discourse by silent-scanning, of face-to-face contacts by more impersonal interactions."[27] Of little devices, Turkle pointed out "we expect more from technology and less from each other" and "we are changed as technology offers us substitutes for connecting with each other face-to-face. . . . As we instant message, e-mail, text and Twitter, technology redraws the boundaries between intimacy and solitude. . . . Tethered to technology, we are shaken when that

world 'unplugged' does not signify, does not satisfy."[19] Texts are now preferred to calls by the majority of Americans and are wildly more popular
among teenagers, with the oft-cited reason of keeping one's feelings at a
distance. The changes in interpersonal interactions that have been induced
by both books and smartphones have had extraordinary societal impact,
though not all of them are viewed as positive.

Promoting Creativity

Spreading ideas and stimulating creativity in the APP period is probably best exemplified by the birth of modern science. Until a scientific experiment, its results, and its interpretation are published, reviewed, and
confirmed by others, one is hard-pressed to accept any advance. This time-
honored path of establishing and validating scientific facts was only made
possible by printed materials. Books weren't just about the printed word or
numbers, but were progressively enriched by graphic content. Pie charts,
bar charts, and line graphs were eventually added in the eighteenth century.
Graphics weren't even necessary for germinating a whole new discipline of
literary artists "who managed to counterfeit taste, touch, smell, or sound in
mere words [that] required a heightened awareness and closer observation
of sensory experience that was passed on in turn to the reader."[5]

The field of anatomy was an exemplar of one that really took off. In *The
Scientific Renaissance,* Marie Boas Hall wrote "progress in anatomy before
the sixteenth century is as mysteriously slow as its development after 1500
is startlingly rapid."[28] Eisenstein took it a step further: "anatomy as a science (and this applies to all other observational and descriptive sciences)
was simply not possible without a method of preserving observation in
graphic records, complete and accurate in three dimensions."[29]

APP some of the greatest scientists who ever lived could publish their
works and be recognized for momentous insights. At or near the top of the
list was Galileo Galilei, who in March of 1610 published *Sidereus Nuncius.*
It was a booklet of only sixty pages, ten inches tall, seven and a half inches
wide.[30] In it, he refuted the Ptolemaic theory that Earth was the center
of the universe, and debunked Aristotle by sketching the moon, based
on his telescope observations, showing its craters and mountains. A *New
Yorker* article by Nicholas Schmidle entitled "A Very Rare Book" cited an
unnamed historian who said the book contained "more discoveries that

changed the world than anyone has ever made before or since."[30] Rick Watson, an American bookseller, described the moon copperplate etchings, known as the Florence Sheet, as the "Declaration of Independence in the history of scientific discovery."[30] On the page of Galileo's depiction of Jupiter's moons, Owen Gingerich, a retired Harvard anatomy professor, proclaimed it as "the most exciting single manuscript page in the history of science."[30] It was even compared with the Gutenberg Bible itself, so powerful has Galileo's achievement been.[30] Although this example, albeit one of striking historical importance, came from science, the spawning of creativity and idea sharing certainly wasn't limited to science, but has clearly extended to all walks of life.

That little mobile devices have likewise been engines for creativity is not hard to accept. There are now millions of apps that have been specifically designed for smartphones and tablets, markedly enhancing the functionality of these devices. For example, related to astronomy, there are augmented reality apps like Star Chart, which has been downloaded by more than ten million people. By simply pointing your mobile device to the sky, the app tells exactly what constellation you're looking at, with information on 120,000 stars. Later in this book we will get into the full medical package of sensors, lab-on-a-chip body fluid assays, and conversion to high-powered microscope and physical examination tools. All of these innovations were predicated on having a powerful pocket microprocessor, with wireless connectivity to hardware and the Internet. The two big mobile operating system platforms, Apple's iOS and Google's Android, have taken idea sharing to an unprecedented level for developing applications, well beyond science and medicine. The creative outgrowth from smartphone apps has had a profound influence on virtually every sector of industry, including financial, energy, retail, and transportation.

With respect to idea sharing, the numbers from Figure 3.2 indicate an approximately sixfold growth for books produced in Europe and with global smartphones shipped. It took almost four hundred years for this to be accomplished from the time of Gutenberg's invention, but it has only taken eight years for this same relative magnitude of growth to be achieved with smartphones. And the number of units has jumped two log-orders. This equates to about fifty times faster, one thousand times more units, for a population that has increased only twenty-fold. So mathematically the opportunity for idea sharing has been greatly amplified, you could say by

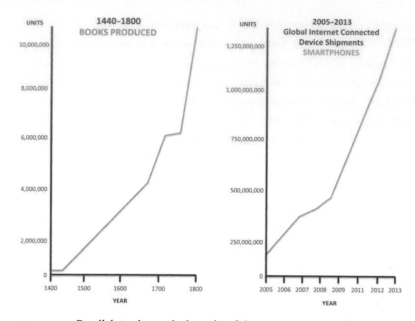

FIGURE 3.2: Parallels in the marked uptake of the printing press and smart-phones, with very different x-axis time intervals.

a million times. And books haven't gone away—they're right on our little devices!

Fostering Autonomy

When we're sharing ideas via print or electrons, there's a lot more chance you can do things yourself. Take Isaac Newton, one of if not the most influential scientists of all time. Amazingly enough he was self-taught in mathematics via books that he either bought or borrowed. Newton him-self was responsible for, as Bernard Cohen wrote in *The Mathematical Papers of Isaac Newton,* "the transformation of a youth who knew no more mathematics than simple arithmetic and who could not read a treatise on astrology for want of trigonometry into the profound creator of higher mathematics."[31] As Eisenstein affirmed, the impact of books to alter the master-apprentice traditional relationship was quite clear, as people could "instruct themselves primarily from books with a minimum of outside help" and "cut the bonds of subordination which kept pupils and appren-tices under the tutelage of a given master."[32] The do-it-yourself (DIY) ca-pabilities took varied forms, from learning to be musicians, self-help in medicine, to autodidact printers like Mark Twain and Benjamin Franklin.

Smartphones have ushered in an extraordinary array of DIY activities. Mobile devices now account for the origin of approximately 80 percent of all Web searches. By searching the web from anywhere, the graphic instructions, usually with video, photos, and audio guidance, pave the way for autodidactic achievement. Whether you're remodeling a home, learning to play a musical instrument, getting into oil painting, making moonshine, or fixing your plumbing, there's an app for that.

How about flattening the Earth? No question that Gutenberg's press accomplished that mission, especially with the prominent force of religion at its origin. "The evangelical urge to spread glad tidings ultimately resulted in establishing presses"[33] all over the world, including Asia and Africa, the Middle East, and Mexico. What started as a European invention quickly spread everywhere, as the "virtuous cycle of literacy" got rooted leading to increasing demand for books.[34]

As for smartphones, they work wherever there is a mobile signal, which is pretty well covered throughout 95 percent of the world's population. There are more than seven billion cellphones on Earth, which is way more than the number of toilets or toothbrushes in the world, making this technology the most pervasively deployed in the history of mankind.[35] The conversion of "dumb" cellphones to smartphones is occurring at a torrential pace, as is the increase in video connects between people via Skype and FaceTime. This sets up the potential to bring multimedia expertise from one place to another virtually anywhere and anytime. Ironically, smartphones and tablets are now helping children learn to read in remote places around the world.[36]

The big social networks that span the globe connect their participants from all 196 countries. Any mobile device app would be expected to work just as well in Bulgaria as it does in Bangalore, in Ronkonkoma as well as in Rio de Janeiro. The implications this has for global medicine are far reaching, as we'll delve into. But certainly leveling the planet for communication and access to technology has been an exceptional outgrowth of little wireless devices.

The ability to reduce costs and archive materials was one of the pivotal outgrowths of Gutenberg's press. As Eisenstein asserted, "Of all the new features introduced by the duplicative powers of print, preservation is possibly the most important."[37] Here we are not just addressing printed materials directly but also, by virtue of word of mouth, amplifying the spread of information. With the skyrocketing of literate individuals, data was being made public rather than maintained as secret, as it was previously. This was especially important for progress to be made in science. Perhaps the most profound impact was the ability to extensively capture the culture, relative to the BPP era, during which such information was remarkably sparse. A note accompanying a gift book from Guillaume Fichet, the French scholar (who arranged the first French printing press) to Robert Gauguin, the French Renaissance philosopher, already reflected this realization in the late fifteenth century: "Bacchus and Ceres were made divinities for having taught humanity the use of wine and bread but Gutenberg's invention is of a higher and diviner order, for it furnishes characters by the aid of which all that is said or thought can be written, translated and preserved to the memory of posterity."[38]

Today smartphones are archiving more data and information than most people generally appreciate: texts, e-mails, and websites visited, pictures and videos taken, social media posts, along with location and time stamping of all activities. And that archiving includes not just what is stored in the phone, but what is in the cloud tracked back to the little device. So while the printing press set up archiving for preservation of materials from cultures and some prominent people, mobile device archiving takes that to an extreme basis on the individual level, an event that will prove as seminal as the archiving of printed material.

Of course, both communications devices can be used to relieve boredom. Although boredom first became a word in 1852, it is not hard to imagine that this emotional state has been around since the beginning of civilization. Indeed the ancient Greek general Pyrrhus, around 300 BC, was said to be desperately bored in his retirement. But he didn't have easy access to books to overcome it. Enter smartphones—if you want to see a smartphone used for treating boredom, all you need to do is watch a couple shopping in a store, with the man sitting in a chair pecking or playing with his phone. Or walk up and down the aisle of a plane midflight and see everyone playing games on their smartphones or tablets.

I saved boredom for last, hoping that this somewhat protracted comparison wouldn't induce it. For many, drawing extensive parallels of smartphones to the printing press will seem far-fetched. If we look back at Figure 3.1, you could say that the historical impact of smartphones is trivial compared with Gutenberg's invention. There may not be another Reformation or Renaissance coming, and perhaps they are not likely to be replicated in the future either. But it wouldn't be overreaching to suggest that smartphones have already been a key contributor to revolts and have helped to fuel the third industrial revolution. Jeremy Rifkin, who is an authority on the latter subject and authored a book with this title wrote: "Communications technology is the nervous system that oversees, coordinates, and manages the economic organism, and energy is the blood that circulates through the body politic, providing the nourishment to convert nature's endowment into goods and services, to keep the economy alive and growing. Infrastructure is akin to a living system that brings increasing numbers of people together in more complex economic and social relationships."[39]

It's important to bear in mind the concept of "incunabula," which has a dual definition: books printed before 1501, and the infancy or earliest stages of something. As we saw with printing, there was a considerable lag phase before much of its effects were manifest. As Eisenstein reminded us, "One must wait until a full century after Gutenberg before the outlines of new world pictures begin to emerge into view."[40] The earliest form of the smartphone was introduced in 2005; the real prototype, the first iPhone, in 2007. So we are at the embryonic phase of evaluating the smartphone's impact, and not even a decade into a new, unplugged world.

The point that Rifkin made about digital infrastructure cannot be diminished. The functionality of the smartphone is the one highly visible, palpable, end-user component, but it isn't worth much more than a glorified music player without the broadband Internet and pervasive wireless connectivity upon which its magic relies. So as we think of little mobile devices, it's useful to acknowledge that they only represent an icon of a much deeper infrastructure.

As I rest my case that there are some noteworthy parallels between Gutenberg's press and smartphones, I now want to narrow things down and get into my central thesis. While it is arguable that smartphones will never wholly simulate the principal "precedent for change," I believe that ultimately they will prove to be immeasurably transformative for the future of medicine. Much more will be covered throughout this book to back up this perspective. And as we look back someday, this innovation may well be considered the Gutenberg of health care.

Paternalism, Priests, and Phones

Realizing that is a bold assertion, now I'd like to get more specific about how we connect the dots from the first chapter on medical paternalism and the current chapter. I've purposely gone in chronological order, as the "doctor knows best" era began around 400 BC, almost two millennia before printing came about. BPP the high priests were among the only people who could read and had access to books. The priests, nobility, and highly affluent were the only literate individuals, an exclusive basis for knowledge and power. Martin Luther authored his *95 Theses* in 1517, profoundly challenging the church's authority.[41] Obviously, he wasn't writing about medicine, but a few of his theses may be considered relevant to the topic at hand: (1) There is no divine authority for preaching that the soul flies out of purgatory as soon as the money clinks in the bottom of the chest; (2) Why are there penitential canon laws, which in fact, if not in practice, have long been obsolete and dead in themselves?; and (3) It is foolish to think that papal indulgences have so much power that they can absolve a man even if he has done the impossible and violated the mother of God.

We've already seen the connection between doctors and God. It's in the original caduceus symbol, the godly nature of medical care; it's in "patients must honor doctors since they have received their authority from God."[42] While God anointed Aesculapian physicians in the ancient Greek era, it's still even strongly implied in the original 1847 AMA *Code of Medical Ethics.*[43]

Accordingly, the power of doctors can be likened to that of religious leaders and nobility. This dominance was derived from knowledge and authoritative control of medical information in general, and each patient specifically. Luther confronted the supreme authority of the church, with over three hundred thousand copies of the *95 Theses* that were widely distributed.[44] We've never seen such a discrete challenge to the medical profession, but we've not had the platform or landscape for that to be accomplished. Until now.

Just as the model of a communications revolution explains the future impact of Gutenberg's press, we are about to see a medical revolution with little mobile devices. For the flow of information will be radically different. Instead of the command ritual of data going first to doctors and trickling down to patients, this deep-rooted practice is about to be turned upside down. Serving as the channel, smartphones will convey all the relevant data pertaining to an individual directly to that individual (or in the case of children, to the parents)—from personal health records, biosensors, lab tests, scans, genomics, and environment. The smartphone readily connects to the cloud and will increasingly connect to supercomputer resources. In many cases, smartphones will play a role well beyond a passive conduit, such as actually performing the lab tests or medical scans, parts of the physical examination traditionally done by a doctor, or processing the data that is graphically displayed or used for predictive analytics.

But the role of smartphones in this electronic communications revolution is not only indexed to the individual. We've already seen the beginnings of managed competition among individuals using their smartphone data from sensors, such as quantifying sleep, glucose, or blood pressure. This can and will be further amplified across a wide gamut of physiologic metrics and through the use of social networks. At a much larger level, the extensive sharing of little device data—from single individuals to create huge population cohort information resources—presents new opportunities for massive open online medicine (MOOM). Conceptually, we're talking about bottom-up medicine, which was never possible until we had the tools and digital infrastructure to pull it off.

Smartphone spread of information isn't confined to transferring medical data. It's a means of rapidly amassing and galvanizing people who are fed up with the current state of health care. Of waiting an average of sixty-two minutes to see the doctor, leading to the full toll of seven minutes of seeing the doctor for a return office visit, often without eye contact (a unilateral sighting). Of experiencing a serious error while in the hospital, such as acquiring a dangerous nosocomial infection or receiving the wrong medication with a critical side effect. Of seeing the hospital bill that reflects the notorious chargemaster with ludicrous fees. Of being responsible for ever-increasing copays for prescription medications, doctor visits, insurance, or any consumption of health care resources. So just as we have seen emotions, ideas, pictures, and videos transmitted via smartphones to prompt political protests, the increasing frustration and vexing aspects of health care today may influence a bottom-up movement, propelled by smartphones and social networks, for improving the future of medicine.

Looking back at Table 3.1 and specifically honing in on the medical smartphone attributes, it is notable that there are already tens of thousands of medical apps that have been developed by a network of worldwide developers. What's most amazing, however, is not the sheer number, but the staggering creativity. Who would have thought we could digitize breath via a smartphone to detect cancer? Or measure critical lung function parameters by breathing into its microphone? Or use a microfluidic attachment to run hundreds of routine lab tests with a drop of fluid? How about repurposing a phone into a high-powered microscope or into multiple physical examination devices, such as an ophthalmoscope or otoscope? Such devices empower both the patient and the doctor.

As we'll see, medical smartphones will create unprecedented DIY applications. Since these devices operate anywhere there is a mobile signal, the chance for egalitarian access to portable medical technology throughout the world is especially promising and exciting—for example, using the camera and text messaging to screen for skin cancer. Ironically, much of the progress in medical smartphone use is occurring in the developing world, which not only starts at a lower tier of technological capability, but also is without the hindrance of perverse reimbursement incentives. The opportunity to lower health care costs with unplugged medicine is starting to get proof of concept, and will be reviewed in depth subsequently. But when the role of hospitals and clinics are challenged via remote monitoring and virtual office visits, it is not hard to envision a major change in cost structure. And major resistance.

So the substrate for a new medical communications revolution is in place. I believe it is inevitable, but the timing of when this will be actualized is uncertain. We know how hard it is to change things in medicine, just as it is extremely difficult for religious rituals to be altered. For example, dating back to the eighth and ninth centuries in Europe, the priest faced the apse, the wall behind the alter, with his back to the people, praying in Latin, which few people in the Mass understood.[45] This particular orientation was known as "*ad orientem.*"[46] That could mean disorientation to the maximus. Although this ritual is still in practice in some churches in Europe today, it has largely been abandoned—since the 1960s. It only took one thousand years for the priests to typically face the people and use the native language. While doctors are not so good at using nonmedical jargon, still write prescriptions in Latin, and due to pressures in using electronic medical records are less good at facing the patient, there is a new path going forward.

A very interesting experiment provides a glimpse into that new path and brings together the primary subjects of this chapter—books and digital devices. Arnon Grunberg is a well-known Dutch novelist, pictured in Figure 3.3, who is trying to understand what emotions his readers will experience when reading his new book, and how those compare with his emotions while writing it.[47] To do this, he writes while wearing an extensive array of sensors, including a cap with twenty-eight electrodes to track brain waves, along with sensors for heart rate and galvanic skin response (a metric for emotional arousal or stress), in front of a camera for monitoring facial expressions. When his book is published, fifty readers will use the same battery of sensors and camera while reading on an e-reader device to correlate how well art is created and consumed—in a way beginning to digitize the creative process. While today it is easy to determine which lines in a book are highlighted by e-readers (e.g., by going to the Amazon Kindle site of the book) so that the author can detect what resonated, this experiment plumbs the question far more extensively. A designer of the experiment, the Dutch neuroscientist Ysbrand van de Werf, asks, "Will readers of Arnon's text feel they understand or embody the same emotions he had while he was writing it, or is reading a completely different process?"[47] Grunberg, who is the subject of this scientific neuroaesthetic scrutiny and known for his antipiety books, said, "I don't think this experiment needs to prove that literature can be good for you. Sometimes, literature can actually be dangerous, if you take it seriously."[47] Taking this another step further,

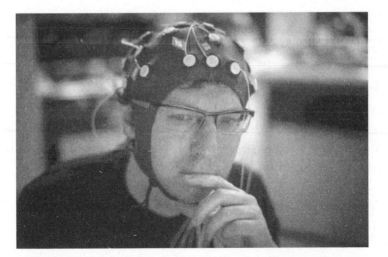

FIGURE 3.3: The author Arnon Grunberg using brain sensors to determine his own emotions while writing, in order to compare them with his readers' emotions. Source: E. Roscow, "The Quantified Writer: Monitoring the Physiology of the Creative Process," Neurogadget, December 10, 2013, http://neurogadget.com/tag/arnon-grunberg.

researchers at MIT have developed a "wearable book" that is loaded with sensors and provides readers virtual experience and feelings as they read the story.[48]

Here, we have transcended the full gamut of two revolutions in communication—from the real origin of literary reading to wireless little device digital technology. We've reviewed the remarkable impact of the former, along with starting to explore the potential of the latter. Grunberg's view of his experiment (the similarity of the name with Gutenberg and his reputation for piety bashing are not to be missed) reminds us that both the old and new technologies can be dangerous. Nevertheless, I believe we can shape the future of medicine in an exceptionally salutary, yet altogether different, way. For just as Gutenberg democratized reading, so there is the chance that smartphones will democratize medicine. That will ultimately be achieved when each individual has unfettered, direct access to all of their own health data and information. Or captured by the popular mantra "nothing about me, without me."

Chapter 4

Angelina Jolie: My Choice

AN AGENT OF CHANGE

"But today it is possible to find out through a blood test whether you are highly susceptible to breast and ovarian cancer, and then take action. . . . Life comes with many challenges. The ones that should not scare us are the ones we can take on and take control of."

— ANGELINA JOLIE[1]

"If people let the government decide what foods they eat and what medicines they take, their bodies will soon be in as sorry a state as the souls who live under tyranny."

— THOMAS JEFFERSON

"It used to be that patients learned about their health only from their doctor. Thanks to mobile health gadgets, apps and services such as 23andMe's, that is changing."

—The Economist[2]

Angelina Jolie was used to leading big screen, big action roles, from swashbuckling archaeologist Lara Croft to being tortured in a North Korean prison as Evelyn Salt to an assassin in *Mr. and Mrs. Smith.* She has been called "the embodiment of physical perfection . . . a fierce, tattooed warrior and seductress with a genuine wildness."[3] One of her tattoos, on her left forearm, is a quote from Tennessee Williams: "A prayer for the wild at heart, kept in cages." Another is the Japanese sign for death. Reflecting about her childhood, she said, "when other little girls wanted to be ballet dancers, I kind of wanted to be a vampire."[4] While her stage name of Jolie means "pretty" in French, she vividly transcended that descriptor and became an icon for exceptional beauty and sex appeal. The number of polls and magazines that have designated her as the, or one of the, most beautiful or sexiest women in the world is too numerous too count. Collectively, this background accounts for why Angelina is one of the most well-known human beings on the planet.

While known for performing many of her movie stunts, collecting knives, having an interest in mortuary science (had a childhood dream of being a funeral director), owning pet reptiles and snakes, few may remember her "bungee jumps" in her house that led to a fire and some burns. But that's probably OK because she's said: "I think scars are sexy because it means you made a mistake that led to a mess." She certainly has to be considered tough.

At the same time, she has maintained a megawatt profile for both inner and outer beauty. Her dedicated efforts as a global humanitarian and particularly a crusader for refugees have been recognized for well over a decade; in 2003 she received the first Citizen of the World award as a goodwill ambassador for the United Nations.

So in May 2013, when she published her *New York Times* op-ed "My Medical Choice,"[1] it was a worldwide whopper. Unless you were living in a cave, you read or heard about *her decision* first to get her BRCA genes (breast cancer, BRCA 1|2), sequenced, second to undergo bilateral mastectomy, and third to make a huge public disclosure. The result has been called the Angelina Effect,[5-16] and it has had a global impact. In my view, the real "effect" has little to do with the media broadcasting a story about genomic screening and a star—this is a huge, landmark story about self-determination in medicine.

First, why did she get her BRCA genes sequenced? Her admixed European ancestry combines Slovak and German from her father (the actor, John Voigt), and French Canadian, Dutch, German, Czech, and remote Huron from her mother. She was very close with her mother, Marcheline Bertrand, referred to as "Mommy's Mommy" in her op-ed, who died in 2007 about 7.5 years after being diagnosed at age forty-eight with ovarian

cancer. Notable from her mother's surname was the French Canadian ancestry, which like Ashkenazi Jewish ancestry is associated with a higher
rate than the general population of BRCA1 mutations. According to Dr.
Kristi Funk, who operated on Angelina, Marcheline also had a history
of breast cancer, and Marcheline's mother had ovarian cancer.[17,18] This
family history in three generations clearly fulfilled the criteria for BRCA
testing. In the general population the risk of a pathogenic (disease associated) BRCA mutation is 1 in 400 (0.25 percent). In Ashkenazi Jews it is
1 in 40 (2.5 percent). In women with a diagnosis of ovarian cancer it is
1 in 8 to 1 in 10 (10–15 percent), highest among those who present at a
younger age. It is noteworthy that French Canadians also carry a higher
rate of BRCA1 and BRCA2 mutations than the general population, due to
a so-called founder effect, as do people from Iceland and Denmark. These
population groups—Ashkenazi Jews, French Canadians, Icelanders, and
Danes—share a common thread: each is a historically closed, restricted
population by virtue of living on an island or marriages only between cou-
ples of like ancestry, so that the founder mutation has generationally been
passed along and perpetuated.

So with a family history of both breast and ovarian cancer in two generations, along with some added risk that can be attributed to her mother's
ethnicity, Ms. Jolie wanted to know her status and had a blood sample
drawn to get her two BRCA genes analyzed.*

As it turned out, Angelina carried a mutation in BRCA1 with an 87
percent risk of developing breast cancer, and 50 percent chance of ovarian
cancer. Of note, to add to the family genetic burden story, just a couple of
weeks after her op-ed was published, Debbie Martin, her mother's sister,
died at age sixty-one of breast cancer.[19] She had been diagnosed in 2004
at (age fifty-two) but only more recently learned that she, too, carried the
same BRCA1 mutation that Angelina did.†

---

   * She became one of about 250,000 women each year who have such testing. At the time
this was done, there was only one company that did sequencing of BRCA genes—Myriad
Genetics—and the cost was between $3,000 and $4,500. Health insurance companies would
have defrayed this cost because of fulfilling coverage criteria. In 2014, with the implementation of the Affordable Care Act in the United States, insurers are now required to fully
reimburse the cost of BRCA sequencing for women with qualifying risk.

   † And while on the subject of family, it will be important for Jolie's three biologic children
to have BRCA genomic screening. Someday one of them, when having children of their own,
could have their eggs or embryos screened for in vitro fertilization to be certain the BRCA
mutation is not passed along.

From Mutation to Mutilation

The second part of "My Choice" dealt with Angelina's decision to have both of her breasts removed and a staged reconstruction procedure. Only approximately 35 percent of women in the United States who have a pathogenic BRCA mutation opt to have their breasts removed. Many have close monitoring via frequent mammography, ultrasound, and magnetic resonance imaging. Others have treatment with the medication tamoxifen, which can cut cancer risk by 40–50 percent, or opt to wait until there is an actual diagnosis and then undergo less invasive surgery, such as unilateral mastectomy, or lumpectomy with radiation. But Angelina chose to go for the most aggressive preventive strategy. And part of her choice was picking Kristi Funk as her surgeon and the Pink Lotus Breast Center in Beverly Hills as the venue.[17,18,20] Her doctor thought out loud about Jolie's choice in an interview, "so when someone who inspires that degree of admiration— someone who's taken seriously and is also a tremendous beauty, arguably the most beautiful woman in the world—removes the part of the body that is symbolic of femininity and sexuality, you have to say "Why would she do that?"[17,18,20]

As she was undoubtedly informed[21,22] this reconstructive surgery is a big deal consisting of multiple operations that span over nine months, even though it was accomplished in Angelina in just nine weeks. There are risks of bleeding, scarring, chronic pain in the back and shoulder, and infection. Infection has been reported in up to 35 percent of reconstructive procedures. Some women have so many difficulties with the procedure that they ultimately undergo yet another operation to remove the implants altogether. Overall, the syndrome known as upper quarter dysfunction, characterized by restricted mobility and reduced strength and sensation in the chest, shoulder, and upper arm, can occur in over half of patients who have undergone breast reconstruction surgery for cancer.

We know from her op-ed that she had nipple-sparing surgery, but with that 25 percent of patients can suffer necrosis of the areola and nearby skin, and even the nipple itself. Even without that complication, there is typically loss of sensation and numbness of the nipples. Then there is the choice of either implants, which can leak or rupture and ultimately have to be replaced, or autologous tissue transplanted from another part of the body. In 2012, in the United States, 91,655 women had breast reconstructive surgery, with most choosing to have implants and only about 19,000 having autologous tissue transfer. Angelina elected to go with implants.[21]

With bilateral breast removal, it is recommended to be done by age forty, and therefore can be deferred until after having children.[23] Angelina was thirty-eight and has six children, three who were adopted (one from Cambodia, one from Ethiopia, and one from Vietnam), and three, including a set of twins, whom she birthed.

Angelina described a three-step surgical approach. The treatment details have been posted via a website blog by Dr. Funk, as promised in her op-ed.[18] First there was the "nipple delay" procedure, which she pointed out caused some pain and bruising. Then, two weeks later she had her breast tissue removed and replaced with temporary fillers in a procedure that took eight hours and she described was like a scene out of a science-fiction film. She ought to know a bit about that. Dr. Funk did a house call three days later and noted Angelina had six drains (that had been put in place at the time of the surgery) dangling from her chest, three on each side, fastened to an elastic belt around her waist. Then, just nine weeks later, on April 27, 2013, Angelina had the reconstructive surgery with implants. Only a couple of weeks later, she wrote that there are only small scars, that "everything else is just Mommy" to her kids, and "the results can be beautiful."[1]

Despite these three operations, she still has a 5 percent risk of developing breast cancer and a 50 percent risk of developing ovarian cancer.[24] As seen below, she will still need to ultimately undergo ovarian removal, as the risk of developing cancer can be markedly reduced with the surgery.[25–27] Unlike breast cancer, which can be diagnosed early via imaging, there is no validated, noninvasive diagnostic test to make early detection of ovarian cancer possible. So the road ahead for Angelina is paved with more surgery, both for removal of her ovaries and likely for replacement of her implants at some point.

Knowing all of this, why did she opt for this aggressive plan? Two out of three American women don't have the surgeries; they choose a more conservative path. Jolie's reputation of being extremely tough, a warrior, may have played a role. Likely related to losing her mother at a young age, she is more in touch with her own mortality than many and once said, "If I think more about death than some other people, it is probably because I love life more than they do."[1]

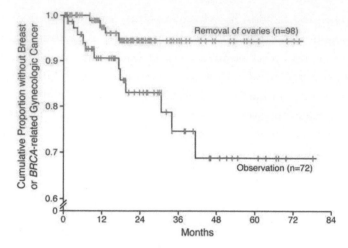

FIGURE 4.1: Risk of developing cancer with surveillance vs. ovary removal. Source: Adapted from N. D. Kauff et al., "Risk-reducing salpingo-oophorectomy in women with a BRCA1 or BRCA2 mutation," *New England Journal of Medicine* 346, no. 21 (2002): 1609–1615.

Going Public

On Angelina's choices, Maureen Dowd wrote, "Yet her courage in going public with the graphic details of her mutilation and reconstruction, even though she's part of an industry that considers a 10-pound weight gain as a career catastrophe, makes her a real-life action heroine."[3]

This was the third major choice. She could have easily kept the whole ordeal private, but instead, just two weeks after the reconstructive surgery, published her piece: "I am writing about it now because I hope that other women can benefit from my experience. Cancer is still a word that strikes fear into people's hearts, producing a deep sense of powerlessness." And further, "I choose not to keep my story private because there are many women who do not know that they might be living under the shadow of cancer. It is my hope that they, too, will be able to get gene-tested, and that if they have a high risk they, too, will know they have strong options."[1] Her doctor was asked, "Was it clear from the get-go that Angelina, as your patient, would make her experience public?" Dr. Kristi Funk responded, "Yes. She waited to find the perfect timing in her personal and professional life, but I think most importantly in her soul. She is intensely private, but she calculated the moment when she would be ready to reveal something so personal. She knew always that in her philanthropic core she couldn't keep this a secret and be who she is. She always knew." Funk described it "as the shot heard around the world" and also said, "The decision to go public came entirely from her. She and Brad (Pitt) hope their situation can resonate with other women."[17,20] There was a lot more than resonating that followed.

There have been many prior examples of the "celebrity medical syndrome."[28,29] For example, in 2000, Katie Couric had a live colonoscopy on NBC's *Today* show, it became known as "the Couric Effect" and led to an increase in colonoscopies. Christina Applegate's diagnosis of breast cancer at age thirty-six popularized the use of magnetic resonance imaging. But none have had anywhere close to the magnitude of impact as Jolie's disclosure.

The Angelina Effect

The public awareness of the link between genetics and cancer, and that it was actionable, was greatly heightened by Jolie's story. As *TIME* magazine put it: "the most stunning woman in the world redefined beauty. That made us all a little smarter."[12] Quantifying the effect has been the focus of some recent studies. In a national online Harris Interactive survey of 2,572 representative American adults, only 3 percent indicated they had read the *New York Times* op-ed, while 73 percent became aware of the story through TV or entertainment news.[8] The awareness of Jolie's prophylactic mastectomy story was 74 percent and half of those knew her estimated 87 percent risk of developing breast cancer. But only 10 percent of respondents had adequate understanding of the risks of breast cancer in women without a BRCA mutation—the knowledge that BRCA pathogenic mutations are quite rare, only in 0.24 percent of the population and they account for approximately 10 percent of breast cancer cases. Another study of 103 newspaper articles in the first month after the op-ed demonstrated the lack of mention of the rarity of Jolie's mutation. The report concluded: "future research is required to investigate whether the media hype has influenced demand and use of BRCA1|2 testing and preventive mastectomies."[30]

As it turns out, the spike in BRCA testing has been rapid, dramatic, and documented globally, including in the United States, Canada, Australia,

Europe, and Israel. Myriad Genetics, despite a June 13, 2013, Supreme Court decision against the company's BRCA sequencing patent (which I will shortly delve into), announced a 52 percent increase in revenue and attributed it to the Angelina Effect.[31] Some clinics in the United Kingdom had a fourfold increase in prophylactic mastectomies.

A page-one feature article in the *New York Times* zoomed in on the impact and status of breast cancer in Israel: "The so-called Jewish breast cancer genes have preoccupied women here for years, but after the actress Angelina Jolie revealed in May that she had undergone a double mastectomy because she tested positive for such a mutation, coverage here exploded, with radio and TV talk shows featuring Israeli women grappling with similar decisions."[32] The picture of a twenty-eight-year-old Tel Avivi who had presented with cancer of her left breast and had a family member with a BRCA mutation aroused controversy.[32] Many readers objected to its graphic nature of showing the incision and her areola. But one graph in the article was especially noteworthy. Because of the Ashkenazi Jew founder mutation, the incidence of breast cancer in Israel is especially high—97 new cases per 100,000 women per year. This compares with 79/100,000 in the United States and 49/100,000 in Poland. But compared with the United States, where there is a 36 percent rate of preventive mastectomies, in Israel the rate is only 4 percent, among the lowest in the world. At least part of the explanation appears to be tied to sexist male doctors who are unwilling to do mastectomies in healthy women. As an example, the article cited the director of oncology at a Tel Aviv medical center who opposes prophylactic mastectomies and claims (despite lack of evidence) a woman cannot have an orgasm once her breasts are removed.

Beyond increasing awareness, more BRCA testing, and preventive surgery, I believe that the Angelina Effect will be seen as a tipping point in medicine. For "My Choice" symbolized the new era of medicine, whereby access to critical information about oneself—in this case genomic information—leads to the individual's empowerment to make a pivotal choice that determines one's fate. Such a decision could hardly have been made a decade ago, since the ability to get or interpret DNA sequencing data was especially limited. It's hard to imagine any set of data being more unique or individualized than one's DNA. It took a massively public figure, with one of the most actionable DNA mutations known, and difficult choices to be made, to come out with her story. This clearly involved a very personal decision with many but no easy options, but the paramount part is that Angelina was in charge. She worked closely with her doctor, Kristi Funk, in a partnership to help select the choice and the timing. And her choice of transparency and willingness to share her experience to teach others is emblematic of what we will likely see in the future of medicine. Had she not gone public, there would have been a giant missed opportunity. This is not just about increasing awareness of the public about a rare breast cancer mutation; it is about having access to one's relevant medical information, enabling the individual to call the shots. If we go back to Gutenberg's press and having newfound access to information via printed materials, there was an "incunabula"—the earliest stages of something. While someday we may not look back on Jolie's story as a movement as big as Luther's Reformation, there is at least one thesis that it advanced—it's my data and my choice. Jolie has forever been transformed from a playing a leading role in action movies to playing a leading role for self-knowledge, freedom of information, and medical information ecology. And the public's heightened awareness of genomics, in particular, represents a key step in the democratization of DNA, just one vital component of our digital identity. There are other complementary forces that are, in parallel, pushing DNA democratization forward—consumer genomics and a landmark decision at the United States Supreme Court. We'll now zoom in on each of these.

The Angelina Effect and Consumer Genomics

On the same morning as Jolie's op-ed, the CEO and cofounder of the consumer genomics company, Anne Wojcicki, had e-mails, texts, and calls pouring into her office. She said, "Angelina Jolie talking about a technical subject and saying, 'I did this, you can do this' is a great thing for us. She did something to prevent disease, and that's exactly what we want people thinking about."[33]

We're going to drill down on 23andMe, whose mission is to democratize genetic information. This was the first direct-to-consumer genomics company; it was founded in 2006 and launched in November 2007 with a $999 saliva test that gave information on gene variants for risk of fourteen medical conditions. Since November 2012, the test cost has dropped to $99 and provides gene variant reports for over 250 medical conditions and for health status that spans carrier status (such as cystic fibrosis or

Tay-Sachs disease) for those planning a baby, ancestry information, your DNA-medication interactions for thirty drugs, and a large number of disease susceptibility reports. It calls this a Personal Genome Service (PGS). The company has 125 employees and has raised over $125 million from Google, Johnson & Johnson, the Russian billionaire Yuri Milner, and several venture capital firms.

In November 2013, the FDA sent a stern letter to 23andMe, which included the following:

> As part of our interactions with you, including more than 14 face-to-face and teleconference meetings, hundreds of e-mail exchanges, and dozens of written communications, we provided you with specific feedback on study protocols and clinical and analytical validation requirements, discussed potential classifications and regulatory pathways (including reasonable submission timelines), provided statistical advice, and discussed potential risk mitigation strategies. As discussed above, FDA is concerned about the public health consequences of inaccurate results from the PGS device; the main purpose of compliance with FDA's regulatory requirements is to ensure that the tests work.
>
> . . . we have become aware that you have initiated new marketing campaigns, including television commercials that, together with an increasing list of indications, show that you plan to expand the PGS's uses and consumer base without obtaining marketing authorization from FDA. Therefore, 23andMe must immediately discontinue marketing the PGS until such time as it receives FDA marketing authorization for the device. . . . Failure to take adequate corrective action may result in regulatory action being initiated by the Food and Drug Administration without further notice. These actions include, but are not limited to, seizure, injunction, and civil money penalties.[34]

The reaction to this FDA notification was intense, not as extensive or global as the Jolie disclosure, but highly charged and polarized.[2,35–77]* Some felt that 23andMe was reckless and arrogant and had overstepped their

---

* A large number of references are provided to demonstrate the intensity and polarization of responses, still representing only a small fraction of the publications in response to this action.

bounds, while others felt this endangered the democratization of health information. Or as a cofounder of 23andMe put it in a tweet: "So much for patient empowerment."[69]

At the heart of this controversy is the issue of medical paternalism, which was reviewed in Chapter 2. Should individuals have the right to *directly* access medical information about themselves? Recall that the American Medical Association, among others, has lobbied the FDA and government to prohibit direct-to-consumer genomic information.

Misha Angrist, a scientist on the Duke genetics faculty, made an interesting analogy: "It reads like the letter of a jilted lover. 'We went on fourteen dates! We exchanged all these e-mails! We held hands in the park! Now you're telling me, "Fuck you," and kicking me to the curb.'"[78] He also told the *New York Times,* "Is the only pathway for me to get access to the contents of my cells via some guy in a white coat? FDA clearly thinks the answer is yes. I find that disappointing and shortsighted and naïve."[35]

Razib Khan, a geneticist and journalist wrote: "This incident highlights the tension between the paternalistic medical establishment that arose to deal with the dangers of nineteenth-century quack medicine, and a 'technopopulist' element of American society pioneering personal health assessment and decision-making by leveraging new information technologies."[40] But David Vallee, a leading genetics professor at Johns Hopkins, weighed in, "No consumer should be left on his or her own to interpret such complicated and highly nuanced data," and that a health care professional should ideally be involved.[63] However, 23andMe's website says, "You should not assume that any information we may be able to provide to you, whether now or as genetic research advances, will be welcome or positive."

Gary Marchant, a life-science law professor at Arizona State University, wrote, "this is the last shoe to drop in the FDA's effort to wipe out the right of consumers to discover their own genetic information, some of the most important, private, useful, and interesting information about our own health and well-being."[79] Another columnist framed it as the FDA waging war against the mind of the individual. The message is: "You're not able to handle the truth. Only we in the FDA can decide what is true and rational. You may think you are proceeding rationally, but that's not good enough. We decide what's rational for you and what is not."[69]

It is also interesting to reflect on the view of Lakshman Ramamurthy, the director of FDA and regulatory policy at Avalere Health, who finds this argument amusing. "If I were to follow that logic, I would say draw-ing yellow lines on highways is paternalistic. I would think having speed limits is paternalistic," he quipped. "I find the argument about paternalism really disingenuous, unless we live in a free-for-all."[38] One can consider this analogy off the mark. While speed limits and lane markings make roads safer, and highway stripes provide information, they don't drive the car. The FDA is demanding sole right to steer the car.

Beyond paternalism, the FDA-vs.-23andMe flap brings out another crit-ical and unresolved matter—validity of the genomic results. Validity can be divided into two categories—technical and clinical. As far as techni-cal, the genotyping for 23andMe is done by state-of-the-art equipment in a clinical laboratory known as the National Genetics Institute, a wholly owned subsidiary of LabCorp. In a replication experiment of 23andMe data performed in 2010, of six hundred thousand genotypes there were only eighty-five that were errors—that is a rate of 0.01 percent,[54] which is as good as any academic genomics research laboratory. So the question about the accuracy of the genotyping is pretty easy to put aside.

Further, in February 2013, 23andMe scientists published, in a well-regarded, peer-reviewed, open-access journal, *PeerJ*, their results of the in-dividuals who had tested positive for their BRCA tests, which are quite limited to the three mutations prevalent in Ashkenazi Jews.[80] There are hundreds of mutations in the BRCA1|2 genes that may be associated with cancer—23andMe only tests for a few of the common ones via what is known as array genotyping, not sequencing. The array method assesses particular bases in the genome rather than systematically looking at all bases in a particular gene or region of the genome. Put quantitatively, it only tests for 0.02 percent of relevant bases known to affect hereditary breast or ovarian risk. But for the three BRCA mutations (185delAG, 6382insC in BRCA1 and 6174delT in BRCA2) the company analyzes, it does so with very high accuracy. (These are different from the well-known French Canadian mutations C446T in BRCA1 or 8765delAG in BRCA2.) It uses the Illumina OmniExpress Plus biochip, which is the same as is used by academic researchers around the world.[68] Of 114,627 customers in the 23andMe database at the time, 204 (130 males and 74 females) tested positive for one of the three BRCA mutations. Of those who were Ashkenazi Jews and were willing to participate in the research study, 32 individuals had unexpected BRCA mutation results that they received directly through their saliva genotyping. They handled this information quite well, without undue anxiety, sharing it with relatives and identifying additional carriers. Furthermore, controls (from the 23andMe database) of 31 Ashkenazi Jews matched for age and sex, but who were not BRCA mutation carriers, did not forego cancer screening, acknowledging that the 23andMe testing is quite limited. Only 1 of the 63 participants reported a negative impact and said, "I would not do it again."[44]

But the clinical validity of 23andMe's reports is quite a different matter. Each customer gets hundreds of thousands of DNA sequence variants assessed for over 250 medical conditions and traits. Some are frivolous like for the type of earwax or whether you are likely to sneeze when you look directly at the sun (this gene variant was discovered and reported by 23andMe from review of their database). But most are for common diseases like heart attack, diabetes, and various cancers, or for DNA interactions with medications. Most of the effect of a variation in DNA sequence—a base (or letter) change or genotype—is pretty small. And nothing is deterministic, just probabilistic. Going back to Jolie's BRCA1 mutation with 87 percent risk of developing breast cancer at some point in her life; it's not 100 percent and who knows when. Consumers typically have a difficult time understanding probabilistic odds.

As Richard Epstein, the noted law professor at New York University, has pointed out, "The FDA should have to show by clear and convincing evidence that 23andMe leads to dangerous results that the FDA claims by surveying customers of the firm."[68,81] Thus far, with over seven hundred thousand customers, there has yet to be any documentation of harm.[82] Our group at Scripps published a *New England Journal of Medicine* study of over three thousand individuals who had a similar consumer genomics assessment to 23andMe's and found no evidence of psychological harm or sustained anxiety.[83] One in 4 participants decided to share their genomic information with their doctor. More recently, Eric Green and colleagues at Harvard studied 1,057 consumers who had a 23andMe test or one from another company. This study confirmed both any lack of adverse effects and the proportion of individuals who shared their data with a physician.[84]

But absence from harm is a far cry from benefit. Some have therefore called this "recreational genetics." I like to think of 23andMe as a starter kit of genomic data, as it is just the beginning of how we will understand human DNA sequence data in the future. When millions of people of diverse medical conditions and ancestries have whole genome sequencing, we'll be a lot smarter. We'll have a much better sense of the magnitude of risk of a change in a letter of DNA code, how the different changes interact with one another, how important rare or low frequency changes are. Today we really only know about common letter changes, which overall have small effects, and we have little understanding of how these common variants interact with one another. But for $99, and for a company that loses money on each saliva kit and analysis that it performs, it's a pretty good deal for consumers. Especially for the reports focused on approximately thirty drug interactions, which typically convey worthwhile information, any one of which might cost $250 or more in a clinical laboratory. It's just the beginning of where consumer genomics can and will get to over time when our knowledge base is enhanced.

23andMe was initially positioned as providing genomics education and research for consumers when it was commercially launched in 2007. But in August 2013, having put two seasoned retail executives in leadership positions, it went into an aggressive marketing mode with a $5 million TV and Internet advertising campaign titled "Portraits of Health."[62] Some of the commercials showed individuals next to a graph of their genomic profile saying things like, "I might have an increased risk of heart disease."[62,85] That 23andMe was "going medical" was also evident in their campaign "Know more about your health!," including new website content with such anecdotes of people getting an unexpected diagnosis that "changed their lives forever." Further, 23andMe started selling their saliva kits and Personal Genome Service via Amazon for the first time.

The marketing was not well received by the FDA. The unfathomable lack of communication over a six-month period, during which 23andMe ignored multiple FDA contacts, only made matters worse. And 23andMe must have known what could happen, given the experience of another consumer genomics company, Pathway Genomics, in May 2010. Pathway was about to launch its saliva test kit at all Walgreen drugstores, when, on the day prior to the national roll out, the FDA sent a letter to Pathway informing the company their test had not been approved. Walgreens precipitously dropped the program. Then, in June 2010, the FDA sent cease and desist letters to all direct-to-consumer genomic companies, including Navigenics, DeCode, Pathway, and 23andMe, which led each to change their model so their tests could only be ordered through a physician. 23andMe was the only one that kept its direct-to-consumer model; they must have known they were playing with fire when they undertook their marketing campaign. Ironically, the cover and feature article of the November 2013 issue (which was published in October, well in advance of the FDA letter to 23andMe) of *Fast Company* called out Anne Wojcicki as "The Most Daring CEO in America" and asked, "Why Are Doctors, Insurers and Privacy Wonks Having a Heart Attack?"[33] It should have included the FDA!

In response to the FDA's shutdown of 23andMe's marketing, there were two public efforts of online petitions, TechFreedom at change.org and We the People at whitehouse.gov, asking the Obama administration to reverse the FDA order.[38] While both were unsuccessful in garnering the requisite one hundred thousand signatures, their statements are worth noting. One was reasonable, when TechFreedom wrote: "The FDA seems to think that Americans can't be trusted with more information about their potential health risks because some people might make rash decisions with it. But banning personal genomics isn't the answer."[38] The other was not, when the "We the People" petition included the following: "we demand that we maintain access to genomics testing services like 23andMe," and "the price of over-regulation is lengthy delays in potentially life-saving medical innovations."[38] The latter claim is clearly off base, since 23andMe, or any other consumer genomics company, has yet to show any evidence of life-saving medical innovation. While much of the information, such as the drug-gene interaction panel or select mutations in such genes as BRCA, may be particularly useful for a given individual, and there are plenty of anecdotal cases to this effect,[86,87] the criteria for "life-saving" (requiring randomized trials or other incontrovertible evidence) have not been fulfilled.

The editors at the *Wall Street Journal* had a strong response, titled "The FDA and Thee," crying foul, that the FDA had overstepped its bounds: "The agency is declaring 23andMe's service an 'adulterated' product under the Federal Food, Drug and Cosmetic Act of 1938, in one more case of twentieth-century law undermining medical progress in the twenty-first."[88] and "The FDA lacks any specific statutory authority to regulate genomic sequencing technologies. Yet in 2010 the FDA simply decreed by fiat that these tests are considered new medical devices that require premarket testing and approval."[88]

The FDA commissioner, Dr. Margaret Hamburg, wrote back, "The FDA appreciates that many consumers would like to be informed about their genomes and their genetic risk for developing certain diseases. I personally share Ms. Wojcicki's perspective that genetic information can lead to better decisions and healthier lives."[89] What she didn't mention was the FDA's insistence that the information pass through a doctor or genetic counselor first.

The final indication that the FDA was preparing for the takedown on 23andMe came just two days prior, on November 20, 2013, when the FDA announced its approval of the first DNA sequencing technology, the so-called MySeq platform from Illumina. To trumpet the approval, the FDA commissioner and the NIH director wrote a joint editorial in the *New England Journal of Medicine*.[90] In retrospect, one could have seen what was in store for direct-to-consumer genomics: "Doctors and other health care professionals will need support in interpreting genomic data and their meaning for individual patients. Patients will want to be able to talk about their genetic information with their doctor. With the right information and support, patients will be able to participate alongside their doctors in making more informed decisions."

Despite these actions against 23andMe and others, there are many glaring inconsistencies in how the FDA treats consumer genomics. Myriad Genetics, for example, has never had FDA approval or clearance for their BRACAnalysis. Indeed, since 1976, the FDA (via the Medical Devices Amendment Act) has given a pass to any diagnostic test that was developed by a single laboratory, and most of these are molecular genetic assays.[91] As a result, of the roughly three thousand genetic tests that are commercially available with physician orders, only a few have ever received FDA approval.[79,91] Other instances of direct-to-consumer sales of genetic testing, for purposes of mapping ancestry and genealogy (Laboratory Developed Tests), have never been subject to FDA crackdown.

Yet the FDA has explicitly approved consumer tests like the OraQuick at-home human immunodeficiency virus (HIV) test, which carries an alarmingly high false negative rate of 1 in 12.[71] Then there's the inconsistency with lack of any regulatory authority of the FDA over the $32 billion per year industry of dietary supplements—there are over fifty-five thousand of these, and only 0.3 percent have yet been studied to determine their side effects, not to mention their purported benefits![92,93]

One additional contradiction that deserves highlighting is how we make use of risk calculators in medicine, and, as Joe Pickrell, a geneticist at the

New York Genome Center, sharply pointed out, traditional epidemiology.[94] At a variety of government websites, you can calculate your risk of a heart attack, stroke, breast cancer, diabetes, Parkinson's disease, colon cancer, or melanoma, based only on rudimentary information such as age, gender, and family history used to calculate the risk. There is a disclaimer at the National Cancer Institute's (NCI) website for breast cancer risk calcula-tion: "There is a small chance that test results may not be accurate, leading to mak[ing] decisions based on incorrect information."[94] This is essentially the same kind of prediction that 23andMe was offering, yet while anyone can use the NCI site alone, 23andMe has been classified as a Class-3 Med-ical Device by the FDA, which means that it cannot be allowed on the market before it has been approved.[94,95] As Michael Eisen, a University of California, Berkeley, geneticist, who is an advisor to 23andMe, nicely sum-marized, "Genetic tests are simply not—at least not yet—medical devices in any meaningful sense of the word. They are closer to family history than to an accurate diagnostic."[96]

While 23andMe agreed to stop selling its PGS, it still will provide the raw genomic data to consumers, and there are free software tools that can be used to get the key interpretative information. So, as it turns out, it is difficult for the FDA to fully regulate consumer genomics. I fully concur with the leading biomedical journal *Nature,* which had an editorial on this matter and concluded that "even if regulators or doctors want to, they will not be able to stand between ordinary people and their DNA for very long."[97] Despite the obstacles, it's just a matter of time before such genomic information is free-flowing to the public. OK, maybe not free, but certainly flowing.

Big Consumer Genomic Data

Before leaving 23andMe, there is one other big thing to note—its ambi-tious strategy to build a database with the DNA data from twenty-five million customers and use it to revolutionize health care. That kind of big data, Wojcicki said, "is going to make us all healthier," because their "da-tabase of information . . . is going to become an incredibly valuable tool for all of research—for academics, for pharma companies." What she called a "massive asset for society" has led to an outcry by others. For example, Charles Seife, author of *Zero: The Biography of a Dangerous Idea,* called it "a front end for a massive information-gathering operation against an unwitting public," and "a one-way portal into a world where corporations have access to the innermost contents of your cells and where insurers and pharmaceutical firms and marketers might know more about your body than you know yourself."[98]

This is not true. When you become a customer of 23andMe, you are asked to opt in to their research and 90 percent of people do that—with the assurance that you will be kept anonymous as the data is amalgamated. The information itself is quite useful to researchers as well. The company's scientists have published seventeen publications in peer-reviewed journals, having discovered novel gene variants on conditions that span from Parkinson's disease to photic sneeze.[82] They have received large peer-reviewed grants from the National Institutes of Health for crowdsourcing data from individuals with such conditions as allergies or asthma. Much of this work has been done with a database of only a few hundred thousand individuals. If the 23andMe objective of twenty-five million customers were ever reached, even with the rather limited part of the genome that 23andMe assays, the opportunity to make discoveries on the root cause of diseases, how our DNA interacts with medications, and enriched understanding of genetic circuitry—how a variant in one gene cancels out the effect of another, for instance—would all be markedly improved.

Creating a massive information resource of millions of customers, and monetizing the anonymized data for pharmaceutical companies or health insurers, represents an unproven strategy, not just because they need customers to buy the data, but because they must protect the data to avoid re-identification. As Seife's criticism makes clear, some people are going to be very uncomfortable with the prospect of selling their information to a drug company. Addressing both concerns is critical, because the promise of massive medicine information resources is so great. This issue is much bigger than 23andMe, and I will discuss it fully in two dedicated chapters later in the book.

The Supreme Court and Genomic Medicine

The BRCA genes that were the key to Angelina Jolie's preventive surgery turned out to be exceptionally important as the test case for gene patenting. Before we get into the details of the case, let me review a bit on the

BRCA genes. The BRCA1 gene is on chromosome 17 and has 81,888 base pairs (coding letters); BRCA2 is on chromosome 13 and has 10,254 base pairs. These genes are critical for the housekeeping of our DNA, both being involved in its repair.[99] When they aren't functioning properly, there is potential for cancer to develop. The genes were first cloned in 1994 in laboratories at both the University of Utah and the company Myriad Genetics. In 1996, Myriad Genetics was granted a patent for the gene sequences, making it the only entity in the United States legally authorized to perform clinical sequencing of the BRCA genes. When other companies, universities, or academic laboratories tried to perform BRCA sequencing, Myriad enforced their patent and notified such entities to cease and desist any such activity. Myriad's own fees were steep, as we've seen, running between $3,000 and $4,000 per sequence.[100]

A limited part of my BRCA1 gene sequence is provided to demonstrate a few key points (Figure 4.2). While this gene has over eighty thousand base pairs, there are hundreds of variations. At the bottom, I have compared a segment of eighty-eight base pairs with the reference sequence for the same stretch. There is one difference between my genome and the reference one here, with an A instead of a G in the lower segment. Just above that is a less-magnified view of 9,024 bases. There are fourteen vertical lines, each representing a variant from the reference genome. The last vertical line on the right with an arrowhead indicates a spot where the difference in the DNA actually causes the code to call a different amino acid (a glycine instead of a serine). The top left section gives the names and locations for the DNA variants that I have in this bit of sequence. This is meant to show that there are hundreds of DNA sequence variants that each of us has in our BRCA genes (and throughout our genome). It could be a substitution, as shown, but also a deletion, or an insertion, extra copy of a segment, inversion, or transposition. Some of these can cause an amino acid change and radically alter the function of BRCA1; most, however, are innocuous, without altering the function of the gene. The importance of these points will become evident as we delve more into nuances of Myriad Genetics' monopoly.

In May 2009, the American Civil Liberties Union and other plaintiffs filed suit against Myriad Genetics and the US Patent and Trademark Office. The lawsuit claimed that the BRCA gene patents were invalid, unconstitutional, and were limiting access to testing. The case was considered by

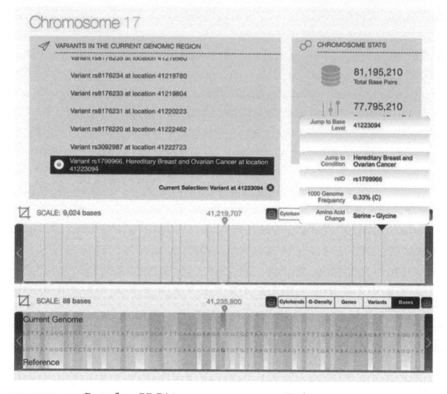

FIGURE 4.2: Part of my BRCA1 gene sequence on my iPad.

many courts along the way, but ultimately was heard by the US Supreme Court on April 15, 2013, just before the Jolie disclosure. The ruling came down on June 13: isolated genomic DNA is not patentable.[101] That is, the Supreme Court held that Mother Nature cannot be patented.[102,103] The proprietary claim of Myriad was equated, among other things, to looking through the first telescope at the planets and their moons and seeking to patent them.[102,104–114]

Soon after the court's decision, a large number of companies, including Quest Diagnostics, Ambry Genetics, Invitae, LabCorp, Gene by Gene, and others, announced they would now sequence the BRCA genes. And in many cases at a cost substantially lower than Myriad.[115–118] So this could be seen as a big step for democratizing DNA information—making the BRCA sequencing tests accessible to at-risk individuals.

Not so fast, unfortunately. Myriad's proprietary database, unaffected by the patent ruling, holds the keys to the BRCA1|2 gene treasure trove. There are several hundred variants in these two genes that collectively cover over one hundred thousand DNA letters like the ones in Figure 4.2. Which ones carry risk, and what is the magnitude of the risk, for a woman that might be considering preventive mastectomy? Over the course of seventeen years, millions of women had their BRCA genes sequenced by Myriad, with a high proportion of these done from patients who had already developed cancer. For each individual, the DNA variations from the human reference genome were identified. Some of these were clear-cut culprits that could induce breast or ovarian cancer, or both. But with over one hundred thousand DNA letters in the two genes, there were an exceptional number of sequence variants that were initially classified as having "uncertain significance" (known to professionals as VUS). For these, Myriad would obtain DNA samples from relatives of the individual in question to sort out if it was the real deal or an innocent change. While still today there are many BRCA sequence variants that even Myriad reports out as VUS, the company has an unequivocal information advantage over new entities that are going into the BRCA sequencing business. Monopolies, in general, are not good for consumers, but monopolies in medicine such as this are totally deplorable. In the three months following Jolie's op-ed, Myriad posted $202 million of revenue, a 52 percent jump from the prior financial quarter, which the company attributed to the Angelina Effect.[31] Myriad is also using the courts to defend its business by suing the new companies sequencing BRCA on the basis of its other ten patents on methods of testing, DNA primers, probes, and laboratory-synthesized DNA (so called cDNA), which, the Supreme Court has ruled, are patentable.[119]

Efforts such as the Sharing Clinical Reports Project, a grassroots, volunteer initiative involving both doctors and patients, are trying to collate the BRCA sequencing results from hundreds of thousands of individuals to fill in the holes in our BRCA knowledge base.[120] Nevertheless, it will likely take a number of years to break Myriad's chokehold on BRCA data interpretative capability.

Despite those remaining issues, the Supreme Court ruling was fundamental for democratizing genomic information. For while it came much too late in the case of BRCA genes to avoid a monopoly of invaluable medical information, there are another nineteen thousand genes in our genomes, 40 percent of which have been patented, the rest of our genome—98.5 percent of which is not comprised of genes but is still remarkably important in defining our unique biology. By striking down the right to patent genes, our DNA has been freed from such constraints in the future. The economics of BRCA sequencing have already been favorably impacted—Medicare slashed the reimbursement by 49 percent in 2014 (from $2,795 to $1,440).[116] For all these reasons, it should be no surprise that for 2013, *Discover* magazine ranked the "Supreme Word on Genes" as the #2 Top Story in Science.[121]

Collectively, in this chapter, we have seen the powerful impact of one individual, one company, two governmental bureaus (FDA and the Supreme Court), and two genes in dealing with public access to genomic information. In the background, there is engrained medical paternalism, while at the same time an ongoing communications revolution bringing unprecedented health data directly to individuals. Now we're ready to move on to the specific types of information that will be increasingly accessible for any individual, and that will irrevocably alter one's medical future.

The New Data and Information

Chapter 5

My GIS

A TEN BY TEN
APPROACH

"The digital traces we leave behind each day reveal more about us than we know. This could become a privacy nightmare—or it could be the foundation of a healthier, more prosperous world."
—ALEX "SANDY" PENTLAND, MIT MEDIA LAB[1]

"Where is the wisdom we have lost in knowledge? Where is the knowledge we have lost in information?"
—T. S. ELIOT

"The goal is to turn medicine into the land of the quants."
—JEFFREY HAMMERBACHER,
MT. SINAI ICAHN SCHOOL OF MEDICINE[2]

Getting map directions from a Google search engine is so quick, you probably don't think at all about what's under the hood. It's a classic geographic information system (GIS) with multiple layers of data—such as traffic, satellite, or street views—superimposed on a map. Although the term GIS wasn't coined until 1968, the first of what would now be considered spatiotemporal applications were developed in the 1800s.[3] They were used to track cholera outbreaks in Paris and London. These days, of course,

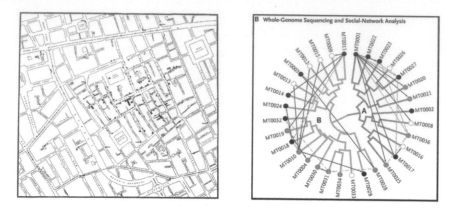

FIGURE 5.1: Differences in our ability to map an infectious disease epidemic. Sources: (left) "1854 Broad Street Cholera Outbreak," Wikipedia, accessed August 13, 2014, http://en.wikipedia.org/wiki/1854_Broad_Street_cholera_outbreak; and (right) J. L. Gardy et al., "Whole-Genome Sequencing and Social-Network Analysis of a Tuberculosis Outbreak," *New England Journal of Medicine* 364 (2011): 730–739.

more people might use GIS on a road journey than in epidemiology, but their medical applications remain very important—although instead of simply plotting places where a cholera epidemic victim died, we can combine modern tools of social networking and whole genome sequencing to pinpoint the strain of the pathogen, the individual responsible, and the precise path of transmission for an outbreak (Figure 5.1).[4] This is because we can now combine and integrate multiple layers of information to essentially create the Google map of you. Much like Angelina Jolie's story, centered on a single mutation in a BRCA gene, showed how preventive medicine can be less about population-wide risks and mass screening techniques, the GIS of millions of human beings is becoming a fundamental application for the future of medicine. This is the first chapter of the "My" section of the book; each one is about different components of *your* information. Later in the book we'll get to the transformative implications of having and owning your GIS data.

The human GIS comprises multiple layers of demographic, physiologic, anatomic, biologic, and environmental data (Figure 5.2) about a particular individual.[5] This is a rich, multi-scale, mosaic of a human being, which can be used to define one's medical essence; when fully amassed and integrated, it is what a digitized person looks like, at least for the sake of how medical care can be rendered.

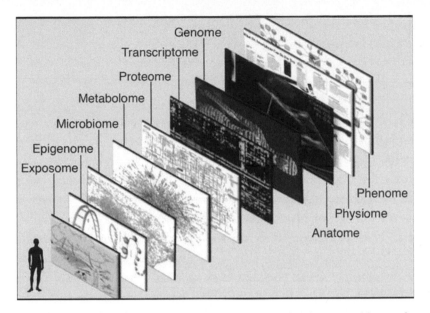

FIGURE 5.2: The human GIS—multiple superimposed and integrated layers of medical information. Source: Adapted from E. J. Topol, "Individualized Medicine from Prewomb to Tomb," *Cell* 157 (2014): 241–253.

The Panoromic View

Let's now unpack the human GIS to define and understand each component. The "ome" attached to each denotes the study of something. The phenome refers to all the phenotypic traits of an individual, such as height, weight, and eye and skin color. I like to combine it with one's social graph, which broadens the "look from the outside" of a person to their social network. The physiome is the collection of one's physiologic metrics, such as heart rate and blood pressure. The anatome is our individual anatomy. The genome refers to the six billion letters that make up one's DNA sequence. Likewise, the other biologic omes are the proteome, all of your proteins; the metabolome, your metabolites; the microbiome, representing the microbes that coinhabit you; and the epigenome, comprised of the side chains of DNA and how it is packaged. Finally, there's the exposome, referring to your environment, all that you are exposed to. Collectively, I have coined the term "panoromic" adopted from the word panoramic, meaning lots of information and covering many topics.[5] A panoromic view of each individual provides a comprehensive sweep across all the omes relevant to health and medicine.

Social Graph and the Phenome

The term "social graph" encompasses a dense package of information, including demographics, location, family and friends, friends of friends, interests, likes, education, pets, pictures, videos, and much more. This is precisely the sort of information stored on sites like Facebook, a fact that hasn't escaped researchers. The prominent mathematician, Stephen Wolfram, the founder of a computation knowledge engine known as Wolfram Alpha, developed a consumer software product known as "personal analytics for Facebook" that within a minute provides a remarkable set of data and graphics about oneself and one's social network—what Wolfram calls "a dashboard for life."[6,7] If you are a Facebook registrant and haven't seen this, I encourage you to take a look at yours for free: http://www .wolframalpha.com/facebook/. What you will see will be a bit creepy, as it extracts all the information that you have ever posted on Facebook, creates a word cloud of your posts, their precise time and patterns, your likes and comments, most-liked post, most-commented post, the demographics of all your friends, including a world map of their locations, their local times and birthdays, and your social network map separating out friends and family, influences, neighbors, social connectors, outsiders, and insiders.

We know that social networks have important relationships for health, as Nicholas Christakis and James Fowler established convincingly in several high-impact publications along with their book: *Connected*.[8] These social scientists and many others subsequently have highlighted the essential influence of our social graphs on obesity, smoking, and most other aspects of behavior and lifestyle. With more kinds of data, as well as greater quantities of data being shared, there is considerable potential for social networks to play a much greater role in the future of health care. Yet the medical community still doesn't generally respect this information as a critical part of an individual's background for health.

Historically, for the phenome, we rely on medical records to provide the demographics and clinical features. This includes age, gender, occupation, family history, medications, medical conditions, operations, and procedures. The chart of a patient also has physical descriptors, such as height, weight, appearance, and vital signs. We essentially get a phenome from this information—"the composite of an individual's observable character-istics and traits."[9] Noteworthy is the point that for any given individual, particularly as we age, there is unlikely to be just one phenotype; instead, multiple conditions are likely to be present, which makes one's phenome not as straightforward as it might appear. For example, blood pressure tends to rise with age, while visual acuity declines. Ideally, someday, we will have all of this data comprehensively collected as the phenome for each individual—the social graph plus the traditional medical record informa-tion—and continually updated. While the social graph is subsidiary to the phenome, there's no question that one's social network plays an important role in health.

Sensors and the Physiome

Perhaps the biggest advance in tracking an individual's information in recent years is the outpouring of an extraordinary number of biosensors. There are now wearable wireless sensors, either commercially available or in clinical development, to capture physiologic data on a smartphone. This in-cludes blood pressure, heart rhythm, respiratory rate, oxygen concentration in the blood, heart rate variability, cardiac output and stroke volume, gal-vanic skin response, body temperature, eye pressure, blood glucose, brain waves, intracranial pressure, muscle movements, and many other metrics. The microphone of the smartphone can be used to quantify components of lung function and analyze one's voice to gauge mood or make the di-agnosis of Parkinson's disease or schizophrenia.[10,11] One's breath can be digitized to measure a large number of compounds, such as nitric oxide or organic chemicals, which could enable smartphones to track lung function or diagnose certain cancers. Beyond all these wearable and noninvasive sensors, nanochips are being developed to be embedded in the bloodstream to monitor the appearance of tumor DNA, immune activation, or genomic signals indicative of a forthcoming heart attack or stroke. Whether such biosensor data were collected intermittently or on a continuous basis, they would provide an exquisite window into the operating functions of the body across virtually every organ system and medical condition. We have approximately four hundred embedded sensors in our cars, more than ten in our smartphones—why shouldn't we have any in our bodies?

Imaging and the Anatome

Magnetic resonance, CT and nuclear scanning, and ultrasound have provided a remarkable capability to define one's anatomy (here called "anatome" to denote the study of one's anatomy)—without surgery. Human anatomy, the population-based average, does not take into account marked interindividual heterogeneity; that's why a precise definition of the anatome of one's body is key. But these traditional methods of imaging rely on access to expensive hospital and clinic-based equipment. The emerging use of pocket devices to obtain high-resolution ultrasounds or X-rays is changing that landscape, making the assessment of an individual's anatomy much easier, faster, and cheaper. Now a smartphone or some other small device can be used both to perform the physical exam of the eyes, ears, neck vessels, heart, lungs, abdomen, and fetus, as well as to share medical imaging, enabling a patient to fully review his anatomy on a tablet or smartphone.

Sequencing and the Genome

The genome refers to our DNA sequence of six billion *A, C, T,* or *G* letters, 98.5 percent of which is not comprised of genes; our nineteen thousand genes that encode proteins take up only approximately 1.5 percent, consist of about forty million letters, and this component is known as the exome.[12]

There has been a more than four-log order, or a one hundred-thousandth reduction, of the cost of sequencing a genome over the past decade, far exceeding the decline in cost for semiconductor chips, which until now has been considered the most formidable pace of technologic progress in history. The cost for sequencing a human genome has dropped from $28.8 million in 2004 to less than $1,500 in 2015.[13,14]

In parallel to the plummeting of cost, the expansion of our knowledge base on root causes of diseases has markedly increased over the past decade. Finding rare sequence variants that explain heritable disease relies on this technology, and the jump in known causes of rare diseases. The ability to diagnose the molecular basis of rare mitochondrial diseases has jumped from 1 percent to 60 percent,[15] giving the sense of the progress that is being made.[5] It won't be much longer until the genetic underpinnings of all seven thousand Mendelian diseases (conditions following the classic inheritance patterns such as autosomal dominant or recessive) are defined.[5]

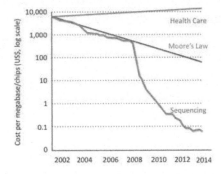

FIGURE 5.3: Cost of sequencing decline is exceeding Moore's law of chips, with cost of health care going in the opposite direction.

Even as we make progress on some problems, we are also finding our genomes are more complicated than we had thought. We all learned in "Genetics 101" that for one individual there was one DNA, that our thirty-seven trillion cells in our body have the same DNA. Well, that turned out to be dead wrong—the simple, seemingly immutable archetype just got mutated. Sequencing the genome of single cells has made it clear that we're all mosaics.[16,17] For example, researchers at the Salk Institute did single-cell sequencing of brain cells from individuals who had died and found striking differences from one cell to the next.[17] Part of this mosaicism is explained by so-called de novo mutations, which occur in cells when they divide over the course of one's life. We've also learned about the remarkable extent of heterogeneity that exists from one cancer cell to another. So moving from the conceptual framework of sequencing an individual's DNA to that of a cell has already taught us some invaluable, disease-relevant lessons.

There are important limitations to acknowledge about sequencing. When a person undergoes sequencing (some are now calling this getting "genomed") there will typically be about 3.5 million variant bases compared with the human reference genome. But, as we discussed with BRCA, Myriad Genetics, and the Supreme Court ruling, most will be variants of unknown significance (VUS). They will become known when millions of people of diverse ancestries, with the whole gamut of medical conditions, have been genomed, and an individual's family members as well. Lastly, not only are we mosaics of DNA that we don't completely understand, we can't even sequence all of it. While the term "whole genome sequencing" is normally used, about nine hundred genes of the nineteen thousand are not accessible due to their location or other technical issues. So there's still plenty to learn about our genomes in the future, and much more than I've touched on in this very brief summary.

The Transcriptome

Before our cells can do anything with our DNA, they must transcribe it to RNA. This has been known for decades, but our respect for the importance of RNA has grown enormously over recent years. Not only have many different forms of RNA been discovered and characterized, but their dynamic impact on the genome's operating instructions has become clearer, too. This is the transcriptome, and the technologies have evolved quickly from the first efforts to detect gene expression across the whole genome to RNAseq, which detects gene fusions and the wide assortment of different RNAs. Many of these have relevance for disease or preserving health.

The Proteome and the Metabolome

We have long assessed the presence of proteins in routine lab chemistries, such as liver or kidney function tests. But now the window into an individual's protein biology has markedly broadened, enabling us to define a person's protein-protein interactions as well as the presence of autoantibodies (antibodies directed against one's own proteins). Similarly, using mass spectrometry, the entire array of metabolites—the compounds resulting from our metabolism—that one produces at a particular point in time can be assessed. The result is a sweeping view that differs vastly from an assay of a single or group of proteins or metabolites, which is how most of our lab tests are set up. Being able to tap into the whole range of an individual's RNA transcripts, proteins, and metabolites at any given moment creates quite an extraordinary opportunity to understand one's instantaneous biology, in an unbiased fashion.

The Microbiome

It's hard for most of us to accept that we are nine parts microbe and only one part human, at least as far as a count of our cells goes. The era of sequencing has been especially instructive about the trillions of microbes (bacteria, viruses, fungi) that live within or on us. The diversity of DNA in us from microbes far outstrips our own DNA, with one hundred trillion instead of thirty-seven trillion cells, over eight million genes instead of only approximately nineteen thousand, and more than ten thousand species instead of one.[18] The microbiome represents the interface between the individual and her environment. For example, one's diet has a strong influence on one's microbiome. And the medical importance of these microbes has escalated far beyond what most of us envisioned, with their influence in obesity, cancer, heart, allergic and autoimmune diseases, and many more conditions, in which the gut microbiome is particularly prominent.

The Epigenome

The side chains and packaging of our DNA, by methylation, histone modifications, and chromatin, represent yet another highly dynamic part of our genomic biology. For example, methylation of a base in the genome can shut down a gene. Assessing a specific region of the genome for epigenomic markers is technically straightforward today. Epigenomic changes can be inherited independent of our DNA sequence, and the "reprogramming" has an impact in a wide range of medical conditions, including cancer, diabetes, and autoimmune and cardiovascular conditions. And like RNAs, proteins, the epigenome is highly cell-specific—the DNA side chain changes in one type of cell may be entirely different from another. Given that there are over two hundred cell types in the body, you can get a sense of how diverse the impact on our biology can be. The whole human epigenome has been mapped, but, unlike the human genome, this is not something that can be done at scale yet.

The Exposome

Our environment, through exposure to things like radiation, air pollution, pollen count, and pesticides in food, has a profound impact on our medical essence. Environmental sensors, many of which wirelessly connect or attach to smartphones, have been and are increasingly being developed to quantify and track such exposures.

Collectively, these ten omes provide the panoromic view of an individual, with an extraordinary breadth of information that will be increasingly accessible and useful as we move forward in medicine. No one human being has had the "full Monty" yet, but the person who has come closest is Michael Snyder, the head of genetics at Stanford University. Snyder had his whole genome sequenced, and, at several points in time his transcriptome, proteome, and metabolome.[19] The benefits became clear after Snyder was diagnosed with diabetes mellitus soon after developing an upper respiratory infection. They might seem unrelated, but the omic data appeared to connect the dots; despite the fact that no one had reported such a relationship before. The diagnosis also led Snyder to change his lifestyle and restore normal glucose homeostasis, and then go on to check this in some relatives who turned out to have unrecognized glucose intolerance, and for whom diet and exercise proved similarly helpful. More recently, Snyder's Stanford forty-member research group has expanded the initial effort with sequencing Snyder's epigenome, gut microbiome, and use of multiple biosensors. Getting this GIS-like information has generated a massive amount of data: 1 terabyte (TB, a trillion bits) for DNA sequence, 2 TB for the epigenomic data, 0.7 TB for the transcriptome, and 3 TB for the microbiome.[5] For perspective, 1 TB would equate to one thousand copies of the Encyclopedia Britannica and 10 TB, which is approximately how much Snyder's panoromic project amassed, would hold the entire Library of Congress. In the world each year about five zettabytes of data—or forty sextillion bits—are generated.[20] If we divided this by the world's seven billion people, this would put an average individual at nearly 1 TB of data generated per year. While there is no such thing as an average person, this calculation gives the sense of how much more data flow can be expected from a human GIS.

The point of reviewing this first foray toward a full human GIS is not to suggest it is yet practical. It is remarkably expensive and the data that are generated far exceeds our ability to interpret it at this juncture. However, it is indeed feasible. It represents just the beginning of how we can actually digitize a human being and set the real foundation for individualized medicine. And remember that not yet practical does not mean it never will be; after all, it took ten years and $5 billion to sequence the first human genome, and now it takes less than twenty-four hours and costs less than $1,500.[5]

Using the GIS to Individualize Medicine

The ten omic tools, in aggregate, set up the extraordinary potential to provide a new, highly individualized form of medicine, from prewomb to

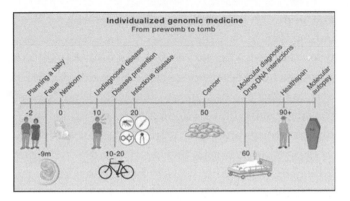

FIGURE 5.4: Individualized medicine from prewomb to tomb.
Source: Adapted from E. J. Topol, "Individualized Medicine from
Prewomb to Tomb," *Cell* 157 (2014): 241–253.

tomb, as schematically illustrated in Figure 5.4. The GIS can be applied
across one's life span. Let's see how.

Prewomb

One of the most far-reaching forms of prevention in medicine is using
genetic knowledge for the purpose of planning a baby. The proportion of
people carrying serious recessive alleles is much higher than generally ap-
preciated. Some examples of the rates are: 1 in 40 for cystic fibrosis, 1 in 35
for spinal muscular atrophy, and 1 in 125 for Fragile X syndrome. Among
Ashkenazi Jews the carrier rate for Gaucher disease is 1 in 15 and for Tay-
Sachs 1 in 27.[5] Prospective parents can be readily screened for important
carrier conditions via a variety of commercial tests; 23andMe screens for
fifty conditions; Counsyl tests for over one hundred. Both these companies
use array chips that only pick up the mutations that have been classically
implicated for a particular condition, however, and as previously mentioned
in the example of the BRCA or cystic fibrosis genes, there are hundreds of
variants in any particular gene that might be pathogenic and are not currently getting screened. Newer approaches involve actual sequencing of the
genes in question, such as those being employed by Recombine, Good Start
Genetics, or GenePeeks. If both parents test positive for the presence of an
important recessive allele, there are many alternatives, including adoption
or electing not to have children. The most popular choice, however, is in
vitro fertilization (IVF) with preimplantation genetic diagnosis. The tech-
nique involves creation of an embryo and determining if it has resulted
in the recessive alleles coming together. It is quite effective for preventing

the condition in the fetus. A recent advance of sequencing human oocytes without destroying them has the potential to markedly improve the success of IVF and avoid having to proceed to the early embryonic stage of the preimplantation blastocyst before determining the genetic diagnosis.[14] Another option is the use of a sperm donor, although sperm banks are completely unregulated for any standard genomic assessment,[21] so donor sperm might create new problems. While some have questioned such efforts, disparaging them as a quest for "designer babies,"[22,23] they represent very attractive, cost-effective but remarkably underutilized means for preventing serious medical conditions.

Fetal Sequencing and Tracking

A revolution in prenatal medicine has already taken off, thanks to the ability to diagnose major chromosomal aberrations like trisomy 21 (Down syndrome), trisomy 13 (Patau syndrome) and trisomy 18 (Edward syndrome), and others including DiGeorge syndrome, Cri-du-chat, and Prader-Willi syndrome, via a single tube of the mother's blood as early as eight to ten weeks of pregnancy. (Previously this required the invasive procedures of either amniocentesis or chorionic villi sampling, which carry a risk of miscarriage in 1 in 400 procedures.)

There are presently four companies that market these new tests, each with remarkably high accuracy.[24,25] They have become the most rapidly adopted molecular diagnostic in the history of medicine, with nearly 20 percent of the four million live births per year in the United States having this prenatal genomic screening in 2014 (Figure 5.5). But it is widely anticipated that this will become common practice in the next few years. Indeed, the state of California, which has the largest prenatal screening program in the world, with more than four hundred thousand expectant mothers assessed annually, already provides these tests to all pregnant women who have increased risk.[26]

Of course, we could also sequence the fetus's entire genome instead of just doing the simpler screens. While that is not a commercially available test, and there are substantial bioinformatic challenges that lie ahead before it could be scalable, the anticipatory bioethical issues that this engenders are considerable.[27] We are a long way off for determining what would constitute acceptable genomic criteria for early termination of pregnancy, since this not only relies on accurately determining a key genomic variant linked to a serious illness, but also understanding whether this condition would actually

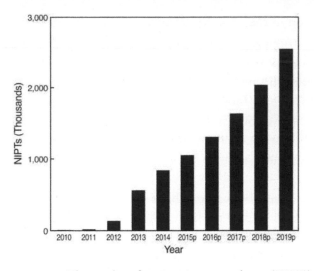

FIGURE 5.5: The number of noninvasive prenatal tests (NIPTs) in the United States and the projection (p) for the next five years.

manifest. The term "patients in waiting" has been applied to individuals who carry a known disease-related mutation, but do not show any signs of the condition.[28] Many, if not most, will never develop the disease due to the presence of such things (that are yet poorly understood) as other genes that modify or epigenomic reprogramming that cancels out the disease risk. Therefore, there is much uncertainty about the limits to prenatal screening—accuracy, boundaries of diagnosis severity, and whether the medical risk of the mutation risk is unequivocal.[27] In the meantime, just being able to screen many critical conditions so early in a pregnancy, without any invasion of the mother's womb, represents a giant step forward in medicine.

Later in pregnancy, a simple wearable sensor for the mother affords the ability to track fetal heart rate and its response to maternal contractions. This can be useful for remote, wireless monitoring of high-risk pregnancies for the earliest possible diagnosis of fetal distress.

Neonatal Sequencing and Tracking

Mass newborn screening with a heel stick began in the United States back in 1963, and has evolved little since that time.[29] It might have gotten worse: an exposé that occurred near its fiftieth anniversary, titled "Deadly Delays," reported on the highly variable time it takes for hospitals throughout the United States to analyze the samples.[30] Although it is very inexpensive and easy to screen for more than fifty rare disorders like phenylketonuria

(PKU) or galactosemia, it takes weeks to accomplish this at many hospitals. This is a travesty, as irreversible damage to the baby can occur without rapid diagnosis of many of these conditions.

To provide a far more prompt and comprehensive approach, the group at Children's Mercy Hospital in Kansas City led by Stephen Kingsmore has shown it is feasible to do neonatal whole genome sequencing in under twenty-four hours, which not only can provide actionable information for the newborn, but also then serves as a resource for the new little person's whole life span.[4]

There are a number of wearable sensors for the newborn, in socks or clothing, including Owlet, Mimo, and Sproutling, that wirelessly alert the parents about sleep, heart rate, or respirations. Concerns have rightly already been expressed about parental obsessive tracking of newborns—that too much information may lead to both undue anxiety for parents and unnecessary medical evaluations of the baby.[31] Even though we know that there are over four thousand deaths in the United States each year from sudden infant death syndrome (SIDS), we aren't smart enough yet to know which babies deserve monitoring. In the future, omic tools may be helpful for guiding the use of such sensors in babies at increased risk.

Undiagnosed Diseases

It has been estimated that there are over one million Americans who are suffering from a serious, disabling, or even life-threatening disease but have been left without a diagnosis. Typically, such individuals get a workup at multiple medical centers and accrue enormous bills that range from hundreds of thousands to even millions of dollars. Now it is possible to use sequencing to unravel the molecular diagnosis of an unknown condition, and the chances for success are enhanced when there is DNA from the mother and father, or other relatives, to use for anchoring and comparative sequencing analysis. At several centers around the country, the success rate for making the diagnosis ranges between 25 percent and 50 percent. It requires considerable genome bioinformatic expertise, for a trio of individuals will generate around 750 billion data points (six billion letters per sequence, three people, each done forty times to assure accuracy). Of course, just making the diagnosis is not the same as coming up with an effective treatment or a cure. But there have been some striking anecdotal examples of children whose lives were saved or had dramatic improvement. Once the root cause of the disease has been established, there is the possibility of repurposing an existing drug or surveying the drugs that are in clinical development for potential use. What has been especially encouraging is the recent willingness of some insurance companies to cover the cost of sequencing and analysis, as they come to understand that the upfront cost of sequencing might preempt a very long and expensive multicenter medical evaluation. With more validation, this could be a prudent and parsimonious strategy for the future.

Prevention of Disease

Breast cancer is not the only disease we can prevent with the help of genomics. There are a number of rare mutations that are highly actionable, such as Lynch syndrome (hereditary nonpolyposis colorectal cancer, HNPCC). It is diagnosed in 3–5 percent of the 160,000 new patients with colorectal cancer each year, and as with BRCA, the genes involved normally repair DNA and have other housekeeping functions important during cell division. The other major form of hereditary colon cancer is familial adenomatous polyposis due to mutations in the gene APC. For both of these hereditary conditions that carry high risk for colon cancer, close surveillance and surgery can be used for prevention. Both are autosomal dominant, appearing in each generation of families, but could be completely prevented by carrier screening and IVF, as discussed above related to prewomb planning.

Many other examples of rare mutations exist that can be paired with a prevention strategy, such as the ion channel mutations that cause dangerous, potentially lethal, heart arrhythmia syndromes. Those individuals found to have pathogenic mutations can be treated with either a medication specifically directed to the ion channel abnormality, or with a defibrillator that continually monitors heart rhythm and provides an electrical jolt when a serious arrhythmia occurs (as discussed in the case of Kim Goodsell).

But these examples are rare mutations that follow simple Mendelian inheritance patterns. Most of the common diseases of man are unfortunately polygenic, with many genes interacting in a complex fashion, and the inheritance pattern is not at all straightforward. Only for a limited number of these have the genomic markers or causative DNA sequence variants been found, not to mention a path to prevention. One positive example is age-related macular degeneration (AMD), a leading cause of blindness.

For individuals who carry genomic risk, there are a number of ways to reduce the chance of blindness, such as cessation of smoking, avoidance of sun exposure, close surveillance with eye exams, and a diet both especially rich in vegetables and fruits and low in saturated fats. Another example of a variant gene with clear-cut elevated risk is the apoε4 allele. Having one copy exposes a person to a threefold risk of Alzheimer's disease (from 8 percent with no apoε4 alleles to roughly 24 percent with one copy); being a homozygote—having two copies—raises the risk to over 75 percent. But unlike the AMD risk gene variants, there isn't yet any preventive strategy that has been validated. With Alzheimer's dementia, such an important, common, and dreaded condition, there are intense efforts for drug development. Some of the large, ongoing clinical trials with novel, experimental medications are specifically designed for individuals who are apoε4 carriers or homozygotes.

But knowing one's apoε4 status may be important long before developing late-onset dementia in the eighth or ninth decade of life. Compared with individuals with apoε2 or ε3 variants, who represent more than 80 percent of the population, apoε4 carriers and homozygotes are especially prone to bad outcomes following head injuries, including prolonged recovery, cognitive impairment, and developing dementia at an early age. Especially worrisome is the risk of traumatic brain injury (TBI), a syndrome that encompasses a range of serious neurologic and psychiatric effects for which there is no known effective treatment. Sports with high risk of head injury, such as boxing or football, are of particular concern, and some experts have even suggested that athletes participating in these sports should be screened for apoε4 variants. As one Alzheimer researcher put it to David Epstein in *The Sports Gene:* "the dementia risk of having a single apoε4 copy is roughly similar to the risk from playing in the National Football League (NFL), and . . . the two together are even more dangerous."[32] In fact, when I watch football and see a player with any head injury, the first thing I think about is whether the player is unknowingly an apoε4 carrier, in which case he might suffer irrevocable brain damage over time. These days, after decades of discrediting the research linking football and traumatic brain injury, the NFL has finally cued into the major risk of concussions. Use of sensors in player's helmets, with impact-sensing accelerometers to quantify the extent of head injury, even without a concussion, are starting to be tested in the NFL. But there has been no genetic screening or evaluation of the large number of former players who suffer traumatic brain injury. Moreover, we have yet to address the issue of screening in children who are considering participation in high-risk sports.

To be clear, however, apoε4 is an outlier gene variant, since it is fairly common (around 20 percent have at least one copy) and carries substantial risk. Most common genomic variants, meaning they are present in more than 5 percent of the population, carry only a small risk. In contrast, rare variants, meaning they are found in less than 1 percent of people, are much more apt to be associated with substantial risk. Because whole genome sequencing has only been performed in a limited number of people to date, without diverse phenotypes or ancestry, we have a ways to go to pick up the important rare variants. Such rare genomic variants of increased risk represent sharp signals that are particularly informative for an individual, and may therefore be useful for prevention of a particular condition.

But just knowing risk is not enough. We need to know when the condition will strike. And here is where biosensors come into play. If we knew, for example, that a child was at high risk of asthma, it would be ideal to use sensors to pick up incipient airway problems long before the first wheeze or symptoms. There are many conditions where we know there is genomic risk, but we have been clueless about when to intervene to prevent the event.

Embedded sensors in the blood, which talk to one's smartphone (or, in the case of children, to the parent's device), may be especially helpful. From genomics, we can identify children who have a high risk of autoimmune (Type 1) diabetes. We also know that it takes approximately five years before a critical proportion of the islet cells of the pancreas are cumulatively destroyed by autoimmune attacks, at which point diabetes manifests. Tiny nanosensors have now been developed to detect DNA, RNA, protein, and autoantibody signals. What if we had a blood-based sensor that detected immune system activation, and at that moment in time the immune system was down-regulated with a suitable drug? Perhaps the pancreas could be saved. This type of intervention is representative of a number of autoimmune diseases with sporadic attacks, such as multiple sclerosis, rheumatoid arthritis, or lupus.

For preventing a heart attack, a genomic signal from the cells sloughing off from an artery lining (known as circulating endothelial cells) has indicated the smoldering process that antedates the actual event—formation of a clot in the artery and stoppage of blood flow to the heart muscle. By knowing precisely when an individual is incubating a heart attack, potent anticlotting medications could be given to block this from happening.

And we know that in individuals affected by cancer, there is tumor DNA present in their plasma. This could be monitored during the course of therapy and prevent the need for expensive PET or CT scans that carry high radiation risk; however, an embedded biosensor could provide much tighter surveillance with the chance of picking up tumor recurrence, or, someday, even uncover the first signs of tumor long before there is a mass detected by a scan.

In a similar vein, the concept of a "molecular stethoscope" is attractive. Beyond looking at cell-free DNA, the cell-free RNA transcriptome has important potential for detecting medically relevant signals, as recently demonstrated by tracking pregnancy and fetal development or diagnosing Alzheimer's disease.[33] From time to time, during an individual's life span, a single tube of blood may be useful for a DNA/RNA screen in the future, serving as another dimension of one's GIS. There will, however, be challenges for interpreting the data. We'll come back to this topic later when we get into predictive analytics.

Infectious Diseases

The use of whole genome sequencing along with mapping social networks has been applied to fighting multiple pathogen outbreaks, including Klebsiella pneumonia, methicillin-resistant Staphylococcus aureus, Clostridium difficile, and tuberculosis. For communicable diseases, this has been an extraordinary development to understand origin and transmission. Equally impressive is the digital science of networking, which has yielded the important metric of "effective distance" as an explanation for contagion spread (and it applies to rumors and innovations, too).[34]

Pathogen sequencing has potential application well beyond determining the origin of an epidemic. Still, today the typical workup of a patient with a serious infection involves taking blood cultures or other body fluids and waiting two days before the culture results come back, and further time to determine sensitivities of the pathogen to antibiotics. During this two to three day period of time, the patient is usually given a blitzkrieg of potent, broad-spectrum antibiotics to "cover" all the possible pathogens that might be responsible for the infection.

To understand the lifesaving power of sequencing for infectious disease, take the story of Joshua Osborne, a fourteen-year-old boy who nearly died of a brain infection. He had continuous seizures but no diagnosis—even though he had a brain biopsy and comprehensive blood pathogen testing.[35] But sequencing of his spinal fluid quickly demonstrated that the cause was leptospira, a rare bacteria, and he was successfully treated with the appropriate antibiotic.

With sequencing, our common practices could be radically altered. There are now lab-on-a-chip sequencing platforms that can be integrated with a smartphone or tablet. Much more rapid, point-of-care pathogen sequencing will likely be feasible in the future. This will hopefully provide far more precise and early treatment of sepsis, one of the deadliest medical conditions.

Cancer

As a disease rooted in genomics, cancer is especially well positioned for an improved understanding and therapeutic approach. Indeed, by sequencing thousands of tumors from patients, along with the germline (native) DNA of each individual, we have identified changes to approximately two hundred genes, known as "driver" mutations, that are crucial for tumor growth.[5,36] The majority of these are called oncogenes; they can directly promote tumor formation and can be targeted by specific drugs. The rest are changes to tumor suppressor genes, such as P53. These are much more difficult to treat since it is their loss of function that enables the tumor to propagate. Drugs to augment a biologic function of cell biology are much harder to come by, so the presence of tumor suppressor genes as drivers usually means a workaround plan is needed on the pathway, rather than revving up the gene directly.

Just as we defined the GIS of a human being, there has been extensive work by the Cancer Genome Atlas, a project that began in 2005, funded by the NIH, to determine the GIS of most common types of cancer. In Figure 5.6, the different layers of information gathered for twelve different types of tumor are shown. The data include the mutations, the structural variants (meaning the change in the number of copies of the gene present), the gene expression, the DNA methylation, the proteins (RPPA stands for reverse phase protein array), and clinical data. From the extensive omic profiling, the principal biologic pathway(s) of an individual's cancer can be defined. This leads to the ability to match up a specific drug that targets a driver mutation or pathway.[5]

While the pairing of a drug to the driver mutation has had remarkable short-term impact, often accompanied by complete dissolution of the tumor in weeks, there is generally a major problem of recurrence between nine and twelve months later. A prototypic example of this phenomenon occurs with a drug directed to a BRAF mutation, present and causative in over 60 percent of people with metastatic melanoma. One important explanation for this recurrence or durable resistance to treatment involves the genetic heterogeneity of the cancer. When different parts of a tumor are sequenced, there are marked differences in the mutations found. This problem gets worse once a cancer metastasizes, as metastatic lesions have different mutations compared with the primary locus. It seems likely that combinations of drugs to target different mutations and pathways, as established by a GIS approach that takes heterogeneity into account, will be necessary to achieve long-term successful therapy. This is akin to the approach that has been successful in treating the viruses of hepatitis C and HIV, whereby three or four drugs in combination have proven to be highly efficacious. But much more work will be necessary to determine if cancer will succumb to combination therapies like viruses have.

At present, most doctors and hospitals only offer spot mutation screening, if anything, confined to HER2 for breast cancer or KRAS for colon cancer, despite the possibilities offered by the GIS approach. Most places that undertake the GIS approach are academic centers and do so as part of a research initiative. Only a few places have begun to offer sequencing for clinical guidance in cancer patients. One company, Foundation Medicine, has initiated a commercial product of limited sequencing of about three hundred genes of the tumor to query the presence of likely driver mutations.[37] Initial results in over two thousand patients have looked promising for finding culprit cancer genes, but clinical trials will be necessary to show that this information leads to improved outcomes compared with the standard, non-GIS approach. Further, given that only a limited number of genes (three hundred of nineteen thousand, or 1.6 percent) are assessed, and the rest of the 98.5 percent of the genome is left as dark matter, we can readily predict this partial GIS approach will likely miss important data. We already know, for example, that there are many noncoding (nongene) elements of the genome that can induce cancer; part of this information could be tapped by performing RNA sequencing. And there is no assessment of the patient's germline DNA. Nevertheless, although Foundation Medicine's sequencing strategy has many constraints, it represents a key direction for the future.

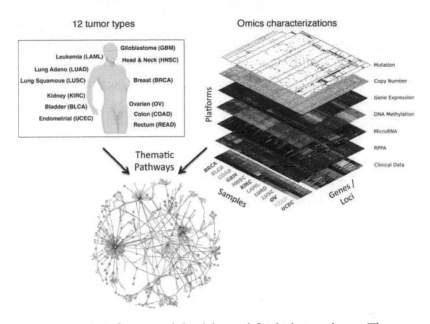

FIGURE 5.6: GIS of cancer and the ability to define biologic pathways. There are twelve different types of cancer represented here, but this approach applies to all. RPPA refers to proteomics. Source: J. N. Weinstein et al., "The Cancer Genome Atlas Pan-Cancer analysis project," *Nature Genetics* 45 (2013): 1113. Reprinted with permission.

There are two other exciting advances in cancer. One is related to tumor diagnosis or tracking, using a "liquid biopsy" of the tumor derived from a blood sample. As previously mentioned, the vast majority of patients with cancer have tumor DNA in their plasma that can be readily isolated from the blood and sequenced. It certainly looks like this will be part of the cancer GIS of the future.

The other area of major progress is cancer immunotherapy, *Science* magazine's "2013 Breakthrough of the Year."[38] Rather than genomic-guided treatment for cancer, this involves revving up the immune system by blocking molecules that ordinarily put the brakes on the immune response. Marked success in clinical trials has been validated in a variety of metastatic cancers, including melanoma, lung, and kidney. But the response rate hovers between 20 percent and 30 percent, so we need to learn what the factors are in a particular individual that will predict benefit. Besides the risk imposed by tampering with the immune system, these immunotherapy agents are very expensive—one drug, ipilimumab, costs over $120,000. Indeed, cost is a major problem: almost all of the genomic-guided drugs for cancer cost over $100,000 per course of treatment. So individualized medicine is imperative from another standpoint—economical use of these new biologically based therapies.

Molecular Diagnosis

Just as a GIS approach is starting to get traction in cancer, the natural extension for this is across all medical diagnoses. Take, for example, "Type 2 diabetes," which is actually an umbrella term for a variety of problems related to glucose: resistance to insulin, failure of the islet cells to make insulin, a defective transporter of insulin, a defective ion channel, an abnormal adrenergic receptor, abnormal sensing of glucose, and so on. It's not just about mechanism(s), but also ancestry can play a role. Recently, common sequence variants in a solute carrier gene (SLC16A11) and a rare variant in another gene (HNF1A) were found to increase the risk of diabetes in Mexicans and Latin Americans,[39,40] and a common gene variant (TBC1D4) in Greenlanders impedes muscle uptake of glucose and carries a tenfold increased risk of diabetes.[41] Yet we do nothing clinically to understand the basis of a person with the diagnosis of diabetes and essentially try "hit or miss" treatments. With fourteen different drug classes to treat diabetes, a more intelligent GIS approach could be quite informative for effective treatment. There are probably at least as many molecular subtypes of diabetes as there are drug classes used to treat the condition. Besides genomic characterization, the use of a continuous glucose sensor, even for a limited time of days to weeks, would provide granular data on the individual's glucose regulation. It's surely not just diabetes that needs a new molecular taxonomy. There have been a number of exceptional omic studies that break down common diseases into discrete molecular subtypes; the list is ever growing and includes asthma, multiple sclerosis, rheumatoid arthritis, and colon and uterine cancer. It's hard to imagine any common medical diagnosis that is not presently an oversimplified, reductionist umbrella term, unsuitable for an era of medicine, that is GIS ready.

Pharmacogenomics

Just as we have oversimplified diagnoses, so have we had little appreciation for the importance of an individual's genome or how it modulates their response to a medication. Presently, there are just over one hundred medications that the Food and Drug Administration labels as having an important, known DNA interaction.[42] This list is likely to grow; in fact, of the more than six thousand prescription medications, virtually all would be expected to have a response that depends on an individual's DNA. Indeed, each part of how each individual responds—absorption, metabolism, binding, transport, excretion—is genetically determined. Even worse than not having this data for 98 percent of drugs is that we do have pharmacogenomic information for some one hundred drugs and we don't use it for the practice of medicine.

Many of the pharmacogenomic interactions are quite pronounced, some of which I have summarized in Table 5.1.[42] The odds ratio refers to the magnitude of the variant's effect. So for lithium treatment for bipolar disorder, the DNA variant is associated with a 120-fold increase in achieving a therapeutic response (the study was performed in a Han Chinese cohort).[43] For treating hepatitis C with interferon-α, there is a thirty-eight-fold efficacy tied to the gene variant.[42] The other three examples relate to major side effects, where the sequence variant has a very large impact on the individual's chance of developing a serious adverse event.

While these are very large effects, none are utilized yet in clinical practice, at least not in the United States. In Taiwan and Singapore a new prescription for carbamazepine cannot be filled until the patient's risk genotype for developing Stevens-Johnson syndrome, a potentially lethal side effect, is ascertained. It is unfortunate that we have a legacy of over six thousand medications that were commercialized before there was the technology or will to determine DNA-drug interactions. Furthermore, and perhaps more disquieting given the current opportunity, there are very few examples of any pharmaceutical or biotechnology company developing a drug with a systematic effort to unravel the pharmacogenomic effects. Ideally, an individual's GIS in the future will include a comprehensive profile of his or her anticipated drug interactions.

Health Span

The human reference genome, which has been regarded as the platinum standard for genomic variation, has a significant flaw—the individuals who were used to construct it were young without any phenotype. So what we consider as the "anchor" may be riddled with disease-related variants. For example, a major predisposition for clotting disorders is attributed to the

Drug and Condition	Gene	Odds Ratio	Comment
Lithium for Bipolar Disorder	GADL1	120 X	Efficacy in Han Chinese
Interferon-α for Hepatitis C	IL28B	38 X	Efficacy to cure viral infection
Carbamazepine for Multiple Neurologic Conditions	HLA-A*3103	26 X	Stevens-Johnson Syndrome
Simvastatin for LDL Cholesterol Lowering	SLCO1B1	17 X	Severe muscle inflammation
Flucloxacillin for Infections	HLA-B*5701	81 X	Liver toxicity

TABLE 5.1: Some DNA-Drug Interactions with Pronounced Effects. Source: Adapted from A. R. Harper and E. J. Topol, "Pharmacogenomics in Clinical Practice and Drug Development," *Nature Biotechnology* 30, no. 11 (2012): 1117–1124.

gene variant known as Factor V Leiden. But if you look up the Factor V gene in the reference genome, it's Factor V Leiden! We need a reference genome with rigorous phenotypic characterization to avoid this problem. By collecting a large cohort of individuals with extreme health span (such as in the "Wellderly" project that we've been engaged in at Scripps for the past eight years) and performing whole genome sequencing, we can have an assured healthy background reference genome for comparison.

But there's another pressing reason why health span genomics will be critical to the human GIS. We have little knowledge about modifier genes and protective alleles—the variants that cancel out the risk or provide actual protection from a disease, respectively. A noteworthy example is the gene APP (amyloid precursor protein). One rare variant of this gene leads to premature Alzheimer's dementia, but another appears to fully protect from ever developing Alzheimer's—even in very elderly individuals with two copies of apoε4. Unfortunately, this protective APP allele is quite rare (less than 0.3 percent of European ancestry), but it may provide an invaluable lesson from Mother Nature for developing a drug to prevent Alzheimer's disease in the future. Similarly, rare variants of a lipid gene called ApoC3 markedly reduce triglycerides in the blood and confer a 40 percent reduction in coronary artery disease.[44] Furthermore, there are unquestionably a large number of rare DNA variants that similarly reduce risk or afford frank protection from diseases—we just need to find them! And eventually get rid of what has been referred to as the "ignorome."[45]

Molecular Autopsies

Every day in the United States there are over one thousand sudden cardiac deaths. Only 10 percent of these individuals are resuscitated.[46] Physical autopsies to determine the causes of death are rare, and even when performed would miss many molecular diagnoses such as genetic ion channel defects like the Long QT or Brugada syndrome. Without knowing the reason for sudden death, living family members are left in the lurch for their own risk profile. Parents of a child who dies of SIDS often suffer profound emotional turmoil and are left without knowing what happened. A molecular autopsy, consisting of the whole genome sequence of the deceased individual, along with some living family members, may be especially informative. Later in the book we will get into the need and opportunity for building such a global information resource for molecular autopsies.

The Human GIS in Perspective

This journey from womb to tomb has given us an idea of what a GIS of the future will look like—massive, multi-scale, panoromic information per individual. Call it ten by ten: ten omic tools and ten stops along the way of one's life span. But this expedition isn't just about *a* GIS, or *anybody's* GIS; it is about *my* GIS. It will be imperative that the GIS is owned by the individual, or in the case of children, by the parents, until handing it off. It will be used by the individual to make critical clinical choices, like Angelina Jolie's.

It is the individual's data, his or her medical essence, what makes him or her tick, and no one has a more vested interest in its proper use. Ownership will be made more obvious by the data flow pattern, as one's GIS will ultimately come through one's little wireless devices. In fact, my whole genome sequence is already on my iPad; all my sensor data flows through and is displayed in my smartphone. The display, however, is just the end-user experience. How will all of this data be gathered, stored, and interpreted? How will it ultimately prove beneficial for any given individual? My GIS will essentially require my cloud. Well beyond capture and storage of data, the capability to perform predictive analytics is paramount. A whole chapter is forthcoming to get into that exciting topic.

But for now we have no real GIS or personal cloud. The sobering reality is that we are still dealing with rather crude, helter skelter data collection, medical records, medications, labs, and scans scattered across different offices. And in today's persistent paternalistic landscape, these are essentially owned and controlled by doctors and the medical community. While we await the inevitability of the human GIS, there are vital ways we can markedly improve and even revolutionize how these traditional components of medical informatics serve the individual. That's what's up next.

Chapter 6

My Lab Tests and Scans

"Equip ordinary people to make their own reliable health diagnosis anywhere, anytime."
—Ariel Sabar, 2014[1]

"I deeply believe it has to be a basic human right for everybody to have access to the kind of testing infrastructure that can tell you about these conditions in time for you to do something about it."
—Elizabeth Holmes, CEO of Theranos[2]

"In every other industry, technology drives down costs and consumers are considered perfectly capable of making decisions for themselves."
—David Goldhill[3]

A *New Yorker* cartoon of a doctor and patient captures their relationship well: "It's a simple stress test—I do your blood work, and send it to the lab, and never get back to you with the results."[4] I know this routine all too well, from both sides of the medical fence, so I was struck when I read in the *Wall Street Journal* about a twenty-nine-year-old Stanford dropout who had formed a company to make lab tests more efficient, accessible, and less painful, for a fraction of the current price.

The dropout was Elizabeth Holmes, who left college after her freshman year to become the founder of the company called Theranos.[2,5-7] She told the *Wall Street Journal,* "The art of phlebotomy originated with bloodletting in 1400 BC and the modern clinical lab emerged in the 1960s—and it has not fundamentally evolved since then." She went on: "they put a tourniquet on your arm, stick you with a needle, take these tubes and tubes of blood."[5] Yup, that's the drill all right.

Roughly ten billion lab tests are done each year in the United States, and they factor into 70 percent to 80 percent of the medical decisions that doctors make.[2,5] Knowing how big a part of medicine this is and that there was something quite innovative going on, I visited the Theranos headquarters, an enormous, modernized, bright-colored warehouse with large pictures of happy kids posted throughout, to interview Holmes.

We started my visit with a light lunch and spoke briefly about her leaving Stanford at age nineteen and spending the last decade building Theranos, which up until quite recently was in stealth mode. Before I interviewed Holmes, I asked her if I could have my blood tested. She was more than happy to accommodate my request. It was a refreshing experience. No tourniquet. No fist pumping or large needles. Instead the young woman drawing my blood put on a finger warmer that dilated the blood vessels in my index finger. Then, without me even feeling the tiny pinprick, she captured a droplet of blood in one of their so-called nanotainers and it was off to the lab they have on premises. Over fifty tests were analyzed (some are shown in Figure 6.1), and I got the results back in just a matter of minutes. Reassuringly, the results were in line with prior conventional lab testing: I had an elevated glucose having just eaten lunch, and my HDL, or "good" cholesterol, was a bit low, which I've known for a long time. What really interested me was how all those results—kidney tests, liver function tests, blood chemistries, lipid panel, complete blood count, and more came back to me so quickly from a droplet of blood. That would normally have taken at least two tubes of blood and many hours before the results were available.

In total, Theranos offers one thousand lab tests at prices that are 50 percent less than what is currently reimbursed by Medicare and 70 percent to 90 percent reduced compared with what hospital labs bill.[2,5] Every test and price is listed on their website.[8] Even more radical is their agreement with Walgreens. We discussed their newly announced Walgreen's contract, in which a pharmacist or assistant would be trained to draw the droplet of blood in a dedicated Theranos corner of the retail store, across all 8,200

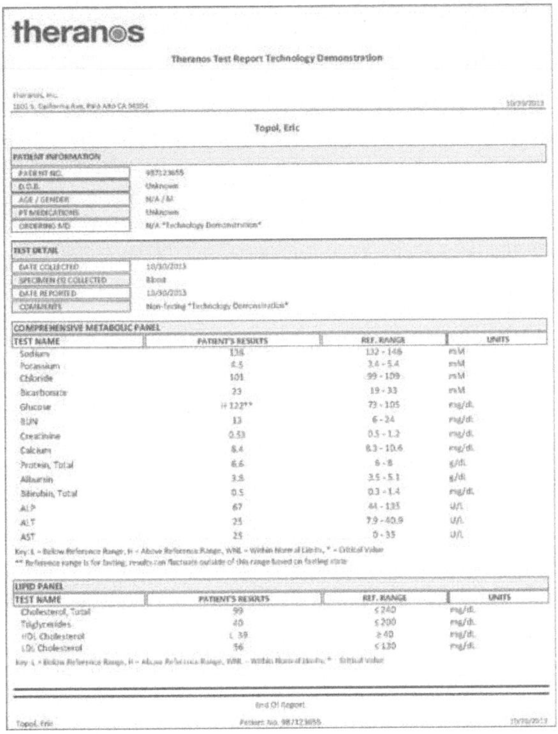

theranos

Theranos Test Report Technology Demonstration

Topol, Eric

PATIENT INFORMATION

PATIENT NO.	987123655
D.O.B.	Unknown
AGE / GENDER	N/A / M
PT MEDICATIONS	Unknown
ORDERING MD	N/A *Technology Demonstration*

TEST DETAIL

DATE COLLECTED	10/30/2013
SPECIMEN (S) COLLECTED	Blood
DATE REPORTED	10/30/2013
COMMENTS	Non-fasting *Technology Demonstration*

COMPREHENSIVE METABOLIC PANEL

TEST NAME	PATIENT'S RESULTS	REF. RANGE	UNITS
Sodium	136	132 - 146	mM
Potassium	4.5	3.4 - 5.4	mM
Chloride	101	99 - 109	mM
Bicarbonate	23	19 - 33	mM
Glucose	H 122**	73 - 105	mg/dL
BUN	13	6 - 24	mg/dL
Creatinine	0.53	0.5 - 1.2	mg/dL
Calcium	8.4	8.3 - 10.6	mg/dL
Protein, Total	6.6	6 - 8	g/dL
Albumin	3.5	3.5 - 5.1	g/dL
Bilirubin, Total	0.5	0.3 - 1.4	mg/dL
ALP	67	44 - 135	U/L
ALT	25	7.9 - 40.9	U/L
AST	25	0 - 35	U/L

Key: L = Below Reference Range, H = Above Reference Range, WNL = Within Normal Limits, * = Critical Value

** Reference range is for fasting; results can fluctuate outside of this range based on fasting state

LIPID PANEL

TEST NAME	PATIENT'S RESULTS	REF. RANGE	UNITS
Cholesterol, Total	99	≤ 240	mg/dL
Triglycerides	40	≤ 200	mg/dL
HDL Cholesterol	L 39	≥ 40	mg/dL
LDL Cholesterol	56	≤ 130	mg/dL

Key: L = Below Reference Range, H = Above Reference Range, WNL = Within Normal Limits, * = Critical Value

End Of Report

Topol, Eric Patient No. 987123655

FIGURE 6.1: My Theranos lab tests via a nanotainer of blood returned to me in minutes.

drugstores in the chain. Recognizing the pivotal role of pharmacists was particularly noteworthy. Such recognition is relatively uncommon among physicians, but Holmes called it "a wonderful application of the talent that exists in these pharmacies."[9] The goal: to be within five miles of every American.

But the critical question for me was the next step—getting the results back to the patient. Holmes argues that a patient's access to their results is *a basic human right.*[2,9] It's the person's blood and their test.[10] Why shouldn't the individual have access to their blood? The only reason Elizabeth and Theranos did not initially provide the results to consumers is that the medical system hasn't been ready for it. That's because we are stuck in the era of paternalism, as exemplified by a commentary that was published in 2011 in one of the leading medical journals that years later is still stuck in my mind: "Should Patients Get Direct Access to Their Laboratory Test Results?"[11]

How can leading doctors today continue to ask whether patients should have direct access to *their* lab tests? Their explanation is that patients will be confused by the results, that this could induce undue anxiety, that only their doctor would really understand the data and put it in context. I don't think so. A lab report always includes a column labeled reference range, and anybody can figure out what is normal or abnormal. To help them, an asterisk or two, or an *H* or *L* designation (Figure 6.1) can highlight anything abnormal. It certainly seems less complicated than looking at a gas bill, or electricity bill, or a credit card statement. As for anxiety, I haven't seen any scientific evidence to back that up beyond the intrinsic belief of some physicians. In fact, a study published in the *Journal of Participatory Medicine* of 1,546 patients who viewed their lab tests online demonstrated little to no indication of worry, confusion, fear, or anger (all less than or equal to 1 percent); 98 percent of patients found this helpful, and the conclusion was: "This study demonstrates that patients who view their lab test results online overwhelmingly react with positive rather than negative emotions."[12] But these results have not yet changed medical practice or the general perception of the medical community. As I've mentioned, health care consumers have truly been the Rodney Dangerfields of medicine: "I don't get no respect."

Despite the unwillingness for the medical profession to let go of lab test results, there are some cracks surfacing to suggest this is indeed going to change. Kaiser Permanente's mobile app and website allow access for their members (note that they are not called patients) to review their lab data. Several health systems are following suit, and a few are even advertising this as a perk. Even Quest Diagnostics and LabCorp, the two largest central labs in the United States, are beginning to make patients' lab data accessible to them via mobile apps. That's assuming they don't live in a paternalistic state; many states require a physician's approval. New online blood labs, such as WellnessFX and DirectLabs,[13] have recently cropped up, allowing consumers to order their own tests. In 2014, Medicare issued a new rule that requires labs to provide patients with copies of their results within thirty days of a request.[14–19a] Instead of an editorial questioning whether patients should have access to their lab tests, there is now a refreshing one urging doctors to proactively counsel patients, remove access barriers, and capture the benefits for a change.[19b] So there is at least movement in the right direction, favoring the rightful owners of the data.

My Smartphone Lab

As far as we are from personal data ownership, we are even further from personal data generation—from the right to order and even run one's own tests. The technology, however, exists, thanks to the next big movement in lab tests—smartphone attachments containing a "lab on a chip (LOC),"[20] "the incredible shrinking laboratory"[20] made possible by the combination of microelectronics and a microfluidic device with a smartphone for its microprocessor and display functions.[21-26] This sets up the perfect point-of-care device for rapidly analyzing digital breadcrumbs from our bodies in the form of tiny volumes—less than ten nanoliters—of blood, urine, saliva, breath, or even DNA itself. That anyone could write an article titled "Microfluidic Technology May Let You Print Out Your Own Health Tests" should give you the sense that something unusual is happening outside the usual place where labs would get done—true do-it-yourself testing.

Smartphones to assay or sequence DNA are in hot pursuit via several methodologies by companies such as Genia, Biomeme, and QuantuMDx.[27] The potential here ranges from a point-of-care, simple genotype for detection of a prescription drug interaction for a patient, to rapid sequencing of a pathogen to determine the cause and optimal treatment for an infection, to actual sequencing of a region of the genome. A little mobile device for such purposes has been described as "a decentralized, universal diagnostic tool,"[27] which could easily interface with the cloud for software interpretative apps.

Here's a partial roundup of some of the remarkably diverse lab-on-a-chip assays that have been or soon will be integrated with a smartphone. For blood, it includes glucose, hemoglobin, potassium, cholesterol, kidney function, liver function, thyroid function, brain natriuretic peptide (used to follow heart failure), toxins, and various pathogens (including malaria, tuberculosis, dengue, schistosomiasis, salmonella, and HIV with a capability of following $CD4^+$ and $CD8^+$ T Lymphocytes and Kaposi sarcoma virus).[28-38] For urine, the list includes a full quantitative analysis, albumin, human chorionic gonadotropin (HCG, for monitoring preeclampsia in high-risk pregnancy), and urinary tract infections.[39] Testing saliva, there is the capability to detect strains of the influenza virus and strep throat.[23] Perhaps most surprising is the spectrum of assays that are emerging from breath—lactate, alcohol, heart failure, drugs (cocaine, marijuana, amphetamines), and even some types of cancer.[40]

That last one may seem strange, but it's been known for some time that dogs can smell cancer.[41-45] It seemed to start in 1989 with a case report in *The Lancet* about a woman whose Collie-Doberman incessantly sniffed a mole, which led to medical attention and the diagnosis of melanoma.[46] By

2004, there were isolated reports of dogs diagnosing lung cancer from breath and bladder cancer from urine. This got more convincing in 2006 when a clinic in Northern California reported on collecting breath samples from fifty-five people known to have lung cancer and eighty-three healthy controls. Three Labradors and two Portuguese water dogs made the diagnosis of lung cancer with 99 percent accuracy! Similarly, dogs were able to detect prostate cancer via urine samples with 98 percent accuracy. At the University of Pennsylvania, there is a Working Dog Center where Dutch and German shepherds have shown 90 percent accuracy in detection of ovarian cancer.[47–50] Dogs have remarkable sniffing capacity endowed with over 220 million olfactory receptor cells, four to five times that of humans, so their ability to pick up the volatile organic chemicals emitted from a tumor— such as alcohols, alkenes, and benzene derivatives—is quite striking. Indeed, it means a dog's olfactory pathways are very powerful LOCs! Building on this exceptional canine capability, multiple companies, such as Adamant Technologies, Nanobeak, and Metabolomx, are testing smartphone "electronic nose" sensors to detect cancer via breath—not just lung cancer, but also ovarian, liver, gastric, breast, colorectal, and prostate.[51,52] One design for a cancer breathalyzer from the Technion Institute in Haifa, Israel, uses an array of forty gold nanoparticles as electrodes attached to a layer of molecules of the known organic compounds serving as sensors; the breath of an individual is introduced and generates a pattern analyzed by software. Using microelectronics to simulate superior sniffing, such smartphone sensors for breath are also being tested to quantify other metabolites that would be linked with particular diseases, such as nitric oxide for asthma.

The lab-on-a-chip work extends beyond the smartphone itself, as wearable patches with microneedles that get just beneath the skin or electrochemical chips adherent to the skin have been shown capable of assaying chemicals such as lactate in sweat,[53] and the real-time data can be displayed via the smartphone. Similarly, contact lenses that can quantify glucose via tears, reflective of what would be level in the bloodstream, are being evaluated for wireless smartphone transmission and display.

Pushing the limits of the lab on a chip is a group at UCLA that uses a 3-D printer to make a lightweight smartphone camera attachment. No ordinary camera, it can photograph a single virus, such as cytomegalovirus, which measures only 150–300 nanometers (a human hair measures approximately one hundred thousand nanometers).[31] So this adds to the ability to rapidly detect a pathogen and could be seen as complementary to a sequencing strategy. As we'll get into later in the book in a chapter dedicated to "flattening the Earth," such smartphone LOC brings highly sophisticated lab testing to anywhere in the world, even in remote places without reliable electricity.

One concern, however, is that whatever is assayed needs to be technically validated to know it is accurate and to be clinically useful for patient outcomes (i.e., actionable) and cost-effective. Even though there are exciting and unprecedented opportunities to measure unique proteins via a smartphone device, such as those indicative of traumatic brain injury or any type of cancer,[54] there is a long history of biomarkers not panning out when rigorously evaluated. Not because the assays are lacking accuracy, but due to the problem of lab assays correlating with clinical events. It's worthwhile to keep in mind the ratio of published papers for a claimed biomarker compared with the number of biomarkers used routinely in the clinic—it is 150,000 to 100.[55] This means there is great potential for false claims or premature uptake of nonvalidated LOC testing in a commercial market.

Nevertheless, we are now getting into the full democratization of lab testing. The goal of Theranos is to get a convenient lab in a retail store within five miles of every home in the United States. The move to smartphone-based lab testing, of course, will preempt the need to go anywhere. This represents the second tier of bypass: first the central or hospital lab, then the corner drugstore. During my interview with Ms. Holmes, I asked her about this eventual next wave of disruption; she said her company is "deeply committed to going in that direction."[9]

Sure, she gets it—she's a digital native. But how their model of lab testing will adapt to one that is based on the consumer's smartphone is not entirely clear. Nonetheless, I don't think there's any question this is where we're headed. Just as the first home pregnancy test of 1978 heralded a new era of consumer empowerment back then, these new products and companies are the precursor to an upcoming, unbridled capability of across-the-board lab testing anytime, anywhere.

Lab-in-the-Body

More distant is the progression from LOC to lab-in-the-body (LIB). As previously mentioned (Chapter 5), this is about embedding a chip into the bloodstream for assaying a wide range of substrates, with the data relayed to one's smartphone.[56,57] At Scripps and Caltech, we've been collaboratively working on a bloodstream-embedded biosensor that picks up genomic signals, for applications in predicting a heart or an autoimmune attack or the earliest diagnosis of cancer. At the University of California, Santa Barbara, an implanted microfluidic-electrochemical sensor has been demonstrated to provide continuous, real-time tracking of drug levels in animals.[58] Another LIB technology is magnetic resonance reflexometry, which uses antibody-coated magnetic particles; it has quantified the biomarkers of a heart attack (via assaying the protein troponin, released from dying heart cells)[59] and the principal adverse effect of the cancer chemotherapeutic agent doxorubicin (which can destroy heart muscle cells). So far all of this work has been done in animals; the sensors were implanted in the subcutaneous space (under the skin in the flank), mirroring the levels of the proteins found in the blood. Implantable optical nanosensors have been shown to continuously and accurately track glucose and electrolytes such as sodium or potassium.[60] Beyond embedding sensors in the bloodstream, wireless optoelectronic chips can be injected or imbedded into the tissue, such as the brain. And a group at MIT has developed a carbon nanotube, implanted below the surface of an animal's skin, which detected levels of nitric oxide for over a year in order to monitor inflammation.[61] Meanwhile, a team of Stanford engineers has created a tiny, wireless chip, 3 mm wide and 4 mm long, that is self-propelled as it swims through the bloodstream using electromagnetic radio waves.[62] Sounds a bit like the sci-fi movie *Fantastic Voyage*? The Stanford group envisioned applications besides lab testing, even getting into drug delivery, zapping blood clots, or removing atherosclerotic plaque from arteries. Georgia Tech's implanted biosensor gets its power from the hydraulic force of the bloodstream. And just in case a chip wasn't needed anymore, dissolvable ones have been developed that can melt away at a time that is programmed when implanted. Surely there are many loose ends before implantable micro- or nano-chips become part of routine medical practice. We need to validate their accuracy, figure out the durability of the sensors, and determine whether continuous sensing or an intermittent readout is optimal. But like smartphone LOC, LIB is eventually going to become commonplace, increasing the proportion of us who are heading toward cyborg status.

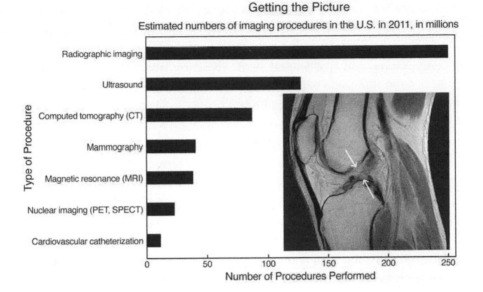

Getting the Picture

Estimated numbers of imaging procedures in the U.S. in 2011, in millions

FIGURE 6.2: Medical imaging in the United States, 2011. Source: Adapted from L. Landro, "Where Do You Keep All Those Images?," *Wall Street Journal*, April 8, 2013, http://online.wsj.com/news/articles/SB10001424127887323419104578374420820705296.

Choosing My Scans Wisely

The number of medical images performed annually in the United States has skyrocketed (Figure 6.2).[63,64] An ultrasound is done half as frequently as a plain X-ray (radiographic imaging). Over the past decade, the number of computed tomography (CT) scans has more than doubled, now reaching almost three hundred scans per one thousand people per year.[64] Most scans, with the exception of ultrasounds and MRIs, bring with them considerable risk of radiation.

To recap on radiation exposure, plain X-rays, mammograms, angiograms (images of arteries), CT scans, positron emission tomography (PET), and nuclear scans all carry the risk of ionized radiation, which is quantified by millisieverts (mSv) units. There is no safe level of mSv, but we know that the higher the exposure, the higher the risk of cancer. Extrapolating from atomic bomb survivor data, there is a sharp increase in cancer risk with exposure of 100 mSv. The average background exposure of a person is 2.4 mSv/yr.[64] But a single nuclear scan can expose a patient to more than 40 mSv, which is the equivalent of over two thousand chest X-rays. A mammogram uses much less radiation, but still is about 0.5 mSv, or twenty X-rays, and like nuclear scans these are frequently repeated from year to year. Radiation exposure is particularly a concern among children, in which the rates of CT scans have climbed in excess of adults, and the risk of cancer is heightened.[65]

In the United States it is estimated that of the four million pediatric CT scans each year, almost five thousand cases of cancers will be induced. Even dental X-rays have been implicated. Brain tumors, while quite uncommon, are more likely among individuals who had "bitewing" annual X-rays, and five times more frequently observed in those who had frequent panoramic X-rays as a child.

An op-ed in the *New York Times* entitled "We Are Giving Ourselves Cancer" pointed out that 3 percent to 5 percent of all cancers may result from exposure to medical imaging.[66] It is unfortunate that the tests are risky. Even worse is that the risk is often unnecessary.[67] Back in 2012, the American Board of Internal Medicine Foundation along with Consumer Reports, a highly regarded independent, nonprofit consumer organization, introduced Choosing Wisely,[68–77] an initiative to reduce unnecessary medical tests and cut costs. When Choosing Wisely was first announced, nine medical professional organizations published their lists of five tests and procedures that they deemed were unnecessary. Of these forty-five recommendations for unneeded tests, twenty-five (56 percent) were related to imaging that uses ionizing radiation (some highlighted in Table 6.1).[70]

This program has now been expanded to nearly fifty organizations, and the lists from many have increased from Top 5 to Top 10 of "Things Physicians and Patients Should Question." Imaging remains the dominant part of the waste and unnecessary medical practices. There are certainly some problems with this initiative, including the lack of public awareness (despite the involvement of Consumer Reports) and that there is no enforcement or "teeth" behind all the recommendations.

Furthermore, Choosing Wisely doesn't emphasize the cumulative *risk* of these scans that involve ionized radiation.[78–81] For example, a typical cardiology practice has its patients who have had a stent or bypass operation; such patients are told to come back for an annual checkup and have

Unnecessary Scan and Organ	Clinical Practice
Nuclear-Heart	Stress testing for screening heart disease patients without symptoms
CT-Brain	Simple fainting (syncope) without neurologic symptoms
CT-Abdomen	Functional abdominal pain syndrome or suspected appendicitis in children
PET, CT, Nuclear of Bones	Staging of early breast or prostate cancer
Nuclear-Heart	Stress testing pre-operatively for low-risk surgery
CT-Brain	Headache without risk factors for structural problems
CT-Spine	Low-back pain
CT-Sinuses	Uncomplicated acute sinusitis
CT, Nuclear-Lungs	Low probability of pulmonary embolus

TABLE 6.1: Some Common Ionized Radiation Scans that Were Deemed Unnecessary by Choosing Wisely. Sources: Adapted from V. M. Rao et al., "The Overuse of Diagnostic Imaging and the Choosing Wisely Initiative," *Annals of Internal Medicine* 157 (2012): 574–577; and C. K. Cassel et al., "Choosing Wisely Helping Physicians and Patients Make Smart Decisions About Their Care," *JAMA* 307 (2012): 1801–1802.

a nuclear stress test. The resulting radiation exposure over the course of a decade is substantial. In a study from Columbia Medical Center of nearly 1,100 patients with heart disease who were serially imaged over ten years, 30 percent had a cumulative exposure of more than 100 mSv.[79–81] That exceeds the A-bomb survivor threshold for high cancer risk. Furthermore, a recent report from the National Academy of Sciences Research Council concluded that a single 10 mSv exposure may be associated with an increased risk of cancer; in 2010, 16.5 percent of American patients who underwent imaging were exposed to a dose at least this high.[63]

As an outgrowth of lack of respect for the risk of radiation in general or just plain medical paternalism, patients are never given information on their specific mSv exposure when referred for a scan.[82,83] In 2013, there was the first sign this might change. Intermountain Healthcare in Salt Lake City, a large health system of 22 hospitals and 185 clinics, launched the first program to measure and report patients' cumulative medical radiation exposure.[84] Here is the response from one of the first patients to get his data:

Mr. Page, a 29-year-old maintenance technician who lives in Clear-
field, Utah, learned that his cumulative exposure from multiple scans
he received at Intermountain was 97.3 mSv. The father of three admits it was "scary" to read a pamphlet telling him the radiation exposure from each scan, but he was comfortable with the idea that the
scans were necessary to monitor cysts associated with his pancreatitis.
He said: "I am aware of the risk but the fact is I'd rather make it to the
point where I might see long-term effects than have a problem now
and not get to that point. But it is good to know the information is
there for the future."[84]

Following suit with Intermountain, the Hospital Corporation of America has announced its Radiation Right campaign, and the American College of Radiology is sponsoring a national initiative to benchmark CT
doses among hospitals.[84] And that issue brings up a critical point—there
is marked variability in mSv dose for the same scan across different hospitals.[64] Precisely for that reason, it is imperative that each patient gets his
or her mSv information specific to the hospital or clinic that is performing
the scan. And certainly these data should be universally available, published, and completely transparent to the public. We are a long way from
achieving this easily attainable and important objective. In the meantime,
doctors should be providing a best estimate of mSv exposure when a scan
is recommended.

For almost any scanning that is done in medicine, there is more than
one alternative, such as using ultrasound or magnetic resonance imaging
instead of a scan that requires ionized radiation. Discussing those alternatives should also be a routine part of the doctor-patient conversation in
deciding who, what, where, how, and when any medical scan is performed.

In rounding out the choosing wisely story of scans, there are three mass
cancer screening imaging programs that deserve scrutiny. First, consider
mammography, a scan that forty million women in America have each
year. In aggregate, all the randomized trials of mammography—with
almost six hundred thousand women—have failed to show any reduction
in death rates from breast cancer in women who get mammograms versus
those who do not.[85-91] For one thousand fifty-year-old American women
screened every year with mammography for breast cancer over a decade,

only five will benefit but six hundred will have a false alarm. That's almost two-thirds of the women screened! The false positives lead to biopsies, unnecessary surgeries or radiation therapy, expense, and untold emotional costs. A three-decade study of mammography in the United States concluded: "Our study raises serious questions about the value of screening mammography. It clarifies that the benefit of mortality reduction is probably smaller, and the harm of overdiagnosis probably larger, than has been previously recognized."[90] A Swiss medical board reviewed all the data and concluded there were more harms than benefits with mammography programs so they should be abolished.[92] The net harm of this mass screening does not jive with the current American Cancer Society recommendation that all women age forty and older should have mammography every year.

Here is the opinion of one physician, David Newman, taken from a *New York Times* piece he authored:[93]

> More bluntly, the trial results threatened a mammogram economy, a marketplace sustained by invasive therapies to vanquish microscopic clumps of questionable threat, and by an endless parade of procedures and pictures to investigate the falsely positive results that more than half of women endure. And inexplicably, since the publication of these trial results challenging the value of screening mammograms, hundreds of millions of public dollars have been dedicated to ensuring mammogram access, and the test has become a war cry for cancer advocacy. Why? Because experience deludes: radiologists diagnose, surgeons cut, pathologists examine, oncologists treat, and women survive.[93]

An even bigger—fourfold—cause of death each year is lung cancer. In 2013, lung cancer deaths occurred in 159,880 individuals as compared with breast cancer's 40,440.[94] We've known for some time that smoking is linked to 85 percent of lung cancer cases. The US Preventive Services Task Force now recommends that all current and former smokers between the ages of fifty-five and eighty should have annual lung CT scans. This recommendation follows from a clinical trial that showed for every three hundred CT scans, one patient life would be saved. But 25 percent of all those who underwent chest CT scans had false positives, prompting unnecessary procedures like lung biopsies. Another flagrant example of net harm.

The third very frequent scan screening for cancer is for the prostate. Even though it has been deemed unnecessary to perform routine PSA screening among men over age fifty, and such practices were called out by the Choosing Wisely initiative as being unnecessary in low-risk patients, most urologists and a large proportion of internal medicine physicians have ignored that recommendation to date.[74] The vast majority of prostate cancers are quite indolent, not aggressive or life-threatening. Nevertheless, the elevated PSA often prompts for nuclear bone scans and CT scans of the abdomen and pelvis to evaluate whether there is any evidence of metastasis. Interestingly, a national effort in Sweden to reduce this imaging was highly successful, disseminating interhospital utilization data among all Swedish urologists, bringing down the rate of low-risk imaging from 45 percent to 3 percent of patients.[95] It is unlikely we'll be seeing such a national program in the United States, although it would represent a solid step toward reduction of unnecessary medical imaging.

So the first step in choosing your scans wisely is to think, "Do I really need it?" Then ask, "Can it be done without ionized radiation?" Then, if a nuclear, CT, or PET scan is truly indicated, ask: "How much mSv will I be getting exposed to?" and "Where can I have this done to have the lowest amount possible with the highest quality scanning?" All of these questions relate to traditional hospital and clinic-based imaging facilities. But that landscape is quickly changing—getting miniaturized.

Pocket Scanning

Of the five major imaging modalities (X-ray, CT, nuclear/PET, ultrasound, MRI), three have now been miniaturized to handheld size.[96–99] Portable X-rays via a smartphone-sized device have been made possible by taking advantage of a natural process known as triboluminescense. Engineers at UCLA reported on the ability to generate X-rays by simply unrolling Scotch tape in a vacuum, akin to what happens when Wint-O-Green Life Savers are pulled apart, separating positive and negative charges and generating a flash of light.[96,98] This technology preempts traditional X-ray's need for fragile glass tubes and high voltage. It is still in the early stages of development for medical diagnostics, but at least feasibility has been demonstrated and there is considerable funding through the Defense Advance Research Projects Agency and venture capitalists.

Miniaturization of the MRI machine, which most of us would conceive of as a monstrous, multiton device, has moved along beyond expectations. The pioneer in this movement has been the German engineer Bernhard Blümich, who back in 1993 had already built what was called the MRI-MOUSE, which stands for mobile universal surface explorer, and was only one foot tall.[100] As the techno-optimist Michio Kaku put in his *Physics of the Future* book, "This could revolutionize medicine, since one would be able to perform MRI scans in the privacy of one's home."[101]

This miniature MRI is based upon a small *U*-shaped magnet that yields a north and south pole at each end of the *U*. As opposed to traditional MRI, it uses nonuniform and weak magnetic fields with computer algorithmic correction for distortion, and has minimal power requirements similar to a lightbulb. Kaku anticipates that "eventually, the MRI scanner may be as thin as a dime, barely noticeable."[102]

In related progress on magnetic resonance miniaturization, a micro-NMR (nuclear magnetic resonance) device with a 10 cm by 10 cm footprint, and operated via a smartphone, has been used to obtain point-of-care quantification of tissue protein expression content from biopsy specimens to rapidly and accurately diagnose cancer.[97] This miniature technology is for molecular profiling, not imaging, but may prove particularly useful for dealing with fine needle aspirates of tumors from outside the body, used instead of a biopsy of tissue, which can make a definitive diagnosis of cancer quite difficult.

By far the scanning technology that has been miniaturized the most is ultrasound. Two different devices have been FDA approved and available since 2010—the VScan (General Electric) and Mobisante. Both are cell phone, pocket-sized devices. A study we conducted at Scripps showed that the image resolution of the handheld ultrasound was as good as the standard, large ultrasound hospital machine that costs over $300,000 for performing heart imaging.[103] With the capability of actually *seeing* all of the heart structure and function—the valves, the heart muscle and all four chambers, the aorta, the sac around the heart—I have not used a stethoscope to *listen* to the heart of a patient in several years. This can be accomplished in a minute or two during the physical examination, and the image video loops can be directly shared with the patient while the information is being collected. Imaging via a pocket ultrasound device decidedly transcends the antique stethoscope from 1816, regarded as the icon of medicine. And of course this miniature ultrasound can be used examining the abdomen, the pelvis (including the uterus and fetus), the lungs, and large arteries such as the aorta or carotids. Reflecting the capability of point-of-care ultrasound, Harvard faculty physicians recently advocated "stop listening and look."[104]

Availability of this technology has led to at least two medical schools in the United States providing a device, instead of the traditional stethoscope, to all of its students on the first day. One health system in Minnesota has recently completed training its primary care physicians with handheld devices to conduct head-to-toe ultrasound physical examinations.

Such safe and informative handheld imaging has many important implications. Recall from Figure 6.2 there are more than 125 million ultrasound studies performed in the United States per year. What proportion of these could easily, rapidly, and accurately be done as part of the office visit physical exam or at the hospital bedside? With an average charge of $800 for the combined hospital and professional fees, ultrasound studies have a cumulative economic hit of more than $100 billion/year in the United States alone. Handheld ultrasound could likely reduce this by at least 50 percent if adoption of this device as the modern stethoscope became a routine part of the physical exam.

What's more, physicians, nurses, or paramedics without expertise in interpretation of the images for a particular patient can do the scan and wirelessly send the video loops to a radiologist or, in the case of the heart, a cardiologist, for rapid feedback, anywhere there is a mobile signal.

Sharing Results

When a patient gets a scan, the results are difficult to access, and it typically requires calling the doctor's office to find out the results. At the time of the scan, the radiology technician or ultrasonographer is not permitted to communicate the results to the patient, because the licensed physician has not yet interpreted them. Patients are often anxious about whether the scan turned up something of concern, and usually have to wait several days before they can hear the results. Not surprisingly, studies have indicated that most patients would prefer immediate access to their results.[105–108] Of course this is preempted with the example of handheld ultrasound, where the physician can perform the scan, show the patient the videos in real time, and provide interpretation. So to be clear, we are talking about access for patients at two levels—getting the results and actually seeing the scan. The latter, at this juncture, is a rarity.

Access to the results of the scan can be readily accomplished through a patient Web portal, as is currently available for Kaiser Permanente members and a few other health systems. But new software technology of mobile medical image viewers, like ResolutionMD, image32, Carestream, and MIM VueMe, has enabled patients to see their medical scans on their smartphones and tablets. The mobile viewers provide exceptional quality of CT, MRI, and nuclear scan images that correspond to the resolution seen in the hospital or clinic monitors. So these pictures, taken of *your* body, can now be fully viewed by *you* on *your* devices. That's a big step. But you may wonder what value this has if you can't actually interpret the images. First, when there is an abnormality, the hope is that your doctor will review the images with you instead of settling with a written report, which in itself is often very difficult to interpret. Second, once you have a high-resolution copy of your image on your device, or readily accessible to your device through your health system's server (or with some of these image-sharing apps through their proprietary cloud storage), you are well on your way for a second opinion if needed. Third, and perhaps unexpectedly, approximately 10 percent of medical imaging is duplicative; that is a redundant scan is performed simply because the physician had no access to the previous image.[63,72,80,107,109]

My Smartphone Physical

The next level of medical scanning takes democratization to new heights—turning the smartphone into an instrument to conduct various parts of the physical exam.[24,110–113] Of course, via a number of apps, you can scan a suspicious skin lesion with the smartphone camera and quickly get a text as to whether a biopsy is indicated. Or get the differential diagnosis of a rash. We've already discussed the ability for the smartphone with hardware "add" attachments or wireless sensor connects to get blood pressure, heart rate and rhythm, temperature, and blood oxygen saturation. But scanning is another dimension. As it turns out, morphing the smartphone to an ophthalmoscope, to fully examine the eyes or refract the eyes for visual acuity, is remarkably straightforward. Similarly, the smartphone makes an exceptionally good otoscope to examine the ears.

I got to try the smartphone otoscope (made by Cellscope) on a most unusual subject—Stephen Colbert. The uproarious, fast-footed comedian had been on vacation the week prior to my coming on his *Colbert Report* show, and he had perforated his eardrum while diving. As a cardiologist, I have to admit I wasn't used to using an otoscope; it had been many years since I had even touched one. So it was amusing to take my smartphone, which I had just used to get Colbert's electrocardiogram, and put on the otoscope attachment and stick it into Stephen's ear. Fortunately, this is really an idiot-proof device that even I could handle, and I was able to get good visualization of Colbert's healing eardrum to show the audience. Surprisingly, the live crowd roared with excitement, to which Colbert exclaimed: "It's my eardrum, not my ass!" And then he quipped, "Hey, doc, can you do a colonoscopy with this?"

When you're not using a smartphone otoscope to check on Colbert, it has immediate applicability to take a look at your child's eardrum should there be uncertainty about an ear infection. The image from both ears can be sent to the cloud and have accurate algorithmic interpretation of whether there is an infection. This could certainly save a trip to an emergency room or an urgent visit to the pediatrician.

But that's just the beginning of what smartphone scanning is capable of with the right add-ons. There is an attachment to scan the mouth and oral cavity for cancer, and responding to Colbert's call, smartphones have now actually been transformed by physicians into mobile endoscopy viewing systems. Turning mobile phones into interactive 3-D scanners through impressive software has been markedly refined, just awaiting medical application. As previously discussed, the microphone of the smartphone can be used to get important lung function parameters. And conversion of the smartphone to a high-powered digital microscope also allows for the diagnosis of several infectious diseases, such as tuberculosis and malaria.[114]

So by minimizing the size of diagnostic medical equipment, it has become eminently portable to do lab testing and medical imaging. If we go back to the Gutenberg press era, miniaturizing the book helped make book reading a way of life. Around the same time, miniaturization of the clock made everyone timekeepers. Now the miniature mobile medical devices pave the way for everyone's medicine. For in medicine's future, there is a powerful common smartphone pathway, not only capable of doing lab tests and scans, but also most, if not all, of the components of the physical exam. We're just starting to get the pieces together for each of our GISs. When combined with our digital infrastructure, this sets the foundation for virtual medical visits that transmit even more information than is obtained during the physical doctor visit of today. But getting to efficient use of smartphone lab tests and scans, along with virtual visits, is not a slam-dunk, by any means. The next step we need to get into is how to completely capture and archive all of these data, from womb to tomb.

Chapter 7

My Records and Meds

"Health information technology (HIT) could save $81–$162 billion or more annually while greatly reducing morbidity and mortality."
—THE RAND CORPORATION, 2005[1]

"We're creating a revolution. Some people are aghast."
ON GIVING PATIENTS ACCESS TO NOTES BY PHYSICIANS.
—TOM DELBANCO, HARVARD[2]

We're all dressed up with nowhere to go. We've got our labs, real-time wireless sensor data, genomic sequence information, and images. Our ability to generate big medical data about an individual has far outstripped any semblance of managing it, and we can't even build the full GIS yet. There is not a single electronic medical record (EMR) system today that is set up to bring all this data together in a meaningful way—not just to aggregate it, but to provide the full analysis of all one's medical information. It's like we invented the printing press but haven't figured out the card catalog. This isn't necessarily because no one has tried; there are plenty of obstacles, but also, in spite of them, some early signs of progress. We're talking about access, not ownership, a baby step in the right direction.

In the ideal world of the future of medicine, you will own all of your data. That's because it will come to you directly, through your little devices. And, of course, you are the rightful owner because you paid (even if indirectly) for *your* tests, scans, office visits, and hospitalizations. And, of course, it's also your body. Is there any other walk of life where services are purchased but the purchaser doesn't take ownership? The typical response from the medical profession for this anomaly is that patients cannot understand the information or will get terribly confused and anxious without proper context and knowledge. Only with spoon-feeding by doctors and health care professionals will these concerns be eschewed. There is also the more self-serving fear that data access might facilitate or even stimulate malpractice litigation. This deep-seated defense of information asymmetry, a patent outgrowth of profound paternalism, will ultimately prove to be untenable.[3,4] The digitization of medical information, and the way it will naturally flow to individuals, will drive information parity and apposite ownership in the future.

That certainly isn't how it works now. Ironically, when you're alive, the medical community owns your records, lab tests, scans, and biopsy and tissue specimens. And when you die, your body becomes the property of your family. You still can't get to your medical records, because you're dead. And perhaps it's not a stretch to say that some people may have even died trying to get access to their medical records.

Access to My Records

Achieving access to one's medical records remains one of the most frustrating experiences in the world of health care today. Typically, getting copies of a hospitalization and operative reports requires contacting the facility, signing a release, paying exorbitant fees for each page of copy, and having the materials sent via fax several days or even weeks later. Access to office visit records is frequently not any easier to come by. Root canal work comes to mind. This will become quite clear from what follows.

Try to guess when this was written:

> Dissatisfaction with the functioning of the medical-care system has become widespread. . . . We believe these problems could be alleviated, in part, if patients were given copies of all their medical records. To a large extent the record embodies the informational product of medical consultation and treatment. In most exchanges in society a purchased product becomes the property of the purchaser, who is then free to evaluate the product on his own, have it evaluated by experts and chose freely among suppliers for any further services.[5]

It was forty-two years ago. The authors were Budd Shenkin and David Warner, respectively, a physician and scientist from Yale, and the paper appeared in the *New England Journal of Medicine* with the title "Giving the Patient His Medical Record."[5] The description of ownership via "purchased product" is indeed hard to miss. To emphasize, these records are rightfully yours—your health, your medical condition(s) and encounters, and you've paid for them. But ownership is simply not honored.

This unwillingness for physicians to share medical information can be traced much further back than forty years, of course. We've already read Hippocrates's advice to "conceal most things from the patient while you are attending to him."[6] Shenkin and Warner proposed legislation requiring "complete and unexpurgated copy of all medical records, both inpatient and outpatient, be issued routinely and automatically to patients as soon as the services provided are recorded."[5]

But that proposal was never adopted, with notable exceptions in a few health systems. Only via the Affordable Care Act has the United States begun a nationwide policy to promote patient access to their medical records.

Open Notes and Closed Minds

An important research project called OpenNotes, first published in 2012, is an opportunity to gather substantive support for the Shenkin and Warner proposal.[7–9] In three highly regarded medical centers in the United States—Geisenger in rural Pennsylvania, Harborview in Seattle, and Beth Israel Deaconess in Boston—over one hundred primary care physicians and more than twenty-two thousand patients participated in an experiment testing the impact of patients getting rapid access to their office visit notes.[7] The physicians, representative of the medical community at large, went into the experiment believing that access to office visit notes might well induce anxiety, confusion, or offense, and that it might have an adverse impact on their busy lives. Just think of all the questions they might have to answer! Indeed, many of the physicians at the three institutions refused to participate, because they believed that their workflow would be seriously disrupted. Further, there was a question as to whether the patients even wanted access, and whether access would promote better patient engagement and adherence with treatment.

The results of the experiment were not what the physicians expected. First, very few physicians experienced any adverse impact on their work.

They also learned to modulate their notes on certain issues such as mental health, substance abuse, obesity, and cancer where they might offend or carelessly upset patients. For example, using the term "body mass index" instead of obesity helped reduce patients feeling insulted, and when there was a suspicion of cancer this was appropriately couched to reduce the chance of worry. They also learned to avoid acronyms like SOB, which doctors use for shortness of breath but which the patient can easily misinterpret. There was no significant increase in e-mail traffic—while some patients required interaction after having read a note, others found their questions answered by having access. Overall, there was no net increase in time required by physicians. One doctor's comment summed it up well. "My fears: longer notes, more questions, and messages from patients," he wrote. "In reality, it was not a big deal."[7] In fact, it was even better, as the doctors saw that their patients were more engaged and satisfied, and their relationships were strengthened.

From the patient's perspective, there was striking evidence of benefit. Surveys indicated that 99 percent of the patients wanted this access in the future, and nearly 90 percent would select their future care based on having open note access. Reading the notes increased their understanding and imbued them with a sense of control, improved adherence to the plans that were discussed at the visit, and enhanced trust of their physicians. There was little evidence of any anxiety, confusion, or offense taken by reviewing the office notes. About 65 percent of patients improved their adherence to medications.[7,9] That is especially noteworthy, because only half of patients demonstrate adherence to prescriptions, and this problem represents an important, if not the most important, reason for failure of management of chronic diseases.

An interesting outgrowth of the OpenNotes experiment was that 60 percent of patients felt that they should be able to add comments to the notes. Imagine that—active participation in one's care and tracking of medical information.[10] Surprisingly, a third of the participating physicians agreed with that idea. This may seem foreign or radical to some, but shouldn't both the physician and patient sign all notes? Physician office notes frequently contain inaccurate or missing data, with, for example, 95 percent of the medication lists having errors.[10] It's long overdue to have patients engaged in the editing process of *their* medical records.

Perhaps the biggest direct impact of the OpenNotes project is that it has become standard practice at the three centers where it was conducted.[7]

All patients have access to all of their office visit notes. But this remains a rarity. In fact, in 2014, only two million patients in the United States were thought to have access to their notes about their treatment.[11]

The reason why is because paternalism has closed the minds of physicians and consumers alike. According to a Harris poll of nearly four thousand doctors and over nine thousand consumers, only 31 percent of physicians believe their patients should have full access to their notes.[3,4]

Correspondingly, only 36 percent of consumers reported full access to their records even though 84 percent believe it is their *right* to have it.[12] Interestingly, over 40 percent of consumers surveyed were willing to switch doctors in order to gain full access to their records.[12] That more than two out of three physicians are unwilling to grant or believe in access of their outpatient notes to patients is in keeping with the use of e-mail in medical practice. Just as many doctors in the OpenNotes project wanted to avoid getting e-mail from patients, more than 60 percent of US physicians do not e-mail with patients, despite multiple studies of how this increases efficiency of medical practice and improves patient satisfaction.[13–15] Physicians argue that there is no reimbursement for this added effort, that privacy and security of e-mailed data cannot be guaranteed, and that such material could be fodder for malpractice litigation.

The Blue Button Initiative

Concurrent with the OpenNotes experiment to advance the case for a fully transparent medical record, there was a large-scale government initiative to promote access. The Markle Foundation, a private philanthropic organization established in 1927, is interested in using information technology to address previously intractable problems. Intractable certainly qualifies here. The Markle Foundation convened a meeting in 2010 with the US government to discuss enabling individuals to download their health data, in line with the foundation's mission to spread "knowledge among the people of the United States."[16–20] The result was the Blue Button program.

Well over sixty million Americans receive health care via governmental agencies, such as the Department of Veterans Affairs and the Department of Defense. Once these consumers were enabled to download their health data, momentum started to extend to the private sector, and major insurers such as United Health and Aetna signed on to provide Blue Button downloads in 2012.[17]

So the good news is that now, theoretically, over one hundred million Americans have access to Blue Button downloads of their medical data. But the data that is downloaded is from an administrative database that is set up to deal with claims, not to provide information in a user-friendly format for patients or their physicians. There are many third-party companies such as Humetrix that work to convert the data files to be more usable with its iBlueButton apps that display the information on a smartphone or tablet.

This gives the individual, family member, or doctor information for the previous three years on the patient's problem list and conditions, medications and supplements, list of physicians and their contact information, lab tests, imaging studies, procedures, hospitalizations, and outpatient visits. This is a great start, but most Medicare beneficiaries have no idea that this information is available and a lot more work is needed to make this easily accessible, especially for individuals not covered by agencies such as Medicare. For example, I am covered via an Aetna insurance plan, which is supposed to be part of this initiative. Despite multiple attempts, I have yet to be successful in downloading my information through Blue Button. So although my friend Dr. Farzad Mostashari, the former US government health information technology (HIT) "czar" (officially known as the head of the Office of the National Coordinator, HIT) said, in June 2013, that within twelve months people would be able to get the same data that doctors send to each other, it hasn't proven to be the case yet.[19] But with over $40 billion that the United States is putting into "meaningful use" of electronic medical records, there will certainly be a push to improve accessibility and usability of the Blue Button program in the future.

The Hits on HIT

OpenNotes and Blue Button are signs of real if uneven progress, but these have also suffered many setbacks. One major problem for health information technology (HIT) has been hype.[15] Electronic medical records have been touted as enthusiastically as initial sequencing of the human genome, which in 2000 led then President Clinton to declare "it will revolutionize the diagnosis, prevention and treatment of most, if not all human diseases."[21] In 2005, the RAND organization projected that electronic records would save up to $160 billion per year.[1,22] That could not be further away from reality.[23,24] More recent reports have indicated that Medicare bills have risen sharply due to "upcoding," whereby the electronic records are systematically used to raise the complexity of a patient's case and put in for higher charges.[25] Computer work annoys physicians and is time consuming: one recent study showed that physicians are spending 43 percent of their time entering data into a computer, and only 28 percent talking to their patients.[26,27]

Nevertheless, a study by Johns Hopkins public health researchers suggested that if EMRs were fully implemented in just 30 percent of medical practices, there would be a reduction in demand for physicians by at least 4 percent and up to 9 percent.[28,29] That projection doesn't take into account the offsetting increased need for other personnel, such as scribes (an interesting throwback to pre-Gutenberg),[30–32] but I don't think it needs to. Once someone develops software that translates the unstructured voice conversation data of an office visit into a useful note for the record, scribes will be unnecessary. Undoubtedly, this can be developed with voice recognition and the machine learning tools that are available and have been successfully deployed for far more challenging undertakings. With such software, suddenly doctors could find themselves with nearly half their time now free.

There is still considerable debate as to whether electronic records reduce medical errors, as mistakes and "near misses" (often tied to medication errors) have occurred with similar frequency in multiple comparisons of electronic and paper records.[33–40] Of course, the EMR is only as good as the data that are entered into it, which is not only subject to human error but also indifferent and inappropriate use at the majority of health systems, which often neglect to input critical data.

Many proponents of electronic records, seeking to explain their problems, make comparisons to the Model T car. Lynne Thomas Gordon, the chief executive of the American Health Information Management Association, said, "We've gone from the horse and buggy to the Model T, and we don't know the rules of the road. Now we've had a big car pileup."[33] And back to OpenNotes, Dr. Jan Walker, one of the project's researchers said, "In a way we feel like we are in the Model T stage of this type of transparency. OpenNotes is like a new medicine that is beneficial to most patients but will harm some; how can we identify those patients and then address the situation openly and honestly?"[11]

The Model T analogy may be too optimistic. At least that car was practical, affordable, versatile, and transformational. It was a single product with interchangeable parts—to reduce waste and make it possible for unskilled workers to mass-assemble cars. In contrast, we have over one thousand certified EMR vendors in the United States, each with proprietary software that usually won't work with records created by different software. With the fragmentation of health care in the United States, the majority of individuals see physicians in multiple health systems with different EMR vendors. Even though in 2015 all doctors and hospitals are required by federal law to use electronic records, we are still in a nascent phase, lacking patient-centric, fully accessible, comprehensive, and easy to use EMRs. We haven't even gotten out of the parking lot yet, no less on the highway. I will return to what the future of medical records could look like after capturing the medication information.

My Meds

Medications are certainly center stage in the narrative of important medical information. You can think of them as a triple whammy—high cost, errors, and problems with adherence. In the United States alone, 3.2 billion prescriptions are written each year, and the cost runs well over $350 billion. Errors are exceptionally common, with over 40 percent of Americans reporting that they or a family member has been a victim of a medication error. Although it is hard to come by high quality data, these errors appear to be linked to well over one hundred thousand deaths and costs that range between $17 billion and $29 billion per year. And then there's lack of adherence to medications with marked adverse impact, representing up to half of treatment failures, 125,000 deaths and $290 billion in costs each year in the United States.[41,42]

Smartphone apps have proliferated to improve adherence, including Mango Health, CyberDoctor, AiCure, Nightingale, MediMinder, MediSafe, and Care4Today.[43-45] These apps help patients track the correct dose and timing of their prescriptions. Some text or call the patient to remind the individual that it is time to take a particular med, and have backups to connect with family members of caregivers to assure adherence. AiCure uses a smartphone camera or PC webcam to track the patient. Nightingale and CyberDoctor capture additional or alternative information

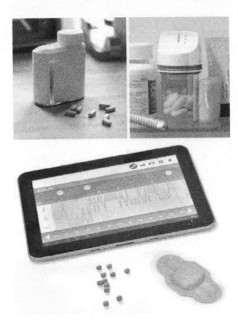

FIGURE 7.1: Medication adherence digital hardware tools including AdhereTech (top left), GlowCaps (top right) and Proteus Digital Health (bottom). Sources: http://www.AdhereTech.com, http://www.glowcaps.com; and Proteus Digital Health. Reprinted with permission.

to understand the patient's schedule or gamify the process, respectively. There are also seemingly countless new "smart" digital pillboxes and bottles.[46] These include AdhereTech and Vitality's GlowCaps (Figure 7.1). GlowCaps and AdhereTech are smart pill bottles that wirelessly track when they are opened.[45] When it's time to take your medicine, GlowCaps start glowing with pulsing orange light and beeping out progressively more insistent arpeggios.[43,47] GlowCaps were used in a small, randomized trial for treating hypertension, achieving 97 percent adherence compared with 71 percent in the control group (a better adherence rate than the oft-cited 50 percent).[47] AdhereTech, which has been dubbed "a cell phone in a pill bottle," measures the contents of what's in the bottle, including sensors that measure humidity and exactly how many pills or liquid doses are left. For reminders, the patient can choose between texts, e-mails, or blinking lights.[45]

The most high tech of all is from Proteus, which got initial FDA approval in 2012 for putting a digestible microchip in each pill. When the tagged pill reaches the patient's stomach the gastric juice activates the chip, sending a signal via an adhesive patch sensor to a smartphone. The pills with embedded microchips can be made for pennies for virtually any medication, and this fairly elaborate technology might be especially well suited

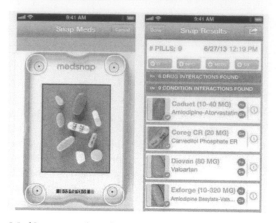

FIGURE 7.2: The MedSnap app identifies a group of pills. Source: https://medsnap.com.

for conditions in which adherence is critical, such as tuberculosis treatment (for which it is being tested).[45]

With many digital strategies for promoting medication adherence, it is likely that some will be validated in the future.[41,45,48–51] Yet the more here and now challenge is just for patients to keep track of each drug and the correct dose and timing that are prescribed. An EMR should certainly provide that information, with every update as any change is made in prescriptions, along with any known allergies and the precise adverse reactions that have occurred with prior medications.

Precision in Prescriptions

One of the explanations for both medication errors and poor adherence is that patients are taking so many medications that they or their doctors cannot keep track of them.[41,48,49] This is especially true for older patients; the average number of prescriptions, often requiring multiple doses per day for each, for individuals over age sixty-five, is six.[41,49] A common scenario for a patient coming in for a clinic visit, when asked about the medications he or she takes, is to take out the pills without knowing their names or doses. One solution is a new app called MedSnap, which can be used to take a picture and quickly determine the identity and dose of various medications (Figure 7.2),[52] much like the popular Shazam app for identifying songs. This should be helpful not only for doctors, but also for patients and caregivers. Such apps, combined with the pharmacogenomic component of the GIS, could go a long way to reduce prescription errors and other problems.

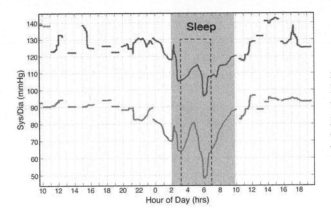

FIGURE 7.3:
Patient-generated data—
thirty-six hours of blood
pressure showing typical
dip during sleep via
wristwatch sensor.

Patient-Generated Data

Patients themselves can generate vast amounts of potentially useful data outside of the clinic. With all the fragmentation that exists with electronic medical records today, perhaps the last thing that is needed is a new, major stress on the system, or a new movement for physicians to resist (just the term "patient-generated" carries a negative connotation to some physicians, as if it were illegitimate or contaminated).[53-55] But this category of medical data will, in the years ahead, become the largest and most diverse of all. It encompasses wearable biosensors, imaging, and laboratory tests, including genomics and other omics.[56,57]

Ironically, given the apparent novelty, patients have supplied substantial data for their medical records all along, as in responses to lifestyle questions or health history. But what's different now is that it's coming via their smartphones. With well over 25 percent of Americans now tracking at least one health parameter on some type of wireless device, and hundreds of mobile apps commercially available to capture user-entered data, this is an area that is ready to explode.[55] Whether it's electrocardiograms, blood pressure continuous readings, glucose or other lab tests (Figure 7.3), it's real data that is providing insights on an individual we've not really had before.

Some health systems are paving the way for the flow of such data. For example, Banner Health in Arizona is using a wireless scale, pulse oximeter, breath flow monitor, blood pressure cuff, and glucometer for some of their patients and has established a portal for viewing the results and providing guidance.[55] Access Community Health Network in Chicago has adopted a similar model. One physician said it was "like having a doctor

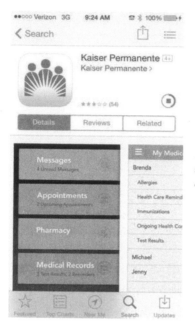

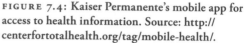

FIGURE 7.4: Kaiser Permanente's mobile app for access to health information. Source: http://centerfortotalhealth.org/tag/mobile-health/.

not only in your house but in your pocket. This is a revolutionary change in medicine."[55]

Despite recent serious issues that have surfaced regarding patient through-put, for over twelve years the Department of Veterans Affairs has been a frontrunner for remote monitoring of chronic conditions. More than its "health buddy," 140,000 veterans were monitored in 2013 for their chronic illnesses, including hypertension, diabetes, chronic obstructive pulmonary disease, and depression, via the VA's "health buddy" system. The technology for the "health buddy" is manual, without sensors or state-of-the art wireless technology, but the patient data are nicely integrated into the VistA electronic record.[55] The pilot wireless device initiatives at Banner and Access are integrating the patient-generated data with the individual's electronic record, and the results have certainly been encouraging for patients.

The Electronic Medical Record of the Future

We are still far away from what could be considered the optimal personal health record.[58–61] While access is the goal today, the end result must be individual ownership. The Kaiser Permanente health system has a mobile app that gives its members access to their medications, records, lab tests,

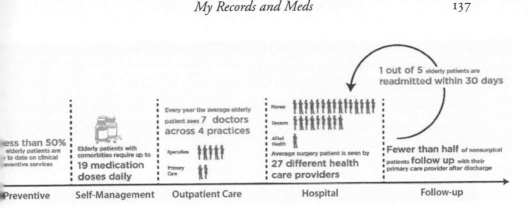

1 out of 5 elderly patients are readmitted within 30 days

Less than 50% elderly patients are up to date on clinical preventive services

Elderly patients with comorbities require up to 19 medication doses daily

Every year the average elderly patient sees 7 doctors across 4 practices

Nurses
Doctors
Allied Health

Average surgery patient is seen by 27 different health care providers

Fewer than half of nonsurgical patients follow up with their primary care provider after discharge

Preventive | Self-Management | Outpatient Care | Hospital | Follow-up

FIGURE 7.5: Source: M. Smith et al., "Best Care at Lower Cost: The Path to Continuously Learning Health Care in America," Institute of Medicine of the National Academies, September 6, 2012, http://www.iom.edu/Reports/2012/Best-Care-at-Lower-Cost-The-Path-to-Continuously-Learning-Health-Care-in-America.aspx. Reprinted with permission.

and results of scans (Figure 7.4). This can be viewed as *de minimis* for what patients should be able to access anywhere there is a mobile signal, but even this level of availability is quite uncommon. The majority of individuals have their medical care by multiple providers that cut across different health systems, markedly reducing the ability to have easy and singular access. For those over age sixty-five in the United States, each individual on average sees seven doctors across four practices per year (Figure 7.5).[62] Beyond the interoperability problem that has plagued electronic health records, this fragmentation interferes with creating a comprehensive, living, interactive record that follows individuals from womb to tomb. As we discussed in Chapter 6, all of one's medical scans need to be accessible, not just their interpretation. All exposure to radiation for these scans must be cumulatively tabulated as well. This may seem a wild dream, but in many ways the technology exists. One medical software expert, Melissa McCormack, suggests "we'd all be better off with our health records on Facebook."[63] She aptly points out the timeline feature, interactivity and sharing that she controls, with status updates to log new medications or diagnoses. Another software model is Evernote, which is an extremely popular data storage tool. Nick Dawson, a leader of the Society of Participatory Medicine, uses Evernote as his electronic medical record, pulling in data from sensors and sharing with providers or family members.[64] Evernote's appealing characteristics include that it is secure, cloud-based, mobile, and has large storage capacity accommodating big files like medical images. It's highly interactive, addressing one of the most glaring shortcomings of electronic health records of today. The input from the individual—its rightful owner—has to be incorporated.

Eventually, these fundamental attributes of an electronic health record will be incorporated and attainable for all individuals. Over one hundred thousand health care professionals and seventy-five million patients have now adopted Practice Fusion, which offers a free electronic health record that includes some of the essential features.[65]

However, even when there is a personal health record that captures one's full GIS, it will still only be regarded as one-dimensional, aggregating data into one cloud server or place. The exciting jump forward requires the ability to do machine learning with the data, understand the multiplicity of interactions, and proceed down the path of predictive analytics.[66] That will fully transform the rudimentary electronic record (even one that assembles massive data per individual) to a preventive medicine apparatus. We'll get into that later, but we need to get closer to the real deal electronic record before that potential can ever be actualized.

Chapter 8

My Costs

*"But the hitherto tranquil life within the walled-off health care for-
tress, protected from the rigors of open price competition, may soon
come to an end."*
—Uwe Reinhardt[1]

"As in any market, when one side has no information, that side loses."
—Tina Rosenberg, "The Cure
for the $1,000 Toothbrush"[2]

*"Everybody focuses on who should pay for the exorbitant cost of health
care. What I decided to do was to ask the more fundamental question
which is why does health care cost so much?"*
—Steven Brill[3]

You're sitting in a comfortable chair, sipping wine, listening to your favorite soft music, and your wrist sensor says your heart rate is 50 and blood
pressure is 110 over 50. You couldn't feel more mellow and relaxed.

But then you start to read a magazine article entitled "The $100,000
Physical" and suddenly you're violently upset, your heart rate jumps to 120
and your blood pressure to 160 over 95. Yes, the issue of cost of American
health care would rile just about anyone up, and it may be the most de-
spicable—at $2.8 trillion or 18 percent of GDP—component of medicine
today. There is much to be angry about, but thanks to the democratization

of medicine, there will eventually be a new cost structure, transparency, and progressive reduction of voluminous waste.

It is hard to believe that it took until the year 2013 for health care costs to become the object of major media exposure. "Bitter Pill: Why Medical Bills Are Killing Us," the longest article ever published in the ninety-year history of *TIME* magazine, a 36-page, 24,105-word opus, written by Steven Brill finally gave the issue the attention it deserves.[3,4] The subheading was: "How outrageous pricing and egregious profits are destroying our health care."[3] After a seven-month in-depth review of hundreds of bills from hospitals, doctors, and medical device and drug companies, Brill performed an especially thorough post-mortem of seven cases. The titles of some of these capture the theme: "The $21,000 Heartburn Bill," "A Slip, a Fall, and a $9,400 Bill," "The One-Day, $87,000 Outpatient Bill," and "$132,303: The Lab-Test Cash Machine." This extraordinary exposé takes on the so-called hospital chargemaster, the mysterious list of what a hospital charges for anything on its inventory or equipment and services. The prices are typically marked up to absurd levels compared to wholesale costs, such as a single tablet of acetaminophen for $1.50 while Amazon sells one hundred for $1.49. Some hospitals charge up to $1,200 for every $100 of their total costs.[5] The one hundred most expensive hospitals in the United States charge 7.7 times their cost.[3,5,6] In 2013, the US government released the chargemaster prices set by each hospital. From them we learned that some hospitals charge ten to twenty times the price set by Medicare. By providing hard evidence of systematic price gouging and lack of rational or fair cost structure, the Brill article certainly provided a wake-up call for the American public. Soon after this publication, the *New York Times* rolled out a series of front-page feature articles entitled "Paying Till It Hurts," which elicited over one hundred thousand comments.[7–20] While the theme was similar for this series, the journalist and physician, Elisabeth Rosenthal, delved into particular topics, including the striking interhospital variability in costs of commonly performed procedures, such as colonoscopy, across the country.[11] Beyond this, the series illuminated the costs of such procedures in the United States as compared with other countries (Figure 8.1)[12,14] or within the United States for the same skin cancer procedure, known as Mohs surgery, across one hundred different medical practices.[19]

As in Brill's article, Rosenthal's series has many similar "sticker shock" examples, such as: the average pregnancy in the United States costs $37,341;[9]

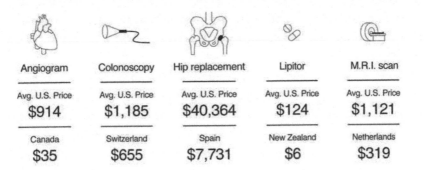

Angiogram	Colonoscopy	Hip replacement	Lipitor	M.R.I. scan
Avg. U.S. Price	Avg. U.S. Price	Avg. U.S. Price	Avg. U.S. Price	Avg. U.S. Price
$914	$1,185	$40,364	$124	$1,121
Canada	Switzerland	Spain	New Zealand	Netherlands
$35	$655	$7,731	$6	$319

FIGURE 8.1: Cost of some medical procedures or items in the United States vs. other countries. Source: Adapted from E. Rosenthal, "The Growing Popularity of Having Surgery Overseas," *New York Times*, August 7, 2013, http://www.nytimes.com/2013/08/07/us/the-growing-popularity-of-having-surgery-overseas.html.

a stent for $117,000;[10] a 15-minute trip to the emergency room for $1,772.42;[16] a knee replacement for over $125,000;[14] the most popular inhaler for asthma at $300 (which costs ~$20 in Britain);[15] $100,000 for antivenin for a rattlesnake bite;[16] and three stitches for $2,229.11.[10] Similar articles have appeared elsewhere, including "The Cure for the $1,000 Toothbrush,"[2] "The $50,000 Physical,"[21] "The Thousand-Dollar Pap Smear,"[22] the "The $55,000 Appendectomy,"[23,24a] the "$300,000 Drug"[24b] and the $10,169 lipid panel.[24c] So even though it took decades to finally be exposed, out-of-control pricing for American health care is now an established fact. That alone is certainly enough to get upset about, but the lesion is much, much deeper.

A Unique, Opaque, Irrational Market

There is no other market like American health care.[25-30] Only rarely will patients have any idea what they have been charged or what their employer or insurer has actually paid. But having paid for the service, the consumer owns nothing. It's "medicine by the yard," where we pay fee-for-service rather than rewards for health preservation. With an employer-based payer system for the majority of consumers, there is an overt lack of incentive for those patients themselves to drive costs down. An unfortunate result is that hospitals, doctors, and labs bill uninsured individuals and insurers vastly different amounts for the same service. Whatever the market will bear is the prevailing business model. In almost all other developed countries the government negotiates and regulates pricing, but not here. The powerful lobbying groups across all sectors of health care certainly wouldn't stand for that!

Overriding all these issues in a democratic society is the ubiquity of secrecy. Like the hospital chargemaster, health care charges in general are willfully kept clandestine. It all fits the model of medical paternalism— why would a consumer need to know this information and why would a doctor bother to discuss it with the patient? Uwe Reinhardt, a leading health economist, compared purchasing health care to "blindfolding shoppers entering a department store in the hope that inside they can and will then shop smartly for the merchandise they seek."[1] Steven Brill concluded that "complete lack of transparency is dangerous when arguably the most important part of our economy deals with life and death itself."[3] We've reviewed the general inadequacy of information that presently characterizes virtually all aspects of medicine, but even against that backdrop costs are the real outlier. This brief look we've had at Brill's and Rosenthal's work is just the beginning of our look at medical cost. After a more complete understanding of the cost issues, we'll come back to the progress that is now being made to promote transparency.

The Waste

The Institute of Medicine put out a 450-page report in 2012 entitled "Best Care at Lower Cost" that tackled the profound waste of our nearly $3 trillion annual health care expenditures.[31] The circle graph (Figure 8.2) shows the different compartments of waste, which comes up to one-third of the annual budget (i.e., more than 6 percent of US GDP). And as we'll review, this surely represents an underestimate.[29,31–33]

We've already touched on prices that are preposterously high. The unnecessary services towering over $210 billion predominantly relates to unneeded procedures and operations.[34] This might be a coronary stenting procedure in a patient without angina, or a lumbar disc operation for a patient with an inadequate trial of conservative therapy. But such a calculation doesn't take into account common surgeries that have been deemed ineffective. A buzzword these days for unnecessary or ineffective medical procedures or care is "low value."[33,35–39] A recent example is arthroscopic (performed via a scope to limit the size of incision) knee surgery known

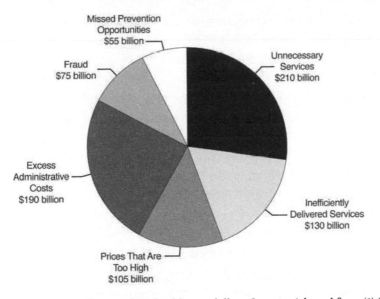

Missed Prevention
Opportunities
$55 billion

Fraud
$75 billion

Unnecessary
Services
$210 billion

Excess
Administrative
Costs
$190 billion

Inefficiently
Delivered Services
$130 billion

Prices That Are
Too High
$105 billion

FIGURE 8.2: Sources of waste of US health care dollars. Sources: Adapted from (1) M. Smith et al., "Best Care at Lower Cost: The Path to Continuously Learning Health Care in America," Institute of Medicine of the National Academies, September 6, 2012, http:// www.iom.edu/Reports/2012/Best-Care-at-Lower-Cost-The-Path-to-Continuously -Learning-Health-Care-in-America.aspx; and (2) D. M. Berwick and A. D. Hackbarth, "Eliminating Waste in US Health Care," *JAMA* 370 (2012): 1513. Note for fraud, which is not discussed further here, the figure ranges up to $272 billion per year. Source: "That's Where the Money Is," *The Economist*, May 31, 2014, http://www.economist.com/ news/leaders/21603026-how-hand-over-272-billion-year-criminals-thats-where-money.

as "partial meniscectomy"—the most common operation in the United States, with over seven hundred thousand performed each year with direct medical costs of $4 billion.[40] In a randomized trial conducted by Canadian researchers, patients with a torn meniscus were randomized to arthroscopic partial meniscectomy or a sham operation, such that the patient or researchers collecting the data for the patients did not know which had been performed.[40] There was no difference in outcomes, emphasizing the profound placebo effect of surgery itself. What makes the trial truly notable is the rarity of such experimental rigor in testing surgeries. Although using sham controls for comparison with actual procedures is the best way to distinguish the placebo effect, surgeons and patients are typically quite reluctant to participate in such a trial design. For this reason, there may well be many operations and procedures that are ineffective, but there have not been any rigorous trials putting them to the test.

Surgery creates another opportunity for waste when complications occur, as complications lead to higher reimbursement in the American medical system. Complications include infections, problems with wound healing, blood clots, heart attacks, and pneumonia. Atul Gawande and colleagues published a report in 2013 on over thirty-four thousand surgeries, of which over 5 percent had at least one complication.[41] The difference in cost was striking. For the uncomplicated operations, the average reimbursement was $16,936, compared with $39,017 for the complicated procedures.[41] A reward incentive for complications is not a rational approach in medicine.

And it's not just profligate surgeries. There are many widely used medication classes that are heavily promoted despite limited evidence of effectiveness—and that may even be hazardous.[42] Over $2 billion is spent on prescription testosterone gels to treat "low T" syndrome,[8,43] even though a risk of coronary artery disease and heart attacks has been established through randomized and large observational studies. Ritalin and other drugs for attention deficit disorder, which were the subject of a 2013 feature exposé in the *New York Times*, "The Selling of Attention Deficit Disorder," now account for over $9 billion per year, most of which is unnecessary or harmful, or both.[44,45] The use of antidepressants is analogous. In 2013, the top-selling drug in the United States was Abilify at $6,460,215,394. Not far below it was Cymbalta at $5,219,860,418. More than 1 in 10 Americans takes an antidepressant and for women age forty to sixty, the rate is 1 in 4. But studies have shown that more than 2 out of 3 of the patients taking these drugs do not fit the accepted criteria. That's especially the case for individuals over age sixty-five, for whom 6 out of 7 taking antidepressants do not fulfill the treatment standards. A new study from a nationally representative sample of more than seventy-five thousand adults showed only 38 percent who were taking these medications met the stipulations for treatment.[46] From a standpoint of waste, these data are enough to make one depressed.

But that's still scratching the surface for waste in prescription drugs. Because we haven't even begun to apply pharmacogenomics, we have ignored one of the biggest opportunities to achieve economic fitness in medications use. Take for example the three top-selling drugs globally for rheumatoid arthritis (and other autoimmune conditions), which are Humira, Enbrel, and Remicade. Together these three drugs account for over $30 billion in annual sales. But at best the clinical response rate is around 30 percent, translating to over $18 billion of waste each year. No significant efforts have been made to find the genomic or biomarker for predicting responsiveness, yet undoubtedly one exists, as is the case for virtually all medications. The flip side is the avoidance of serious, often life-threatening side effects. We know the genomic signals for the dangers of such drugs as carbamazepine (a severe autoimmune condition known as Stevens-Johnson syndrome) or flucloxacillin, which can cause liver failure, but they have not been incorporated into medical practice in the United States. As discussed in Chapter 7, there are over six thousand prescription drugs, but we only have pharmacogenomic information for just over one hundred (2 percent), leaving us in a bleak state of drug darkness. A recent study at Vanderbilt quantified the proportion of patients who would benefit by genotype screening of five commonly used medications.[47] Using such GIS information in the future for drugs that are on the market, and for those being developed, could lead to a turnaround.

Next up for unchecked improvidence is medical imaging.[47–48] The global market for imaging devices in 2014 was $32 billion.[49] The use in the United States for all types of scans—CT, nuclear, MRI, ultrasounds, and mammography—dwarfs their use in any other country in the world. Both MRI and CT scans in the United States exceed 250 per 1,000 people.[50] Over five hundred million medical scans were done in the United States in 2014; assuming a conservative $500 charge per test, this calculates to roughly $250 billion.[49] How many of these scans were necessary?[38] Moreover, an estimated 3 percent to 5 percent of individuals getting scans will get cancer because of the cumulative exposure to ionized radiation, as highlighted in the *New York Times* op-ed "We Are Giving Ourselves Cancer."[51] These induced cancers are not included in the economic toll of medical imaging. Also not included is all the medical imaging that is not supposed to be done according to the Choosing Wisely initiative,[52] discussed at length in Chapter 6, further confirming those recommendations were not aggressive or far-reaching enough, given the evidence base.

Unproven, high-tech therapies represent further waste. At the top of the list are robotic surgery and proton beam radiation, two interventions that have no data to support their use compared with standard therapies. Take robotic surgery.[53,54] There is only one general robotic surgery vendor in the United States, Intuitive Surgical, which charges between $1.5 and $2.2 million per da Vinci robot (that doesn't include the proprietary disposable equipment used for each case). Use of robotic surgery has grown exponentially across America with 1,370 hospitals (approximately 30 percent) buying at least one da Vinci in 2013.[53,55] They are used for procedures as diverse as hysterectomy, open-heart surgery, and prostate removal, with well over 1.5 million robotic-assisted surgeries performed worldwide. Another manufacturer, MAKO, makes a robot that is used for orthopedic procedures. In contrast to the lack of competition among robotic manufacturers is the fierce marketing by hospitals in the United States to promote their robots. Beyond the widespread television, radio, and billboard blitzes, one surgeon said, "I've seen hospitals bring their robots to halftime shows at sporting events."[55]

Proton beam radiation, the latest entry into high tech seduction, is an even bigger ticket item. Proton beam accelerator centers cost about $200 million to build,[56] and growth in the United States[57] is disconcerting, since there are no data that this form of radiation therapy, which supposedly is more precise, has any advantage over conventional radiation treatment for cancer. Not only are the centers exceptionally expensive to build, but also each procedure costs about 2.5 times what conventional therapy does. As of the end of 2013 there were forty-three such centers in the world, and, unsurprisingly, a disproportionate number are located in the United States—the world's capital of technology use, whether or not there exists any data to substantiate it.

And then there's more unwarranted medical stuff that doesn't necessarily involve high tech. Like annual physicals. Each year approximately 255 million Americans, or about 81 percent, go to see their doctor.[45,58,59] Many of these visits, such as for babies or pregnant women, are certainly important. But the last estimate for the number of people in the United States who get an annual physical dates back to 2007, and that number was 44.4 million. Back in 1979 a Canadian government study recommended giving up annual physicals, but it took until the last couple of years in the United States before this policy was advocated. Elisabeth Rosenthal wrote, in the *New York Times*, "So why do Americans, nearly alone on the planet, remain so devoted to the ritual physical exam and to all of these tests, and why do so many doctors continue to provide them?"[7] Not only do the unnecessary annual physicals cost more than $7 billion per year, but they also lead to all sorts of incidental findings—and more tests, more scans, more procedures, and more operations. A systematic review of all the studies of annual physicals concluded that they were wasteful and should be abandoned.[60] But despite this there is heavy promotion of executive physicals throughout the country, such as the Princeton Longevity Center's $5,300 comprehensive exam that will take "your health beyond the annual physical."[45]

On the flip side of the waste on physicals that are supposed to be preventative and have backfired are missed prevention opportunities, which cost $55 billion (Figure 8.2). Of the $3 trillion spent each year on health care, 84 percent is spent on treating chronic illness. What's more, 5 percent of patients, the so-called hotspotters, guzzle 50 percent of what the health system spends per year on chronic illness.[61] The top 1 percent account for 21.4 percent of expenditures, averaging $87,850 per patient.[62] And yet we haven't instituted any innovative digital technologies to deal with chronic diseases or the key individuals who are driving costs. Simple mobile device tracking of blood pressure, glucose, heart rhythm, lung function, and many other metrics tied into the common chronic conditions might prove useful, no less much tighter surveillance and guidance for the hotspotters.

We haven't even mentioned end-of-life care, which is yet another runaway expense portion for the United States. Medicare spends 28 percent of its budget, more than $170 billion, on patients' last six months of life.[63,64] The end-of-life treatments, including intensive care unit stays, aggressive use of procedures and operations, are not factored into the unnecessary calculation (Figure 8.2). But given the lack of effect on life span or quality of remaining life, those treatments are almost always unnecessary.

The result is that my estimates for unnecessary care or waste are considerably higher than what has been published by the Institute of Medicine. I'm guessing that waste—as I've defined it here—may actually equate to a half of American health care spending.

Outsourcing Health Care

We spend at least twice as much per capita per year—approximately $8,500—as any other developed nation. Yet the 2014 Commonwealth Fund report ranks the United States last of the eleven wealthiest nations for overall health care; the average spending per capita for the other ten countries is $3,100, or 63 percent less.[65,66] One of the results of the high cost of care in the United States is that patients are going outside the United

States for care.[67,68] The average cost of a day in the hospital in the United States is $4,287, compared with $853 in France or less than $500 in the Netherlands, but we don't need calculus to know that care in the hospital is not five to eight times better in the United States.[65,69] Prices can be even lower elsewhere, and this has certainly propelled medical tourism in many parts of the world, including such destinations as India, Thailand, Indonesia, Mexico, Dubai, and South Korea, as well as Europe. When Michael Shopenn needed a new hip and he was given an estimate that it would cost nearly $100,000 at his hospital in Boulder, Colorado, he used the Internet to find a full package cost of $13,660 near Brussels, where he had the surgery done.[14] That price included airfare and all-in medical and travel expenses. It nearly boggles the mind that the price could be so different. Part of the difference is the price of the hip. In Europe, an artificial hip can be purchased for $4,000 while the exact same model would cost $8,000 for an American hospital. But that's just the beginning, since in Europe the markup might be $200 but, in the United States, it could be at least ten times this figure.[14] Not surprisingly, Europe is quickly becoming a prime venue for medical tourism because of its price competitiveness.

Like with prescription medications, the US government does nothing to regulate the cost of medical devices or use any of its potentially enormous bargaining power to reduce costs (see Figure 8.1, which quantifies the impact of this policy). So it defaults to pricing whatever the American market will bear. But in virtually every other developed country, it's just the opposite. Elsewhere, the government has a strong influence on what any drug or device costs, and appropriately uses its muscle unimpeded by lobbying groups or special interests. That's why I like the acronym "NICE" in the UK—the National Institute for Health and Care Excellence. It isn't "nice" to industry, it dictates what costs it will accept, and it has rejected out of hand several new drugs when the companies were not willing to negotiate to an acceptable price. In contrast, the United States has no teeth.

In the "Paying Till It Hurts" series, Elisabeth Rosenthal pointed out that medical tourism doesn't have to be international. An example is a health plan in New York City that transports patients to Buffalo by limousine to achieve marked reduction in cost.[12] Similarly, Premera Blue Cross Blue Shield, which is Alaska's biggest health insurer, flies patients to Seattle for some procedures to reduce costs, such as knee surgery for half the price including transportation expenses.[12] Walmart has a Centers of Excellence program that provides access for its 1.1 million employees, on a voluntary basis, to one of six health systems in the United States for certain types of surgery. That is without cost to the employee and undoubtedly reflects a good deal the mammoth store chain was able to negotiate.

Some things are hard to outsource, like delivering a baby. The average total price in the United States charged for pregnancy and newborn care for a vaginal delivery is $30,000; for a C-section it's $50,000.[9] In either case, insurers pay out about half of these amounts charged. But in Europe, for most countries, the costs are just a small fraction—20 percent to 30 percent—compared with what US commercial insurers typically pay. Here the intercontinental differences are not accounted for by the cost of a device or drug, but simply hospital charges and the absurd markup of each and every item via the chargemaster, so nicely unmasked by Steven Brill.

Who Knows the Cost?

When I was training in internal medicine in the early 1980s, one of my attending physicians, Dr. Stephen Schroeder, gave repeated talks to the interns and residents about the critical importance of knowing the cost of everything that was ordered for each and every patient—lab tests, medications, procedures, scans, the works. He predicted thirty-five years ago that this was an essential practice for new physicians because we were headed to a health care financial debacle. Of course, he was indeed right; he was way ahead of his time, and, as with many visionaries, he was ignored.

Fast forward to the present. In 2014, a very interesting study by a group of orthopedists was published in *Health Affairs* titled "Survey Finds Few Orthopedic Surgeons Know the Costs of the Devices They Implant."[70] A total of over five hundred orthopedists at seven academic medical centers were asked to estimate the costs of commonly used devices and were only able to do so accurately (within 20 percent) less than 20 percent of the time. That was in spite of the belief by 80 percent of the orthopedists that knowing the cost information was important. The lead author, Dr. Kanu Okike, complained, "We never see the cost displayed anywhere, and even if you were interested, there's no great way to find it."[71] He's right about that: the US medical device world is characterized by purchasing groups that make private deals with hospitals, requiring nondisclosure agreements. As stated in the conclusion of the paper, "Medical device manufacturers strive to keep their prices confidential so that they can sell the same implant at a different price to different health care institutions."[70] In commenting on their results, Okike cited the lack of price transparency as medicine's biggest problem. However, there are other major factors that need to be acknowledged.

Back in the late 1990s, I instituted a program in the cardiac catheterization laboratories at Cleveland Clinic to track costs in real time. A stent procedure to de-block a coronary artery involves the use of many catheter types, including those with a balloon at their tip, and wires, as well as the stents. Each of these supplies is expensive, and there is considerable variability in their costs between manufacturers. Cumulatively, in difficult procedures, the tally can be four to eight times greater than the cost for equipment during an average procedure. For Medicare and many private insurers, there is a fixed, lump-sum payment for the procedure irrespective of what equipment is used. So we set up a system with a bar code on each device package that would be scanned and the cost would be displayed on the screen where the vital signs and X-ray pictures were displayed. As each catheter or piece of equipment was opened up, prices were displayed like when you are checking out at the grocery store. I thought it would be a great tracking method for our cardiologists—not only to have awareness in real time but also to take steps to be economical. But it was quickly rejected—the physicians did not want to have to factor in cost data to their decisions of how the procedure was performed. Some doctors think it is frankly unethical, violating the physician-patient relationship. The credo for many, if not most, is to deliver the best care irrespective of cost. The result, however, is that procedures and their equipment cost $150 billion each year, when they could surely be less.

That's a bit like the FDA in America, which reviews new drugs or devices for approval on the merit of safety and efficacy, without any regard for their costs. This compartmentalization of cost information by doctors and regulators has certainly contributed to our health care economic crisis— not knowing or not wanting to know isn't going to help. An uncoupling of medical care and costs may be considered unhealthy.

With electronic medical records, it's possible to display the real-time cost of lab tests (and many other costs) for the doctors at the time they are ordered. One recent study, which incorporated this display, showed only a modest improvement for this strategy—"up to" $107 per one thousand visits per month—compared with not having this cost data available.[72] The explanation is likely similar to the failure of real-time cost display in our cardiac cath labs: many physicians see the information as inappropriately interfering with their style of medical practice, their judgment, and their control. Unfortunately, this represents a dissociated, bubble mentality that is not consonant with what is going on in the world. One extreme response came from a Forbes columnist, Tim Worstall, who wrote "Bending the Health Care Cost Curve: Fire the Doctors."[73] He brought up the principle of Baumol's cost disease, or more simply the empirical notion that services employing personnel get progressively more expensive. He suggests that the best way to deal with this problem would be to have machines replace doctors.[73] I don't believe this is right or an acceptable solution for addressing the resistance that doctors have for heightened awareness and their practice being influenced by cost.

Two other strategies may ultimately be more promising. In 2014, Massachusetts rolled out a transparency law that requires a health care provider to disclose the allowed amount or charge an admission, procedure, or service within two working days.[74] Two days to get the data is not particularly helpful when you're in the midst of a heart attack and need a stent placed on an emergency basis. Indeed, a delay of up to two days is hardly comparable to any other service or goods that are purchased in the world, but it can be seen as a first step of legislation to provide medical cost information to consumers.

Education is another approach, and medical schools like Yale have put emphasis on knowing and sharing everything related to costs in their curriculum.[75] In "The Thousand-Dollar Pap Smear," Cheryl Bettigole zeroed in on the key Q&A: "What is the biggest driver of health care costs in the hospital? Answer: the physician's pen" (or a mouse or keyboard).[22] Clicking on a box such as a Pap smear in an electronic medical record is typically thoughtless and reflexive. It is also the norm of medical practice. In fact, clicking a mouse, instead of the old requirement to fill out forms, probably makes it easier. Certainly it is imperative to teach students, physicians in training, and those in practice, to get with the program, that calling for tests with little thought is no way to practice medicine.[76] It is hard to believe it has taken all these decades for this to get started. But when you put medical paternalism in context, why would a doctor need to have to deal with such a mundane, lowly topic?

Peter Ubel of Duke University has been a leading voice for full disclosure of costs to patients, with essays such as "Doctor, First Tell Me What It Costs"[77] and "Full Disclosure—Out-of-Pocket Costs as Side Effects."[78] Moriates, Shah, and Arora have also advocated this sentiment in "First, Do No (Financial) Harm."[79] Their argument is straightforward. With the high costs of medical care, proactively sharing this information and avoiding unnecessary tests or treatments are major professional responsibilities. Not only do patients go bankrupt from the costs of care, but even more often they cannot adhere to a treatment plan because it is not affordable.[18,79–83] Now medical costs are intertwined with one's medical condition; the stress and anxiety related to high deductibles and out-of-pocket expenses can have a significant emotional toll. Unfortunately, however, the complexity of health care insurance in the United States preempts the ability for a doctor to know what would be the actual, out-of-pocket costs for any given patient. We need to see what's behind the curtain on that in real time, the exact cost burden to patients, for any goods or services. There's no longer any room for opacity on the part of health insurers.[84–87]

The Drive to Transparency

For over five years, the Surgery Center of Oklahoma has set a sterling example to its peers. With forty surgeons and anesthesiologists in Oklahoma City, this group has posted pricing for all their operations and services, all inclusive, on their website. Need a pacemaker—it'll be $7,600. Rupture your Achilles tendon?—it costs $5,730. This has attracted enormous attention because it's such an outlier. As Tina Rosenberg aptly put it, "What's remarkable is that this is remarkable."[88] Imagine having the same transparency in your costs for a medical procedure as anything else you purchase in your life!

The implications are huge. Just like the Best Buy chain store guarantees that if you find a better price, they'll match it, the Surgery Center of Oklahoma's website has enabled patients to leverage better deals all over the country. The impact locally is noteworthy, as the pressure mounts for others to follow suit in order to be competitive. Many other medical facilities in Oklahoma are now posting their prices for the first time. It's not the only example of transparent pricing in the country, since drugstores like CVS Minute Clinics and local urgent care clinics post their prices. But it's just the beginning of health providers, on their own initiative, driving cost transparency.

That's just one of the forces that are surging to blow this wide open. In 2014, Medicare released all of their detailed payment data for 880,000 physicians and health care providers.[89,90] More than thirty states in the United States are either considering or pursuing legislation to increase price transparency. Through the provision of the 2014 Affordable Care Act, the federal government requires all health care exchanges to post out-of-pocket cost data for many medical services on their websites. Some health systems, like Intermountain Healthcare in Salt Lake City, with a network of 22 hospitals and 185 clinics, has committed to posting on its website all of its cost data for 25,000 total items in its cost master. The big insurers, including United, Aetna, and Blue Cross Blue Shield, all have developed cost estimators that give approximate data for total cost and out-of-pocket expense for hundreds of common services. In the past few years there has been an inundation of new companies dedicated to providing transparent cost data to consumers.[6,91–101] Venture capital firms have invested over $500 million, and some of these companies have progressed to initial public equity offerings.[92] The list includes Castlight Health, pokitdok, Doctible, GoodRx, Health in Reach, eLuminateHealth, Change Healthcare, HealthSparq, SnapHealth, ClearHealthCosts, Healthcare Bluebook, and many more. Brighter and other new upstarts are opening up the dental cost landscape. Each of these companies differs in many ways—how they estimate pricing information, how they present the data, who can access the site, and what exactly is provided.[102a] The Healthcare Bluebook, which is freely available to consumers, provides the "fair price" by zip code for physician and hospital services by averaging the costs in a particular area. Doctible is crowdsourcing patient medical bills and out-of-pocket costs so the public can see them. Using proprietary software that analyzed claims data, Castlight Health provides employers and their employees (not the general public) price data by individual doctors and health systems and is beginning to add quality metrics. It is also introducing reference pricing, which is the maximum price an insurer will cover. Any difference would theoretically have to be paid by the consumer. This additional strategy may apply pricing pressure beyond transparency per se. Indeed, the California Public Employees Retirement System (CalPERS), the second largest benefits program in the United States, has successfully used a reference pricing initiative to lower costs. Patients who opt for hospitals that do not meet the CalPERS cost threshold take on cost-sharing responsibility.

There are more consumer-centric websites, such as New Choice Health, to find out all of the comparable costs in any particular city or region; Medibid's data is intended for patients to set up a bidding process.[102b] It works just like Priceline. As an example, using this bidding site, a patient from Seattle needing knee surgery went to Virginia to reduce his cost from $15,000 to $7,500. Just like Kayak, Travelocity, and Expedia disrupted the lock by travel agents many years ago, and Zillow and Trulia took on the real estate brokers, and Edmunds or Autotrader exposed car pricing, we have finally seen the opening of medicine's kimono.

Taking lessons from the travel and real estate price comparator websites that provide all their data for mobile device access, the companies removing the shroud of secrecy from medical costs are doing the same with smartphone and tablet apps (Figure 8.3). As a result of this widespread disruption, Reinhardt believes we're now moving into a new phase in the fight over pricing transparency. He said in an interview, "You lived in the secure castle with complete price opacity, no one knew what anything cost, which worked well for you. But you now have these insurgents at the gate, beating at the door, and they're even getting help from the inside. Pretty soon you'll be fully transparent."[103,104]

All this looks promising, but there are still plenty of challenges that lie ahead. Owing to the historical pattern of patients not questioning their doctors, only 32 percent actually ask any questions about what their medical services will cost.[104] It remains to be seen, especially among the aged, who are the most likely to need health care, whether immediate access via wireless devices to cost information (as opposed to having to ask doctors or other health care professionals directly) will have an impact. Likely their children and the digital natives will drive the use of point-of-need price data and provide teachable moments for those requiring significant medical tests or interventions.

It is interesting that the majority of consumers will research the costs for prescriptions but that this doesn't carry over to other medical services. The likely explanations are multiple, including that medications involve out-of-pocket costs or co-payment, that pharmacy costs have been set in a competitive marketplace with information that is easily accessible via the Web, that consumers find it easier to discuss costs with their pharmacist

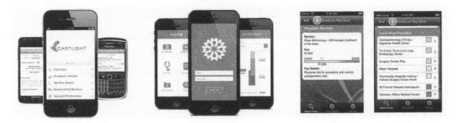

FIGURE 8.3: Examples of mobile apps that display health care pricing. Sources: (left) B. Dolan, "Castlight Health Takes Cost, Quality Measures Mobile," *MobiHealthNews*, March 29, 2012, http://mobihealthnews.com/16804/castlight-health-takes-cost-quality -measures-mobile/; (middle) E. Garvin, "Can Medlio's Virtual Health Insurance Card Im- prove Patient Engagement?" *HIT Consultant*, September 16, 2013, http://hitconsultant .net/2013/09/16/can-medlios-virtual-health-insurance-card-improve-patient-engagement /; and (right) M. Hostetter and S. Klein, "Health Care Price Transparency: Can It Pro- mote High-Value Care?" Quality Matters, The Commonwealth Fund, April 25, 2012, http://www.commonwealthfund.org/publications/newsletters/quality-matters/2012/april -may/in-focus.

than to have to deal with their doctors. It appears that all of these factors will come to bear on other medical costs, since the transparency will rev up competitiveness, the questions will typically bypass physicians, and the marked increase in out-of-pocket consumer costs will strongly encourage the need to know. Over the past five years, the average deductible per em- ployee has more than doubled; this big shift from the employer to employee will undoubtedly promote the access and use of the cost information.

Let's say, hypothetically, that patients become accustomed to investi- gating prices. The next question is whether this will lower costs.[105] Expe- rience from other transparency initiatives suggests that lower costs are not of absolute certainty. Millions have been poured into the campaign for restaurants to show the calorie data for all the items on their menus, but there is no evidence this has changed selection, food intake, or the weight of consumers. When New York State provided the public data on outcomes for bypass surgery in all their hospitals way back in 1996, my colleagues and I published an analysis showing the unanticipated outcome: high-risk patients were referred out of state.[106] Later, *New York Magazine* published an exposé of the adverse effects of such transparency.[107a] Four out of five cardiologists felt that report cards affected their decisions to perform an- gioplasty on patients. Ironically, as the magazine pointed out, "the very system designed to make heart surgery safe may be convincing surgeons to turn patients away."[107a] So it will be important to establish whether having the data accessible and used actually favorably impacts health care costs in the future. One recent study involving medical imaging provides some encouraging support for this effect. When the prices of MRI were made transparent to patients, this induced significant competition among providers and led to markedly lowered costs. [107b,107c,107d]

However, another difficulty is that even though study after study has shown that there is no relationship between cost and quality of care, the public believes there is. An interesting experiment conducted by Hibbard and colleagues, published in *Health Affairs,* showed that a substantial proportion of 1,432 individuals "shied away from low-cost providers and viewed higher prices as a proxy for higher quality."[108] The same way that many people choose bottles of wine! A more recent study of high- versus low-priced hospitals also showed that, with respect to the consumer's view, the reputation of a high-priced health system can override substandard objective measures of quality. From a prospective patient's perspective, there's a tendency to accept "you get what you pay for," even though the totality of data doesn't support that principle in health care at all.

An even more vexing issue is that it is extremely difficult to adjudicate quality in health care. For a specific operation with critical outcomes, such as open-heart surgery, and whether the patient survives, quality may be easy to assess. Indeed open-heart surgery is the exemplar case, because data for millions of patients are available through the thoracic surgery society's database, making adjustment possible for age and forty-four other important risk factors and co-existing conditions. On the other hand, for most medical conditions the outcomes are not easy to define or quantify, and making adjustments based on various other factors is more difficult. Alternative metrics like patient satisfaction surveys are used, and although these are important, they cannot equate to the actual outcomes of a surgery or procedure. My patients who have undergone open-heart surgery typically evaluate their operation by the look of their incision, which is not reflective of what happened inside the chest. With all the drive to cost transparency, there is not only little emphasis to make quality-of-care data available, but also it is extremely hard to come by. That's why the call of Guest and Quincy from *Consumer Reports* that "consumers should have better information about hospital and physician performance than they can glean from user reviews on Yelp, Zagat's, Angie's List, or other such sources" is such a tall order.[109,110]

Nonetheless, we have strong indicators, for the first time in the history of medicine, that cost data will be widely available to each individual. That sanguine sign of democratization of health care financial information is just one of many that a veritable shakeup is in the making. In one sense, it doesn't matter whether it lowers cost in the long run, even though it likely will. It will be a big deal simply when each person gets long-overdue access to relevant data to which they are entitled.

Chapter 9

My (Smartphone) Doctor

"I am more certain than ever that iDoc is the future of medicine in the digitalized world. Doctors had their chance to lead medicine, but they didn't take it."

—FROM ROBIN COOK's *Cell*[1]

"mHealth is about fundamentally changing the social contract between patients and doctors. Physicians are likely to resist the loss of power implicit in greater patient control."

—ERIC DISHMAN, INTEL[2]

"Today the ASK WATSON button provides a second opinion for oncologists. But as it grows more reliable, might it replace some of them entirely?"

—JESSI HEMPEL, *Fortune*[3]

How can we expect radical changes that are occurring everywhere besides medicine to leave the health care landscape untouched?[4] W. Brian Arthur, a researcher at the Xerox Palo Alto Research Center, rightly says "It will change every profession in ways we have barely seen yet."[5] You can just take lessons from history to see how technology radically affects what people do. For example, in 1900 41 percent of Americans worked in agriculture; this has been profoundly reduced to 2 percent a century later. Or Americans employed in manufacturing, which has declined from 30 percent in the 1950s to less than 10 percent today, due to automation. There is indeed now a "race against machines" that is pervasive, and it would be naïve to think that medicine is immune from the impact.[6]

The medical thriller novelist and physician Robin Cook wrote *Cell,* his thirty-third book, about iDoc—"a smartphone functioning as a twenty-first-century primary-care physician,"[7] an avatar doctor equipped with algorithms to "create a true ersatz physician on duty twenty-four-seven for a particular individual, truly personalized medicine."[7] Each individual signing up selects an avatar doctor, choosing their gender, attitude, whether they are paternal or maternal in tone, and how they want to be notified.

The system involves a remote command center staffed with hundreds of physicians who work four-hour shifts to keep them mentally crisp, and a supercomputer that, in real time, continuously monitors extensive physiological data on all iDoc users. Here is an excerpted dialogue from *Cell* between two doctors:

> "It's simple. iDoc is able to titrate lifesaving medication according to real-time physiological values rather than trying to treat symptoms, which is the old 'sick' care medical paradigm. iDoc is the perfect primary-care doctor since it is based on an algorithm that is capable of learning and will be continually upgraded as new medical information is incorporated."
>
> "I'm concerned it can't handle what's on its plate now."
>
> "You know what a Luddite doctor is, George? I run across them all the time. MDs who have been dragging their feet in the acceptance of digitalized medicine, even something as intuitive as electronic records. Come on! This is a no-brainer!"[8]

Unfortunately, an insurance company (called Amalgamated Healthcare) acquires the technology and hijacks it, killing off individuals who have been newly diagnosed with a fatal illness in order to cut costs.

A nonmedical version of this narrative, with some common threads, is the sci-fi romantic comedy movie *Her* in which Joaquin Phoenix falls in love with his computer and smartphone avatar, whose advanced operating system (iOS 10) voice is played by Scarlett Johansson. Here the monitoring capability coupled with machine learning sets up a progressively stronger, intimate relationship culminating in love (and later tragedy).

The book *Cell* and movie *Her* are not at all far-fetched. All of the technology to do this exists today. Robin Cook just went a bit fast-forward to portray the command centers equipped with massive computing capability and hundreds of doctors. Although it may not be the precise configuration for a future health system, it certainly represents a likely scenario. Unfortunately the risks are real, too, even if they probably won't involve murderous insurance companies. While Robin is as enthusiastic as I am for digital medicine to be transformative,[9] the potential for misuse and exploitation must always be kept in mind. As he explained to me, his winning formula for a medical thriller obligates there being a big-time villain. In this case the health insurance company, an easy target, since many have long viewed these companies as villains. The security and privacy of digital medical data, and its potential for misappropriation, are not to be underemphasized, and we will review these issues later. For now, I want to set the stage for the future smartphone doctor era of medicine. You may have noticed that I have put *smartphone* in parentheses in the title of this chapter. That's because smartphone-mediated medicine offers two possible smartphone doctors. Users may be engaging with a real doctor, but they may just as likely be calling an avatar or algorithm with a connection to the cloud or supercomputer.

The Warm-up

For a variety of reasons, between 2009–2011 in the United States, the number of physician visits fell 17 percent among privately insured patients.[10] And that decline is continuing despite the aging of the population and their high density of comorbidities. One of the reasons may be cost, but surely a contributing factor is that there are many emerging alternatives, from retail clinics with nurses to do-it-yourself (DIY) care. Precivil Carrera, a physician in the Netherlands, defined modern DIY medicine as "a form of self-care involving the use of consumer-directed health informatics technologies and applications that allow consumers to track and manage their health by themselves or together with professionals, and that guide consumers' use of health care."[11]

There is considerable evidence that deeper engagement of consumers in their health care yields superior results. For blood pressure, a review of fifty-two prospective, randomized studies showed that people who took self-measurements had better blood pressure management versus those whose only monitoring came through usual care (e.g., at the doctor's office).[12] Beyond self-care, those who interacted with a pharmacist via telemonitoring also showed superior blood pressure control in a randomized trial, with 72 percent of patients achieving controlled blood pressure as compared to only 57 percent with usual care (the national norm is 50 percent).[13] Furthermore, the blood pressure control advantage in the pharmacist arm was quite durable, extending many months after the random assignment of the intervention. Blood pressure is not the only condition successfully treated this way. Using mobile phones to engage adults with diabetes in a randomized trial, researchers at the University of Chicago showed superior glycemic control compared with usual care, at lower costs and higher satisfaction.[14]

Better outcomes have been demonstrated for engaged, activated patients as compared with usual care for a wide variety of conditions, including hypertension, diabetes, obesity, multiple sclerosis, hyperlipidemia, and many types of mental health disorders. Based on this sort positive data, Leonard Kish, a health information technologist, has rightfully called the engaged patient the "blockbuster drug of the century."[15] These successes subsequently led the journal Health Affairs to have a dedicated issue on "the new era of patient engagement."[16–18] Engagement can be conceived as patient activation—"understanding one's own role in the care process and having the knowledge, skills, and confidence to take on that role."[16]

Besides self-care, there is the link to nurses. There are approximately one hundred million outpatient visits in the United States per year, with over six million in retail clinics that typically employ nurse practitioners.[19–22] Clinics in pharmacies, like the Minute Clinics at CVS, or in chain stores like Walmart, Kroger, and Target, cropped up about a decade ago and have cumulatively accrued twenty million patient visits in now over sixteen hundred sites. CVS has plans to double their Minute Clinics to be at fifteen hundred by 2017; Walgreens is adding one hundred more clinics this year to get to five hundred total. Both the difficulty involved in getting conventional physician appointments and the convenience for patients that retail clinics afford have been well documented.[23]

Nonetheless, there are regulatory limits on the practice of nurses in many states, and there is reduced insurance reimbursement for nurses as compared with doctors. Moreover, there is considerable tension between physicians and nurses about delivery of care. For example, after Walgreens announced the expansion of its 330 Take Care clinics, which are staffed by nurse practitioners, the American Academy of Family Physicians claimed the development would ultimately "lower quality, increase costs and pose a risk to patients' long-term health outcomes."[24] In 2014, the American Academy of Pediatrics was up in arms about retail-based clinics and issued a statement that they "are an inappropriate source of primary care for pediatric patients, as they are detrimental to the medical home concept of longitudinal and coordinated care."[23,25] Indeed, the American Medical Association and many other physician groups have issued restrictive policies and regulations about the "scope of practice" available to nurses, dictating what a health care provider can do based on experience, education, and training.[24]

This is not a problem confined to outpatient clinics; the tension extends to hospital services. Even though there have been studies that have shown no differences in outcomes for patients having their anesthesia administered by an anesthesiologist or a nurse anesthetist, the American Society of Anesthesiologists (representing over fifty thousand doctors) has issued warnings that quality of care may be diminished by care provided by nurse anesthetists.[26]

Independent assessments make such criticism look more like turf protection than patient protection. For example, a group of experts from the Institute of Medicine studied the problem and issued a report that provided backing for nurses to practice "to the full extent of their education and training" and called for eliminating regulations that suppress their role.[27] The National Governors Association and the Federal Trade Commission reinforced these recommendations, but the turf battle between physicians and nurses remains unsettled.[26,28–30]

There is only 1 licensed doctor for every 370 people in the United States. In most of the one-quarter of the United States that is considered rural, there is less than one doctor per thirty-five hundred people.[31] The average wait time to see a primary care doctor across the country is about 2.5 weeks, and as high as 66 days in Boston (Figure 9.1).[32,33] That's now, but by 2023, with the baby boomers coming to age, there is a projected 40 percent increase in heart disease and 50 percent increase in cancer and diabetes, which should make competition for appointments even fiercer. And these

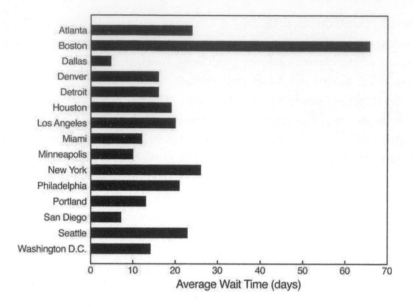

FIGURE 9.1: The average wait time for a new patient to see a doctor for family practice (nonemergency issues) by city. Source: Adapted from "How Long Will You Wait to See a Doctor?" *CNN Money*, accessed August 14, 2014, http://money.cnn.com/interactive/economy/average-doctor-wait-times/.

statistics don't even take into account increased access for forty million citizens who were previously uninsured. Although self-care and physician extenders, including nurses and physician assistants, can help, surely they won't be the whole solution. New tools must be brought to bear. While the medical community is slow to embrace digital and network solutions, these solutions are nonetheless erupting. Take the online health communities like PatientsLikeMe, CureTogether, Insight, and countless others, which provide peer-to-peer connectivity for patients with similar conditions. Many participants say they put more trust in their peers of these communities than in their doctors. In just a span of five years, these eHealth networking sites have attracted millions of consumers and are continuing to grow as a prominent medical information resource. Remarkably, this is certainly one key component of the movement toward the democratization of medicine.

Another emerging digital solution is the advanced Siri for medical guidance—the emergence of virtual health assistants (VHAs).[34,35] AskMD is one of the first Siri-like entries for this concept. A free smartphone app is downloaded, allowing the consumer to enter symptoms, either by typing them in or by voice recognition–embedded software, and tap into its pattern recognition database for feedback. When I visited the *Colbert Report,* Stephen Colbert had already caught on. He said, "I have a smartphone. Am I a doctor? How can my smartphone tell me about me? Is Siri a doctor?" Then he held his smartphone to his chest and asked "Siri, am I dying?" And Siri responded, "I really can't say."

While that got plenty of laughs, virtual health assistants should be taken seriously. Given a device with access to a large database as well as machine learning capabilities, surely we can see an effective, intelligent VHA developed that integrates the individual's medical record, medications, and relevant data monitoring. It would not take much to see a device help guide medication adherence, coach a healthy lifestyle, and respond to questions customized to the individual patient's circumstances and needs.

The Outpatient Visit of the Future

It seems like every week there is a new headline for an article related to who will see you (the smartphone, robot, avatar, algorithm, or Dr. Siri) for medical care or how you will be seen (cellphone, smartphone, Skype) (Figure 9.2).[23,36-49] *Fast Company* had an article titled "Could ePatient Networks Become the Superdoctors of the Future?" and asserted "the idea of going down to your doctor's office is going to feel as foreign as going to the video store."[50] That may seem bold, but they got that one right. Physical office visits are on their way out. Cisco surveyed over fifteen hundred Americans and found that 70 percent prefer virtual rather than physical visits with

The Smartphone Will See You Now
The Avatar Will See You Now
The Robot Will See You Now
The Doctor Will Skype You Now
How Smartphones Are Trying to Replace Your Doctor
The Doctor Will See You Now—On Your Cellphone
When Your MD Is an Algorithm
Dr. Smartphone: 5 Ways Your Doctor Can Diagnose You
Paging Dr. Siri: How Your iPhone Can Diagnose Disease
Can a Smartphone Replace Your Doctor?

From *Macleans, MIT Technology Review, The Atlantic, TIME, Gizmodo, Mashable, Wall Street Journal, Popular Mechanics, The Telegraph, Euronews,* respectively

FIGURE 9.2: Headlines of various articles in the past two years related to smartphone office visits.

their doctors.[51] That's not too surprising, given that the average return visit in the United States lasts seven minutes and new consultation twelve minutes, and that only after an average wait of sixty-two minutes to get into the exam room and be seen. Or not being seen because the doctor is predominantly looking at the keyboard to type into the electronic medical record.

Insurers are taking the lead in expanding these services.[37,52–54] Health Partners, a health insurer based in Minnesota, conducted a study of virtual visits using their web-based Virtuwell platform. They showed that virtual visits not only were substantially preferred, but they also reduced the average cost by $88 compared with physical visits, likely related to increased efficiency and reduced ancillary testing.[37] The University of Pittsburgh compared more than eight thousand e-visits ("Anywhere Care") and office visits and also found virtual connects cheaper, without compromising of quality according to key measures such as misdiagnosis, and considerably more popular among its patients. United Healthcare, one of the largest private insurers, started the NowClinic to give individuals immediate access to physicians for ten-minute secured live chat by phone or webcam. Wellpoint operates LiveHealthOnline, which charges $49 for a videoconference with physicians. Kaiser Permanente has been using virtual visits for several years, predominantly by secure e-mails and telephone calls and a minority of video encounters.[55] For the eight thousand doctors and 3.4 million members of Kaiser Permanente Northern California, virtual visits grew from 4.1 million in 2008 to 10.5 million in 2013 and are projected to exceed physical visits by 2016, according to Kaiser.[55,56] Nevertheless, while it appears that there has not been a decrease for in-person visits, more recent data that accounts for membership growth shows an inflection to be the case. Members strongly preferred virtual visits, while the "physicians have been slow to integrate new technologies into their practices, and most are leery of moving in this direction."[55]

There are many new players that are offering immediate virtual visits,[57] including Doctor on Demand, MD Live, American Well, Ringadoc, Teladoc, Health Magic, MedLion, InteractiveMD, and First Opinion.[58–75] You can hardly miss the pitches: "For $69 and your smartphone in hand, a board certified dermatologist will look at your rash" (from Dermatologist On Call) or "For $49, a doctor will see you now—online" (from American Well). Some of these connect for only telephone or text consults; a few of these companies offer secure video encounters. First Opinion is a text-only service that keeps the user's identity anonymous, circumventing the need for HIPAA approval.[68] There is a subscription fee of $9 per month after the first consult, and assurance that the same doctor will be linked for all subsequent consults. Google Helpouts, which are secure video meetings that are fully HIPAA compliant, have been adopted by One Medical Group, a very progressive, boutique medical practice based in San Francisco that received $40 million of investment from Google.[76-78] There are other very interesting entries to virtual video medical visits, including Verizon and the Mayo Clinic.[79-83] The latter is through a mobile health startup company called Better, which links the user to a Mayo Clinic nurse and charges a $50 monthly fee per household for unlimited access.[79-83] Its website bills it as "Your Personal Health Assistant" and having a nurse in your pocket.

One of the largest outpatient telehealth providers, Teladoc, published in 2014 on its 120,000 consults. It charges $38 per visit, operates 24/7, and the top three reasons for visits were acute respiratory illness, urinary tract symptoms, and skin problems. Overall, the cost for a video visit for most of these services is about $40, lasting from fifteen to twenty minutes. That is noteworthy, since a co-payment to see a doctor physically costs about the same. But there is 24/7 availability, wait time is zero, and it's as simple as tapping your smartphone to get connected with a physician.[51,84a] In some ways it can be likened to Uber as we get used to on-demand service via our smartphones.

Indeed, two companies have now launched the real equivalent to Uber for medical house calls. In select cities, Medicast and Pager offer doctors on demand on a 24/7 basis. It's just like summoning a car via Uber or Lyft, but instead of seeing information about the driver and car on your smartphone screen, you see the doctor's picture, his or her profile, and the length of time it will take him or her to be at your house. It's no surprise that these companies are so similar to Uber—Pager was started by one of Uber's co-founders.[84b]

There has also been the emergence of health visit kiosks. One, called Healthspot, looks like a hybrid of a sleek, futuristic phone booth and automated teller machine (ATM). In these kiosks, which are appearing in department stores like Target, a medical assistant escorts the consumer into the private booth for a secure video visit with a physician. The kiosk is equipped with some of the tools to obtain metrics such as blood pressure. Lee Schwamm, a physician proponent of telehealth, has pointed out that its implementation is much like ATMs for banks. The latter had a shaky start in the 1970s when they were expensive to manufacture, a loss leader for the banks, and quite clunky with limited capabilities.[85] Over time, however, they became fully integrated with global banking and financial services and remarkably consumer-centric. It has become unimaginable to have a bank without full ATM services for 24/7 access anywhere in the world. Dr. Peter Antall, a medical director for American Well compared the new phenomenon of telehealth to that of online banking: "Patients do have to get comfortable with this, but I remember a time where we were worried about electronic banking, and we got over that."[61] Now, of course, most of us do some banking online. Similarly, Randy Parker, the CEO of MDLive said, "Within the next few years, no consumer will even remember not being able to be connected to their providers through telehealth."[86a] The projections from the Deloitte consulting firm support Parker's assertion that telemedicine is growing rapidly. By the end of 2014, nearly 1 in 6 doctor visits in the United States will be virtual, and it is expected that the increase in over one hundred million virtual visits will potentially save $5 billion compared with traditional physical office visits.[86b,86c]

An unexpected example of the efficacy of teleconsults was demonstrated with genetic counselors. A randomized trial was undertaken of 669 women receiving new data on their BRCA gene mutations who were assigned to either an in-person or telephone consult. Extensive evaluation after the information was reviewed showed the telephone consults were just as effective.[87,88] With less than three thousand genetic counselors for a population in the United States of 330 million, surely this is good news for fixing the incongruous mismatch between the supply of this expertise and its increasing demand.

Nonetheless, there are significant obstacles for the widespread adoption of telemedicine. For one, there are archaic state laws for the practice of medicine that restrict a physician's practice to be limited to the state where he or she is licensed. They are a throwback to the late nineteenth century in response to unrestrained entry of medical practice during the Civil War! As a result such laws reflect none of the changes that medical training has undergone. For example, all MD physicians have to take the US Medical Licensure Examination (USMLE), and all medical education and training is set by national standards, which means state-by-state licensing is pointless.[89,90] Another obstacle results from state laws mandating that a patient has to have a physical visit with the doctor before a virtual visit is allowed.

So in order for these companies to operate, it has been necessary to enlist doctors in all fifty states, or restrict their practice to particular states that are covered by licensed physicians. It remains unclear when these antiquated state laws will be overridden. But at least in 2014 former Senator Tom Daschle formed a group known as the Alliance for Connected Care to address the need for a federal telemedicine law.[91] Building on that, the Federation of the Medical Boards have recently drafted into legislation to "create a new pathway to speed the licensing of doctors practicing medicine in multiple states."[92a] Known as the Interstate Medical Licensure Compact, the legislation is expected to be approved by many states in 2015 and "herald a major reform in medical licensing."[92b]

Telehealth will certainly not solve every problem facing medicine. Many of the models for these telehealth providers are fee-for-service, representing an extension of the pervasive and perverse way that American medicine is practiced. While they provide the foundation for a technology to reach remote areas that are medically underserved, the problems accompanying reimbursement and the medicine-by-the-yard model mean that telehealth won't necessarily help move us toward a health system motivated to preserve health, provide broad access to quality care, and avoid fees for episodic evaluation or treatment. Large employers in the United States have been embracing telehealth. Many reimburse the cost of such consultations, and the number offering access to them grew from 12 percent of companies in 2012 to 17 percent in 2013. An upbeat perspective on these developments comes from Dr. Zachary Landman, chief medical officer of DoctorBase. Landman tells the story of when his grandfather had a heart attack in 1950; the doctor tended to him at his home and charged $3.50.[93] He wrote about mobile health now letting doctors practice like it's 1950: "the mHealth movement has democratized mobile-based secure healthcare communication allowing every electing doctor to work in teams, message, share photos, and exchange files on HIPAA-secure mobile platforms."[93]

That indeed may be true one day, but we've already seen how doctors are reluctant to adapt the technology. Half of American physicians are over age fifty-five, far removed from digital native status (under age 30) and any propensity for adopting little wireless devices for their practice of medicine. Nevertheless, innovations abound, and a virtual physical may not be close to common but it is very close to possible. We've already covered a range of apps and hardware extensions—call them add-appters—that enable checking everything from pulse to breathing to eardrums with smartphones, and new devices, such as one from the Israeli company Tyto, which have tiny cameras and microphones that "can perform almost a complete checkup of the body."[94,95a] Besides the virtual physical during a one-off visit, there's remote monitoring of all vital signs and a range of important physiologic metrics, as we've already reviewed.

This is really transformative, multidimensional information—in time, space, and person. First, there's a much higher frequency of data that is gathered in the individual's "wild" rather than in a strained medical setting. That could be either continuous or intermittent, but often data that are being captured were not previously attainable. Examples would be blood pressure or blood oxygen saturation during sleep, or quantitative physiologic metrics (like HRV, GSR) during a traffic jam or an argument with one's spouse. Soon most and someday all the blood tests that would normally be done in a hospital or clinic laboratory will also be obtainable by smartphone add-appters. Second, the individual is looking at all this data on a frequent basis, in contrast to not even having access to it previously. This provides precious contextual insight. For example, some patients of mine tell me their blood pressure is invariably in the normal range except for Monday morning when they go back to work, or that the new medication that was added is not having any effect, or that "long acting" medicines taken in the morning seem to be wearing off by the evening. Patients with a history of heart rhythm abnormalities can see their ECG on the phone screen along with its computer reading. From that they can begin to learn what symptoms are the real deals, significant arrhythmias, as compared to innocent extra beat clustering. Individuals who are at risk for diabetes learn, for the first time, what particular foods or activities lead to better or worse glucose regulation. There could be a much longer list here but hopefully this conveys the power of critical data, simply and graphically displayed on the smartphone screen, to be uniquely and highly informative to the individual.

Third, there's the doctor's enhanced window to the patient's information, much of which wasn't available before, now contextualized by real world experience. Add to that the enhanced engagement of the patient and we begin to see how powerful an enabled patient can be. Let's consider a patient with depression, a condition for which mobile apps are already starting to make a difference.[95b] A medication has been prescribed and there is a question as to whether it is working. The patient reports feeling subjectively better, but all of the objective indices—tone and inflection of voice, frequency of communication, activity and movement, breathing pattern, facial expression, vital signs, HRV and GSR—show no sign of improvement whatsoever. Does this diagnose a placebo effect of the medication? The patient looks at the integrated data and notes a dissociation of symptoms and the metrics. A whole new discussion can ensue as to whether a medication is necessary, whether it's really working, and the potential to explore other alternative nonmedical treatments. Or another patient with a history of frequent asthma attacks is now using the lung smartphone add-appter, which gathers environmental exposures that include pollen count and air quality, ambient temperature and humidity, along with activity, vital signs, lung function (forced expiratory volume in one second via the microphone), chest movement, and breathing pattern. The integrated asthma dashboard shows that the combination of cold air and exercise, on days with poor air quality, explains nearly all of the exacerbations of asthma. Now the patient and doctor can come up with a new plan of anti-attack—with emphasis of preventive inhaler use (and specific types of inhalers) timed to this individual's exposure triggers. That also allows for reduction of medications for the rest of the time, reducing the chances for side effects and expense.

So the real office visit has a whole different look, highly enriched by data that was patient-generated, but also visualized and, at least to some extent, processed by the patient. This sets up an opportunity to strengthen the bond between the patient and doctor. The activated patient has now assumed the role of "data-gatherer" who sends this trove of information for additional guidance and input to the physician. The data can be sent ahead anytime, either during or before a virtual or real office visit. Indeed, the data might even preempt the need for a "visit," and when they do prove necessary, they will no longer be visits or appointments but informative, data-driven discussions. There you have my sense of why recommending medical apps and add-appters makes for such an exciting and intimate way to practice medicine. Perhaps that's why even back in 2012 England's National Health Service (not known as the most progressive health system in the world) requested general practitioners to recommend apps to their patients for managing conditions ranging from diabetes to depression "in an attempt to give patients more power and reduce visits to doctors."[96,97]

For this initiative, the health secretary, Andrew Lansley, said: "I want to make using apps to track blood pressure, to find the nearest source of support when you need it and to get practical help in staying healthy the norm. With more information at their fingertips, patients can truly be in the driving seat."[96]

As we reviewed in Chapter 7, we will get away from keyboards in the office, also known as "death by a thousand clicks," and replace them with computer processing of natural language into notes.[98–100] This sort of data, combined with a machine-learning powered app to turn spoken words into notes, will truly revolutionize the doctor's visit of the future—assuming, of course, that we need the routine visits at all.

Doctors Disintermediated?

We've already seen some examples of how physicians react to the threat of being marginalized, along with their general reluctance to adapt to new technology. Now we get into the "Second Machine Age"[101] question as to whether the new digital landscape will reboot the need for doctors and health professionals. Kevin Kelly, a cofounder of *Wired,* has asserted: "The role tasks of any information-intensive job can be automated. It doesn't matter if you are a doctor, lawyer, architect, reporter, or even programmer: The robot takeover will be epic."[102] An emergency medicine physician likened the current practice of medicine to a Radio Shack store in his piece "Doctor Dinosaur: Physicians may not be exempt from extinction."[103] In late 2013, Korean doctors threatened to go on an all-out strike if the government went ahead with new telemedicine laws that would support clinical diagnoses to be made remotely. Their fear of losing fifty thousand jobs was articulated by one of the medical group leaders: "The government's plans will only bring the collapse of the country's healthcare system and polarization between large hospitals and small clinics."[104] When Johnson & Johnson introduced a computerized conscious sedation machine called Sedasys, the company proclaimed: "This is truly a first-in-kind medical technology that has the potential to redefine the way sedation is administered" and "is a great way to improve care and reduce costs."[105] In contrast, a physician leader of the American Society of Anesthesiologists responded, "Everyone is so hot on technology, but you have to balance the fiduciary duties of the company with the physicians' interest in ensuring the highest quality and safest care for the patient."[105] The founders of PatientsLikeMe, the largest online health community, have asked, "Who will be the best to interpret your MRI? A radiologist? Or a computer?"[106a] It's just a question of time. You can only imagine how radiologists react to robotic replacement affirmations. Or oncologists after reading a *Fortune* magazine feature article on IBM Watson that has been deployed in several cancer centers asking whether cancer doctors will be replaced by a supercomputer.[3] Add to that psychiatrists who read an article in *The Economist* that a virtual shrink may be better than a real one, reviewing a study that showed that patients are more apt to confide and be open and honest with a computer avatar than with a counselor.[106b,106c]

The need for doctors will be reduced, so there certainly is reason to question the projection of a profound shortage of doctors that looms ahead. Already in 2015 it is estimated by the American Association of Medical Colleges that there are almost 63,000 less doctors than needed in the United States. This figure jumps to over 130,000 short in a decade (Figure 9.3).[106d] The shortage is not confined to the United States—the World Health Organization claims there is already an alarming worldwide shortage of 4.3 million doctors and nurses of the 27.3 million combined global workforce.

In 2014, the Institute of Medicine issued a report on medical education, assessing the physician workforce with a key conclusion about the looming shortage: "does not find any credible evidence to support such claims."[106e] Echoing this conclusion, a most unlikely bipartisan combination of

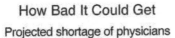

How Bad It Could Get

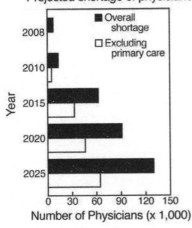

FIGURE 9.3: Projection by American Association of Medical Colleges of physician shortage in the United States. Source: Adapted from "Physician Shortages to Worsen Without Increases in Residency Training," American Association of Medical Colleges, 2014, https://www.aamc.org/download/153160/data/physician_shortages_to_worsen_without_increases_in_residency_tr.pdf.

authors—Scott Gottlieb and Ezekiel Emanuel—representing extreme views of the Republican and Democratic parties, respectively, wrote a pointed piece, "No, There Won't Be a Doctor Shortage."[107] While acknowledging the aging of the population and the increased demand related to thirty million newly insured Americans via the Affordable Care Act, they declared: "The road to Obamacare has seen its share of speed bumps, as well as big potholes. But a physician shortage is unlikely to be one of its roadblocks."[107] Beyond echoing the use of nurses, pharmacists, dieticians, health aides, and other nonphysicians, and the profound waste in American health care (as reviewed in Chapter 8), they aptly point out: "Innovations, such as sensors that enable remote monitoring of disease and more timely interventions, can help pre-empt the need for inpatient treatment."[107] And that is just the beginning of how innovative technology and unplugged medicine can markedly improve the efficiency of physicians.

Smartphone Medicine to the Rescue?

Unfortunately, most physicians don't get it yet and are somewhat vulnerable to being marginalized or disintermediated. They haven't gone digital. Jay Parkinson, who originated and runs a progressive primary care physician practice, wrote in the *New Yorker*, "I've hired two generations of doctors—one from my parents' generation and one from my own. The differences are striking. One feels right at home, empowered and enabled, and the other thinks she's going to break something. The older physician still loves what she does, and enjoys learning out of curiosity, but computers just aren't hardwired into her brain like the younger one."[108]

Earlier in the chapter I mentioned that about half of the physicians in the United States are over age fifty-five. Two out of three won't e-mail with their patients, which has been proven in multiple studies to markedly improve efficiency of practice.[109] To this end, *Consumer Reports* in December 2013 had a digital doctor's office feature, "The Doctor Will e-mail You Now" with a key projection: "You may find your doctor actively encouraging you to send her an e-mail."[110] That does seem quite logical. But a Price Waterhouse Coopers report on mHealth suggested otherwise, headlined "42% of Docs Fear mHealth Will Lessen Their Power Over Patients."[111] (That's engrained paternalism, and we hit that hard in Chapter 2.) There's also the fear of malpractice, which was picked up on by *The Economist*:

"The irony is that a doctor is more comfortable with the liability in a system that does not have rich data than in a system that does have rich data."[112]

Sometimes it takes a fresh, outside view to provide insight and impetus to change. At a meeting of the Semiconductors Industry Association of America in late 2013, I had the opportunity to meet Mike Splinter, the chairman of Applied Material, one of the largest chip manufacturers in the world. He asked me, "Why are doctors still using the stethoscope and manila folder?" I said he was asking the wrong guy but turned it back to him to write it out, which he did, here excerpted:

> And while the tubes have transformed from wood to rubber, and sensing plates are now metal, not much else has changed in this pre–Civil War medical instrument. As my granddaughter would say, "Are you kidding me?" Even though we call the stethoscope a scope, it does not scope anything. It simply is a little amplifier analogous to the Edison phonograph or a Victrola—like the ones you see with big horns in the old-time movies. Sadly, I am not joking. This is a truly archaic device, and yet we trust our lives and health to it in a way that is out of touch with the world we live in today. The stethoscope has no ability to record information; it has no ability to analyze information. Its successful usage depends totally on the practitioner at the moment.[113]

But age and the medical community's resistance to change are certainly interdependent, major factors. New technology just doesn't go over well. I took a hit on this topic with a "white coat lecture" by Donald M. Knowlan, MD, at the Georgetown University School of Medicine in 2013.[114] A white coat lecture is a tradition at medical schools on or around the first day, when a faculty member gives an inspirational talk. For anchoring, please remember that Georgetown was the home of Dr. Proctor Harvey, one of the most well-regarded bedside cardiologists. Here is what Dr. Knowlan, age eighty-six, included in his address to the incoming students:

> But what can you, the class of 2017, expect? In a recent thought-provoking book, *The Creative Destruction of Medicine* . . . [Topol] anticipate[d] future changes in the health care delivery system. He commented on changes such as use of smartphones for complex

diagnostic challenges and personalized medicine with use of genetic information. He even suggested that the stethoscope, so revered here at Georgetown, will be replaced by a handheld ultrasound device. He admitted to not using his own stethoscope for over 2 years, which suggests to me he never learned to use it properly and appreciate its value. Despite all these future advances, he probably hardly scratches the surface.[114]

I've never met Dr. Knowlan, and he has no awareness that one of my favorite things in medicine for decades was to teach the bedside cardiovascular physical exam to medical students, residents, and advanced trainees. Indeed my idol in cardiology is Kanu Chatterjee, a master clinician like Proctor Harvey who emphasized the intricacies of the bedside exam as he taught my fellow students and me at UCSF. Most of that centered on the stethoscope, learning how to hear and interpret the whole gamut of subtle heart sounds—well beyond lub dub. But unfortunately that is old history now.[115–119] That physicians like Dr. Knowlan still emphasize the old ways is no doubt a result of having trained before ultrasound was standard. But for many, such resistance can be, as Drs. Nelson and Narula put it, a part of a "philosophical and practical gap between comprehensive imaging by a consultant and bedside physical examination."[118]

Another eminent, elder statesman, Dr. Arnold "Bud" Relman, former editor of the *New England Journal of Medicine*, who recently died at age ninety-one, also expressed his concerns about the future of medical care highly influenced by digital devices.[120] He believed my view was "much too sanguine" and "not sufficiently concerned about its limitations." These views that challenge the active role of consumers, social networks, and technology that would dare to replace the treasured medical icon are to be expected. While they come from physicians of advanced age, they are indeed representative of the majority of doctors today.

But doctors are facing unprecedented pressures coming from all directions, many of which we have already reviewed (Figure 9.4).[111,121–133] This has understandably led to marked disillusionment, which has been amply documented. When I talk with many of my colleagues about this oppressive squeeze, diminishing reimbursement for their work often crops up in the discussion. But there's something about what motivates physicians that is more compelling than financial incentives.[134–136] Jonathan Kolstad,

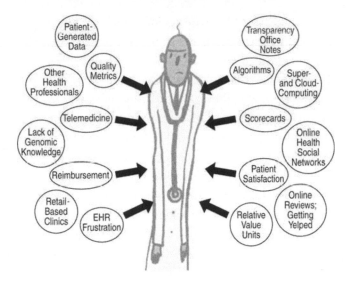

FIGURE 9.4: Doctors are getting squeezed like never before.

a Wharton health economist, received the prestigious Arrow Award for a study that showed what really drives physicians is their performance compared with their peers—that was four times more powerful than financial incentives. He used the report-card system for cardiac surgeons in Pennsylvania as the basis of understanding physician behavior.[134–136]

That's an important finding that certainly resonates with me and can be the basis for adaptation to the way medicine will move forward. Physicians generally want to be the best performer among their peers; they are inherently competitive and data-driven. There isn't any question that, with rare exceptions, they're deeply committed to their patients. So how do we use this lever?

Online evaluations of physicians, like Yelp!, Vitals.com, Healthgrades, RateMDs, and Angie's List really don't achieve this goal.[137–141] While they can provide some objective assessment for metrics like waiting time and parking conditions, much is subjective, such as how friendly and courteous the office staff is, or the communicative skills of the doctor. This information is certainly very useful for consumers but doesn't get to the quality of medical care,[142–144] even though many physicians are responsive and do whatever they can to ameliorate their ratings.[145] Similarly, patient satisfaction surveys, which are widely used for rating physicians and hospitals and are embraced by the US government, have major flaws.[146] It turns out scoring is highly influenced by the patient getting a prescription, such as an antibiotic or narcotic pain medication, or a scan—even though this is all too often contraindicated.

But what if physicians incorporated the powerful microcomputer to decompress their dispensable duties, transferring responsibility for generating data, surveillance, and much of disease management to patients?[147,148] The term *letting go* in medicine usually refers to end-of-life care, and willingness to stop resuscitation or heroic efforts. But here I am invoking *letting go* to denote readiness of physicians and the medical community for patients to take charge. The opportunity now is for physicians to compete for performance—adapting to a democratized form of medicine—fostering e-mail communication with patients, supporting use of mobile device add-appters, patient-generated data, and online social health networks, sharing and co-editing office notes, and all aspects of consumer-driven health care. Off-loading data and information is liberating for the physician, just as it is empowering to the patient. This is not about letting go of the importance of human touch and compassion, which can never be trumped by technology.[132,149–151] When I gave a medical school commencement address in 2014, I spoke about artificial intelligence (which we'll get into in Chapter 13) and real, digital intelligence in medicine, as measured by the "DQ"—digital quotient. Here were my five questions for the DQ of the new physician graduates:

1. Can you see every patient as an individual—learn everything possible about what makes them tick with our new digital tools of sequencing, sensors, imaging?
2. Are you going to advocate patient-generated data so each of your patients is using his or her smartphone or tablet to capture essential data, relevant to his or her medical condition?
3. Will you be fully supportive of activating your patients, getting them maximally engaged in the new form of consumer-driven health care that is just starting to take hold?
4. Will you share all your notes with your patients, and treat them with the utmost respect as a partner for whom you will be giving advice, counsel, and most importantly providing exquisite communication, empathy, and compassion?

5. Will you keep up with all the new information, such as following trusted medical sources on Twitter? And challenge existing dogma and guidelines when it comes down to the unique patient in front of you?[152]

The smartphone is just a pipe, a conduit of flowing data. On either end of it are intelligent human beings who are ready to assume quite different roles from what the history of medicine has established. Patients will always crave and need the human touch from a doctor, but that can be had on a more selective basis with the tools at hand. Instead of doctors being squeezed, resorting to computer automation can actually markedly expand their roles. As Kevin Kelly wrote, "the rote tasks of any information-intensive job can be automated. It doesn't matter if you are a doctor, lawyer, architect, reporter, or even programmer."[102] *The Economist* weighed in on this too: "The machines are not just cleverer, but they also have access to far more data. The combination of big data and smart machines will take over some occupations wholesale."[153] But smart doctors need not feel threatened, for their occupation is secure. Letting go and competing on embracing digital medicine may turn out to be the best way to prevent disintermediation and disillusionment in the long run.

The Impact

Chapter 10

The Edifice Complex

*"Start delivering healthcare farther and farther from the hospital set-
ting and even out of doctors' offices."*
—George Halvorson,
former CEO of Kaiser Permanente[1]

"The hospital of the future will not be a hospital at all."
—Deborah DiSanzo,
former CEO of Philips Healthcare[2,3]

*"In a typical hospital, overheads account for 85 to 90 percent of total
costs because of the complexity of offering a 'one size fits none' offering.
It turns out there are three different business models inside a hospital,
and those three business models are incompatible."*
—Clayton Christensen[3]

When I was training to be a cardiologist in the 1980s at Johns Hopkins,
it took three hospital days for a patient to undergo a cardiac catheterization. Each patient was admitted the day before the procedure to have a
full evaluation, which consisted of a history and physical, chest X-ray, an
electrocardiogram, and the routine laboratories. An intravenous line was
placed to give fluid in preparation for the exposure of contrast dye, which
can harm the kidneys if a patient is dehydrated. A blood type was obtained in the event there was significant hemorrhage requiring transfusion.
On the second day, the patient was brought to the cardiac catheterization

laboratory. After prepping and draping, there was extensive numbing of the skin of the upper thigh or groin area, which overlies the femoral artery. Then a catheter—a small hollow tube—was threaded up the aorta via X-ray guidance, and dye was injected through it to map the three arteries that supply the heart muscle (hence the term cardiac catheterization). A high dose of the blood thinner heparin was administered by vein to prevent clotting in either the catheter or the patient. Multiple views of the arteries were taken by moving the X-ray beam. Additional pictures were taken of the heart to assess the strength of contraction, along with measurements of pressure in the main pumping chamber, the left ventricle. Then the catheter was removed, and manual pressure was applied at the groin site for twenty to thirty minutes to help the femoral artery begin to seal, reducing the chance that bleeding would occur. Since it was assumed the artery required at least twenty-four hours to seal, the patient was returned to his hospital room to stay flat and recover until the patient could be discharged on the third hospital day. After review of the pictures obtained, if an angioplasty procedure were considered necessary to unblock an artery, it would be scheduled in the days or weeks ahead. The same was the case for a bypass operation if that was deemed appropriate.

Now let's jump forward to the current day, thirty years later. This procedure is not only performed as an outpatient one but is also usually done via the artery in the wrist rather than the leg, and the patient can get up and walk right from the cardiac catheterization lab table. More importantly, the angioplasty or stent(s), if necessary, is incorporated during the same procedure and the patient goes home a few hours later.

Such progress would have been unthinkable just ten years ago. But little by little the fear was titrated and the boundaries of what could be done without hospitalizing the patient pushed back. This was achieved without any major jump in technology; instead the evolution can be accounted for by a combination of low-tech things such as use of aspirin, different blood thinner protocols, smaller catheters, the preferential use of the wrist instead of the leg artery, and lower profile, slicker balloons and stents that can more easily reach and cross the blockages. All analog stuff; nothing digital on the list. Nevertheless, the effect has been huge. Coronary angiography, the other term for cardiac catheterization, is one of the most common procedures in medicine: over two million, of which several hundred thousand require combined angioplasty procedures, are performed in the United

States each year. To have now become a quick outpatient procedure for most of these patients represents a radical change, even if it took decades of gradual and persistent tweaking, with a bit of bravado along the way, to accomplish.

This is just one of hundreds of examples of procedures or operations—including organ biopsies, spinal disc operations, hernia repairs, gall bladder removals, and a very long list of surgeries—that used to require hospitalization but now are routinely being done on an outpatient basis, unless an unanticipated complication occurs. For those operations that do require hospitalization, the typical length of stay has dropped dramatically. Open-heart surgery used to lead to a two-week hospital stay in the 1980s, and now it is often just a few days. In the late 1980s, when we did a randomized clinical trial of early discharge after a heart attack—three days instead of seven to ten days—many of my medical colleagues thought this was completely far-fetched, dangerous, and out of touch with the serious nature of a heart attack.[4] An interesting picture cropped up as a result of our aggressive reduction of hospital stay (Figure 10.1).

Nevertheless, the relentless reduction in hospital stays, as inpatient procedures become outpatient ones and inpatient visits become shorter, continues. When our daughter gave birth to our first grandchild, she was in

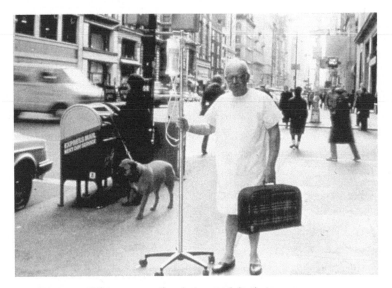

FIGURE 10.1: The concept of early hospital discharge.

and out of the hospital in just over twenty-four hours, with most of that taken up by a tough birthing process.

These factors, at least in part, account for the marked reduction of hospitals in the United States, which peaked in 1975 at 7,156 and has steadily reduced to 4,995 in 2013, representing over a 30 percent decline.[5] But that is just the beginning of hospital attrition. That's because hospitals, as we know them today, will eventually be extinct.

The Harm Factor

In 1999, an Institute of Medicine report shocked me with the finding that ninety-eight thousand people died each year due to hospital-related and preventable *lethal* events. Updates suggest things may have gotten even worse. In 2013, John James, of the organization Patient Safety America, published a systematic review in the *Journal of Patient Safety* of the four "modern" studies that were conducted and published subsequent to the Institute of Medicine report and concluded there are approximately 440,000 lethal, preventable events each year from care in hospitals, or "roughly one-sixth of all deaths that occur in the United States each year."[6] The magnitude of harm, which only began to be disclosed at the turn of the millennium, bespeaks the silence of the medical community. It is indeed characteristic of the deep-seated and pervasive paternalism. Something drastic needs to be done to protect patients from this harm.

I am not alone in my dismay of the current state of affairs. Peter Pronovost, a physician at Johns Hopkins, wrote in *Consumer Reports* that he was appalled that there was no government tracking of hospital deaths, despite its prevalence—he estimated medical harm as one of the top three killers in the United States.[7] His colleague Marty Makary compares hospital deaths to airplane crashes.[8] Crashes make media headlines, followed by a thorough investigation meant to promote future airline transportation safety. Despite the fact that hospitals kill, as he pointed out in his recent book *Unaccountable: What Hospitals Won't Tell You and How Transparency Can Revolutionize Health Care,* the equivalent of four jumbo jets worth of patients each week, there is neither public notice, nor any substantive investigation of medical practice.[9] He wrote "hospitals as a whole tend to escape accountability, with excessive complication rates even at institutions that the public trusts as top-notch."[8] Makary isn't alone in seeing the problem, however: a recent survey of sixty highly ranked United States hospitals asked their employees whether they'd feel comfortable receiving medical care in the unit in which they work. The response at more than half the hospitals was a resounding "No!"[10]

The two primary factors in these deaths are nosocomial (hospital-acquired) infections[10,11] and medical errors.[12] A 2014 *New England Journal of Medicine* review of in-hospital infections in 183 US hospitals showed that the most common types of infection were pneumonia, surgical-site wounds, and gastrointestinal infection, especially by the bacterium C. difficile, which is typically related to liberal antibiotic use.[13] Over 25 percent of these infections were device-related (such as from a catheter or ventilator). The authors estimated that there were nearly 650,000 hospitalized patients per year suffering such infections, which works out to a new infection rate of 4 percent per day.[14] Of these patients, 1 in 9 will die as a result. The hospital-acquired infections are notoriously very difficult to treat, and as time has gone on with progressive worsening of antibiotic resistance, this challenge has been made even more formidable. Beyond the troubling data about infections and the persistence of serious medication errors in hospitals, there was a report on the extensive and perilous problem of misdiagnosis in intensive care units, such as missing a heart attack, pulmonary embolism, or pneumonia, leading to over forty thousand deaths annually.[15]

Such reports have led to strong efforts and pockets of success in some American centers and health systems, but it is hard to see any overall improvement in patient safety. *ProPublica* rightfully asked, "Why Can't Medicine Seem to Fix Simple Mistakes?" in reporting on some hospitals that were publicly flogged for very serious or fatal errors but still could not get on track to avoid these subsequently.[16] The patient perspective is especially poignant and well represented by Mary Brennan-Taylor, who works at the YMCA in upstate New York. Brennan-Taylor lost her mother and has become a national advocate for hospital safety. Her lessons of overriding medical paternalism, and the need to inspire patients to assert themselves are well stated: "I felt responsible for not being able to protect her. I was totally trusting. I never asked the doctors and nurses coming into her room to wash their hands. I never checked her medication."[16]

In an article entitled "Survive Your Hospital Stay," *Consumer Reports* rated 2,591 hospitals for safety, with quite striking findings.[17] The differences in death rates for common diagnoses or surgery were analyzed as a function of low or high rating. The ratings factored in mortality, readmission to the hospital within thirty days from being discharged, infections, communications of the staff, and the use of medical scans. The results were not good, even at the best-rated hospitals. Ironically, this appeared in the same issue with the feature article "Break Free from Cable." Perhaps the cover could have been "Break Free from Hospitals."

Compounding the potential for errors by individual doctors or nurses is the fact that in-patient care is provided by a rotating cast of workers. Dr. Janice Boughton, a hospitalist in Idaho, wrote an essay for the American College of Physicians entitled "Hospitals Are Still Awful" about day-to-day dysfunctions, highlighting the remarkable problem of miscommunications that occur due to involvement of so many different players on different shifts.[18] This surely doesn't help promote patient safety in the hospital setting.

The Cost Factor

The problems with modern hospitals are not confined to harming patients. There's the profound cost, too: hospital costs total more than $850 billion per year, almost 33 percent of all US health care spending, with bills averaging $4,300 a day for hospitals in the United States. (As a reminder, that's nearly threefold the next-highest country's average cost—Australia at $1,400/day.) For over $4,000 per night, one might expect the presidential suite at a five-star hotel, and indeed as the prices of hospitals and luxury hotels have converged, so has there been likeness in design cues. To that end, the *New York Times* published a pictorial quiz for its readers to view photos and decide whether it was a hospital or a hotel.[19] The cost of building modern hospitals is unthinkable. At Scripps, due to state laws that require meeting code for seismic safety, the main hospital had to recently be rebuilt at the tune of approximately $700 million. It doesn't have the hotel look on the inside, but certainly it is a massive investment in an edifice that will likely morph in its primary purpose over the years ahead.

The enormous expenses involved are leading several insurers to push back. With the Affordable Care Act, there is substantially less reimbursement by Medicare for hospital stays, further disincentivizing the use of the traditional edifices of medicine. Until recently, hospitals were routinely reimbursed for readmissions, many of which could be attributed to premature hospital discharge or suboptimal care, and there was, ironically, a financial reward of higher net profit margins for many of the complications that occur during a patient stay. Going forward we're headed to a whole new system of reimbursement for hospitals, from a medicine-by-the-yard model to a "no outcome, no income" one. What was fee-for-service is now changing to fee-for-value. Eric Dishman, global general manager of health and life sciences at Intel, said, "The moment you signal pay for performance, people start thinking about how we misuse hospitals every single day."[20] As a result of this shift, the majority of hospital CEOs think a hospital-building bubble has popped, with marked over-capacity—at least 40 percent to 50 percent excess of beds—left in its wake. The result is a hospital financial squeeze that is compounded by the major movement toward hospital pricing transparency. I think the bubble's aftermath will be even worse than the CEOs anticipate, as the analysis still does not take into account how digital medicine technology will reduce the need for hospitals.

The Hospital of the Future?

As they contemplate their troubled futures, there has been considerable work done by hospital architects and designers on what a hospital *room* of the future will look like. The nonprofit design firm NXT, with support from the Department of Defense and collaboration with thirty industry partners, designed a prototype—the first major attempt of change since World War II—that engendered quite a bit of controversy.[21,22] The project colead, David Ruthven, said, "Technology has to become the connective tissue that holds together the continuum of care."[21] The *Wall Street Journal* coverage of the prototype labeled it "a patient-centered design [that] could reduce infections, falls, errors—and ultimately costs." The design has some interesting elements. The vital signs of the patient are displayed on the wall behind the head of the bed. A cocoon above the patient's head, called the patient ribbon, is meant to block out unwanted noise. A halo light box can be programmed for mood or light therapy. A footwall with a large screen provides both entertainment and video consultation with doctors. Rubber floors and Corian solid room surfaces serve to reduce the risk of infection. Also included is gamification and managed competition—the stats of the doctors and nurses are tracked to determine who helped the most patients in a given day.

Then the critics weighed in. *Wired* magazine described it as "the nicest hospital you will never visit" with design features that "make it feel like an iPhone."[23] The architect Benjie Nycum ripped the design apart for not including any input from patients.[24] He stressed the importance of building a "patient environment that supports and promotes the individual's physical, emotional and psychological healing" and that "being efficient, cost-effective and minimizing the incidence of hospital-acquired infections should be the framework for patient-centered design. With the increasing body of evidence pointing to the health benefits of biophilic design, the absence of natural products, daylight, views, nature, or any kind of softness in this prototype seems like a huge oversight." I especially liked this part of his critique: "The only thing missing from the NXT room is an automatically triggered laser beam to kill fresh flowers brought by unwelcome visitors."[25] In general, although the designers sought to put technology at the center of the room, I think they missed technology's most promising offerings.

In striking contrast with the NXT room-centric design for a hospital future, the Asan Medical Center, the largest health system in South Korea, has not only proposed but also now initiated a number of digital components that cut across the hospital.[26] The mobile apps called "Smart Patient" and "Smart Hospital" (Figure 10.2) are used extensively to provide immediate access of information to both the patients and health care professionals.

Both these divergent views of the future of the hospital miss something major—the lack of need for hospitals! A large poll conducted by Intel on the future of hospitals of 12,002 adults from eight countries and four continents was noteworthy: 57 percent of people believe that traditional hospitals will be obsolete in the future.[20,27] In Denmark, where remote monitoring and video conferencing play a large role in end-of-life care, there has been a huge shift: more than half of patients used to die in the hospital; now over 92 percent die at home. Some American hospitals are in fact in front of the trend, despite the overall hospital-bed bubble.[28] The new hospital at the Navy's Camp Pendleton base, for example, has only sixty-seven beds in its 497,000 sq ft hospital. Even more noteworthy is the new Montefiore Medical Center in the Bronx, New York City, which has 280,000 sq ft, eleven stories, twelve operating rooms, four procedure rooms, an advanced imaging center, laboratory, and pharmacy services— and no beds! Its CEO, Dr. Steven Sayfer, proclaimed, "We are reshaping

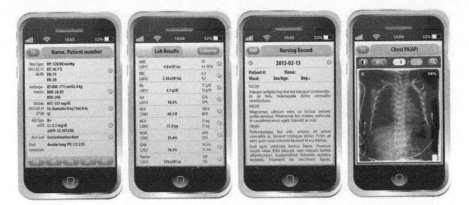

FIGURE 10.2: Mobile apps for the Asan Medical Center: (A) basic information; (B) lab results; (C) nursing records; and (D) scans and images, with interpretations. Source: Adapted from J. Park et al., "Lessons Learned from the Development of Health Applications in a Tertiary Hospital," *Telemedicine and e-Health* 20 (2014): 215–222.

outpatient care and establishing leading practices that provide [healthcare services] through multidisciplinary teams at a hospital without beds."[28]

The result of this trend will be that the hospital room of the future will be the bedroom. Biosensors can record continuous vital signs and any other relevant physiologic metrics; little mobile devices and smartphone physical exam add-appters can enable both communication and examinations. Smart pillboxes and other tools can monitor treatment adherence; personal emergency response systems can summon an ambulance; and the floor can even monitor one's gait. A smart medical home can easily be designed. For elderly individuals who are living alone, frail, or prone to falls, this system could also incorporate personal emergency response systems, medication adherence sensors, and tiles along with motion sensors that monitor gait. Indeed, a smart medical home can easily be designed. A research group in Sweden conceived the sensor architecture for remote, long-term medical monitoring at home[29] and has already tested this for over a year with nearly one hundred thousand sensor data days from almost fifteen thousand distinct sensors. These included sensors under the mattress, motion sensors in each room of the home, and many sensors to monitor everyday activities apart from health and medicine.

Although the Swedish team describes their monitoring system as eminently scalable, there is certainly no shortage of challenges facing at-home hospitals. A comprehensive system that uses many, if not all, of the digital medical tools would lead to a deluge of data that would need to be integrated and processed. The individual, caregiver, or doctor cannot be bombarded with various alarms, except when there is unequivocal need for an alert. The relative ease of collecting the data is in stark contrast to the exceedingly difficult mission of contextualizing it, extracting all the salient information, providing it to multiple parties (such as the individual and doctor) with great visualization and just the right level of notifications. Clearly, such a smart medical home would have to be individualized for the parameters that are of particular interest or concern, and for what hardware is necessary. Unlike many home entertainment systems that have multiple remote control devices that most people can't figure out, it needs to be exceptionally easy to use. And it must cost less—far less—than today's outrageous hospital bills. For the more than $4,000 per day that is charged for a non-ICU hospital room, one can afford to do a lot of remote monitoring in the convenience of one's own home, a sanctuary away from serious, nosocomial infections.

The data collected have to be secure and the systems must safeguard privacy and identity. The privacy story goes beyond protecting digitized medical data from being hacked or put up for sale for thousands of potentially interested vendors. When or if *any* data is collected must also be in an individual's control. Many might appropriately feel as if they were invaded if they are required to wear sensors around a home that is always tracking them. For this reason, a fully equipped smart medical home should not be used for long periods of time. There might be limited periods of long-term use of a couple of biosensors, or extensive monitoring but for a short duration of a few days or a week. So the modular and temporal aspects are key. Most folks wouldn't want their home to become a digital dystopian environment, but to preempt a hospital stay they would likely be willing to have Big Medical Brother peering in. How Orwellian! And to think it was George Orwell who called hospitals "the antechamber to the tomb."[30]

If one accepts that these challenges can be met and the smart medical home becomes a reality, then we can see that the recent hospital-building bubble has led to a far worse allocation of resources than most hospital systems realize. There is no replacement for the acutely ill patient who would be admitted to an intensive care unit (ICU) or the emergency room where the initial assessment for such a patient would be made. Likewise, surgeries and procedures, medical imaging, and laboratory facilities would still have a place in the hospital of the future. But that's about it. All the non-ICU hospital rooms, which represent the majority of most hospitals' floor plans, would no longer be necessary. Patients who used to be housed in these rooms would simply be remotely monitored from home. Perhaps the homeless represent a singular exception.

So what do we do with the bulk of current hospital space when the transition to smart medical homes is accomplished? Some might close or become part of the ongoing and extensive consolidation of hospitals, with more than two hundred such deals occurring in 2011 and 2012.[31,32] Some may choose to add more ICU beds as well as operating and procedure rooms like the Montefiore center that was recently opened. But one significant new opportunity is for the hospital to become the data and information resource center. If we go back to Chapter 9 and the data center in the book *Cell,* it turns out that Robin Cook described such a monitoring center quite well. While such centers could be quite remote from the patient, and alternatively be run by large dedicated companies, there is considerable appeal and advantage for having the data center proximal to the patient. There would be familiarity with the patient via the doctor and staff who are caring for the individual, be it during a recent hospitalization or by providing primary care. The staff of such a monitoring center could represent the future "hospitalist"—not likely to be called a "home-ist"—a physician particularly trained and adept at the interface of machines and people. You might describe them as geeks with compassion, not necessarily an oxymoron.

Just as we flattened the Earth with digital tools, we can flatten these typically tall edifices. Hospitals as they exist today are set up to fail. Their fiscal future is beyond bleak; their paradoxical harm instead of heal potential cannot be dismissed or substantively diminished. Surely hospital consolidation will not remedy the situation.[33] Except under special circumstances, we'd be far better off to have such services performed in the comfort of our own homes. Seeing our own data, on our own devices. In charge.

Chapter 11

Open Sesame

THE OPEN⁵
MOVEMENT

"In addition to professional obligations to patients and society to share knowledge, we may also have an obligation to share anonymized clinical knowledge in a more general manner to meet the human obligation of beneficence."
—NIMITA LIMAYE AND CAROL ISAACSON BARASH[1]

"That's how revolutions gain their power, not from leaders or even ideas, but when ordinary men begin to imagine that they could become kings."
—GREG SATELL, *Forbes* MAGAZINE[2]

"The implications for Big Data in healthcare are huge and exciting. From shortening the feedback loop on adverse drug interactions to identifying the next Patient Zero."
—MICHAEL HARDEN, ARTIS VENTURES[3]

"When you have gigabytes of data, perhaps hundreds of gigabytes, for each patient, that's more data than has existed in all clinical trials combined up until a couple of years ago."
—MARTY TENENBAUM[4a]

The magical phrase in the famous Arabian folk tale *One Thousand and One Nights* is "Open Sesame." When uttered, it opens the cave where the poor woodcutter Ali Baba accesses the treasure of gold coins that the forty thieves have hidden. In medicine today, we are all like Ali Baba, but the treasure that has been hidden away is not gold; it's information. The question now is whether we, like Ali Baba, can breech the gate that keeps us from the data, to a new world of openness and transparency. There is a long history of medicine stymying public and consumer access, of keeping us in a closed cave, but the walls are starting to coming down. Data is flowing more freely than ever before. The digital era has enabled open platforms, open access, and open science. It is now time to realize the benefits of open medicine.

Let's start with the open source software movement. People have been sharing software for decades, but the movement really accelerated around the turn of this century when Netscape Navigator, which was made free as Mozilla Firefox, and the open source Linux operating system became more mainstream. Among the many companies that provided part of their source code to build upon, Apple, Google, and IBM all leveraged open source initiatives. When Apple opened up its iOS to a worldwide developer network, this rapidly led to the creation of hundreds of thousands of apps and markedly expanded functionality of the iPhone and later iPad. My first direct encounter with this culture was in June 2012 at the Apple Worldwide Developers Conference in San Francisco. It was striking to see several thousand people in their twenties, mostly guys (increasingly being referred to as "brogrammers"[4b]), mostly geeky, dressed in T-shirts, jeans, and sandals, from all over the world, whose main occupation was to develop apps for the big Apple. Their world of writing code, using things like APIs (application programming interface)[5] and STKs (systems tool kits), is a relatively new profession. They have become a veritable army of high-energy, talented youth who are symbiotic with the company. They are not commensals, for that would denote that the developers benefit without affecting the company (or vice versa). Rather, Apple's critical decision to open up its iOS has created a true interdependence between the developers and the tech behemoths. Google followed suit with this model for Android apps and has even made its Android operating system open source, available for anyone to build on. IBM has now opened Watson to developers, and the company offers certification to freelancers to build Watson-based apps. Add Facebook, Twitter, Amazon, and a long list of others to the list. It's now hard to imagine a tech company not leveraging an open platform and developers. We have learned that to be really successful, it's not just about hardware and software, but also about achieving a colossal crowd-sourcing network effect.

During the same period, a second major driver of open knowledge has emerged. These are MOOCs (massive open online courses), which broadcast lectures to tens of thousands of people who have an Internet connection and want to sign up. This isn't your grandparents' correspondence course! MIT's OpenCourseWare initiated the movement in 2002 and the MOOC term was coined in 2008, but this really took off in 2011[6–11] with a Stanford University artificial intelligence class: 160,000 people signed up from 195 countries after one public announcement and 23,000 finished the course.[7] (Talk about flattening the Earth, which only has 195 countries.) By 2012, the field was dominated by three big organizations—Coursera, Udacity, and edX (formerly MITx)—in what became known as the year of the MOOCs. Udacity's first introduction to computer science course enrolled 270,000 students, and the numbers have continued to scale in recent years. Coursera has over eight million registered users.[10,11]

The MOOC movement has several important lessons for medicine. Clearly, this platform democratized the educational process by bringing high quality lectures from top universities to anyone in the world. It did this at remarkably low cost and high velocity.

As Andrew Ng, one of the founders of Coursera, put it with some understatement, "When one professor teaches 50,000 people, it alters the economics of education."[7] A MOOC-based master's degree in computer science at Georgia Tech costs a student $6,600. The traditional on-campus-experience degree costs $45,000.[12] Besides this, there is a new phenomenon known as "flipping," whereby students can listen to lectures at home or on the go, but come to class for an interactive, non-lecture experience. Further, the Internet connection is a two-way street, meaning that the MOOC has granular data on each student. The Coursera platform monitors every mouse click a student makes—quiz submission, forum posts, when and where a student pauses a lecture video, or rewinds, or moves to 1.5 speed. Roy Pa, of the Stanford Center for Professional Development, said, "We can have microanalytics on every paper, every test, right down to what media each student prefers."[13] In fact, this ability to virtually track each student sets up the new field of "big-data science for education" or "learning informatics."

As would be expected with any new, radically different model, there are detractors and controversy—about the difference between an online and in-person experience, about assessment and evaluation, and about the commoditization of leading professors and ultimately the degradation of higher education.[8] These detractors raise legitimate and important issues that must be kept in mind, but there are good reasons to treat MOOCs as models for how to change medicine.

Both education and medicine are going through an economic crisis, and neither have sustainable archetypes. Both have the potential to be broadly democratized by piggybacking on the extraordinary digital infrastructure that is in place and is continuing to evolve. Both stand to realize enormous benefits through immense data capture from each individual. Both must reckon with new tensions, including the risk that the virtual world could depersonalize the experience, the need to demonstrate that digital methods do in fact lead to improved outcomes, and the need to overcome considerable resistance from steadfast, vested constituents. College professors and physicians, and their respective communities, are threatened. Ironically, MOOCs may turn out to save the day for doctors, as they could close the huge gaps in medical education for such topics as genomics and digital medicine. And those professors who don't make the cut to produce MOOCs may need more doctors for stress-related illnesses.

I've coined a term to describe these opportunities: MOOM, for massive open online medicine. But MOOMs are about more than just continuing education for physicians or extending medical knowledge to the public. While data collection in MOOCs occurs, massive distribution of lectures is the primary focus. But with MOOMs, the collection of data, and the distribution of the analyzed data, is the primary focus; learning what is already known is of secondary importance. It is about doing what was never possible before. To create a MOOM, a prerequisite is for data to be shared. At the TED meeting in 2014, Google's Larry Page declared, "Wouldn't it be amazing to have anonymous medical records available to all research doctors? Making our medical records open for sharing will save 100,000 lives a year."[14-16] I am not sure how he derived that number (it's certainly not available through a Google search), but he's on the right track: there are enormous potential advantages to medical data sharing.

The first step is to see if individuals are willing to share their data. Two recent surveys reveal an overall high level of willingness to share their medical record data on an anonymous basis. For 1,396 UK adults, 21 percent were very willing and 39 percent were fairly willing—or 60 percent were "willing."[17] The Intel Healthcare survey of 12,002 people from eight countries showed that more than 76 percent were willing to share health data anonymously.[18] Interestingly, the propensity for sharing was more likely outside the United States (especially high in India and Indonesia), was highest among those with higher income, and was increased when associated with potential for research to help others or reduction in their health care costs. Overall, 84 percent would share their sensor data or lab tests, and 70 percent would share information collected from a smart "toilet" (how kind and altruistic to share one's waste—not that we have a way to do that yet!).[18] A third survey, with over a thousand individuals found 90 percent willing to share their data,[19] and a smaller survey by the California Institute for Telecommunications and Information Technology of 465 individuals in the United States also found a similar 77 percent willingness to share health data anonymously for research purposes.[20,21] PatientsLikeMe reported that 94 percent of American social media users would share their health data, with appropriate de-identification.[22] Extrapolating from these surveys, with the caveat that they may not be fully representative, suggests that the majority (about 75 percent) of people are currently willing to share their medical information, provided it is done on an anonymous basis.

We also know that some people are willing to share such data even when they are not anonymous. Some research programs, like Harvard's Personal Genome Project (PGP), actually require the individual to consent to non-anonymous, public sharing of their data in order to participate.[23,24] This "open consent" framework of non-anonymous data donation is a novel, if extreme, form of participatory research, but it does not seem to have deterred participation or interest, as the PGP has been rolling since 2005 and counts more than thirteen hundred enrollees, and includes disclosing of the individual's whole genome sequence along with many other features of the medical GIS. The PGP has leveraged online forums, LinkedIn and Facebook, along with annual meetings, to provide a highly interactive experience and education for the participants who are largely without any background in science.[23]

Sage Bionetworks, a research institute dedicated to promoting open science, has come up with Portable Legal Consent,[25] which enables any individual who signs up to participate in a clinical trial to also agree to sharing his genomic and health data with all scientists who agree to stipulated terms. This is essentially a commitment from the participant to be part of "open source" data, although, unlike PGP, it is done anonymously. Anonymity is still not certain; as we'll discuss in the next chapter, there is the potential of reidentifying an individual via one's genomic data, so anonymity cannot be guaranteed.

Other initiatives pay individuals to share their data. The website of one such group, Datacoup, declares, "Our mission is to democratize personal data by establishing an open, fair marketplace for individuals to sell their personal data. While large enterprise gets wealthy from monetizing our personal data, we as consumers, are left with little more than a targeted ad. The consumer has been completely lost in the shuffle of advertising, technology, and big data."[26] Another alternative known as DataDonors, a non-profit organization run via The Wikilife Foundation, promotes data sharing on an altruistic basis and has accrued data donations from over 500,000 individuals.[27]

Now that we've established that most people would indeed share their medical data, and that there are other mechanisms to incentivize this willingness, the question is: Would it do any good? Let's start with the diagnosis and treatment of cancer, then move on to other ways that it might work.

The Cancer MOOM

Back in 2012, TechCrunch published an article "The Cloud Will Cure Cancer."[28] It seemed like overreaching. But just a year later, what I would classify as the first cancer MOOM was formed. It wasn't called that. It was headlined as "Patients Share DNA for Cures."[29] Four different institutions came together with different, complementary roles: Oregon Health and Science University as the coordinating academic unit, the Leukemia and Lymphoma Society as the grantor and patient advocacy group, Illumina for the sequencing, and Intel for the data processing and information resource development. With an $8.2 million grant over three years, this consortium is enrolling nine hundred patients with leukemia or lymphoma (known as "liquid" tumors) to have their cancer cells sequenced; all that data, combined with their clinical, treatment, and outcome data, will form a new information resource. This is graphically represented in Figure 11.1,

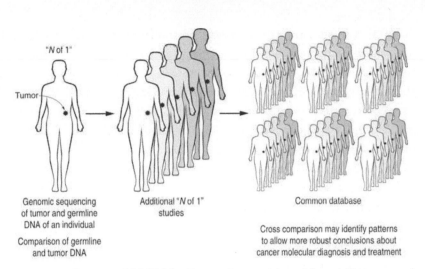

FIGURE 11.1: Creating a MOOM for Cancer. Source: Adapted from A. Brannon and C.L. Sawyers, "'N of 1' case reports in the era of whole-genome sequencing," *Journal of Clinical Investigation* 123 (2013): 4568-4570.

which is meant to portray a tumor that is sequenced, along with the individual's native DNA, and this is compared to the database of nine hundred affected patients. The point is that when patient number 901 comes along, his or her physician can tap into the database to see what treatments worked best for patients with the same or similar tumor mutations, filtering the information according to age, gender, and other potentially relevant characteristics.

Now several more cancer MOOMs are taking hold. The Multiple Myeloma Research Foundation has organized a similar one-thousand-patient study with $40 million support.[30] The American Society of Clinical Oncologists is supporting such initiatives, and its director, Allen Lichter, said, "There is a treasure trove of information inside those cases if we simply bring them together."[31] Their project, called CancerLinQ, is culling records of treatments and outcomes from one hundred thousand patients with breast cancer from twenty-seven oncology groups around the country.[31,32a] While it does not yet contain genomic information, the project reflects the "recognition that big data is an imperative for the future of medicine."[31] Within just a few years, Flatiron Health has quickly been able to access data from over two hundred US cancer centers with over 550,000 patients, with the intent to analyze and share data for improving treatment decisions.[32b,33] Although the information resource does not include tumor-sequencing or omic data, the software company has substantial investment by Google Ventures and plans to incorporate this in the future.

Indeed, a cancer MOOM isn't just something that could add extra value to medicine. It is necessary to make the promises of genomic medicine a reality. When cancer tissue is sequenced, thousands of mutations are found. Ideally, the individual native DNA is sequenced, too, and that also identifies millions of variants as compared with the reference human genome. Sorting through all these variants to find the signal—the mutations driving the cancer—is impossible if you only look at one tumor genome, which will have many mutations that are not causative. That makes it impossible to tailor the therapy genomically. All of these challenges can be best addressed by an information resource that has all the data. In 2014, a global crowdsourcing initiative, called the DREAM Somatic Mutation Calling Challenge, was launched to tackle this complexity.[34,35] Using the Google Cloud Platform and its Compute Engine, the goal is to create a "living benchmark" for mutation detection. But that's just one component of the package. Indeed, a platform is only as strong as the information on mutations, treatments, and outcomes, coming from the largest sample of people possible, that it has to work with. And as exciting as these various small-scale MOOMs are, open medicine could be considerably more powerful still.

Imagine that all the patients who have a diagnosis of cancer become part of a global knowledge resource. Each patient's GIS, scans, treatments administered, and outcomes were all entered into this MOOM. There would be hundreds of thousands and then millions of individuals of diverse ancestry and baseline features with granular, essential information on each one. Every different type and subtype of cancer, every mutation and pathway and their combinations would be represented in the resource, and it would be automatically updated and upgraded as each individual, her treatment and outcome, is entered. We've moved from the N of 1 to the global population of all people who develop cancer and, by developing and maintaining the MOOM, we've now doubled down on the democratization of cancer: N of 1 ➔ N of millions. Yes, a MOOM knowledge base might serve as a momentous advance for improving the outcomes of patients. Lives are never saved; we're all mortal. But precision treatments anchored in this way might be far more effective in preserving the quality and length of life.

Yes, this is a fantasy, a dream that is unlikely to ever get fully actualized. It would require taking all the walls down between countries and cultures, and there's not a real precedent for this kind of global cooperativity and data harmonization. (For tearing down walls, we have certainly seen it with MOOCs, which have enrolled individuals from every country on the planet.) We can't even effectively deal with the many centers in the United States that aggressively sequence tumor tissue from cancer patients. An article in the *New York Times* titled "Cancer Centers Racing to Map Patients' Genes"[36] (using tumor sequencing to identify driver mutations and tailor therapy) told the story: "Major academic medical centers in New York and around the country are spending and recruiting heavily in what has become an arms race within the war on cancer."[36] As Susan Desmond-Hellman, who chaired the National Academy of Sciences' panel on precision medicine opined, "With advances like electronic health records and low-cost, high-throughput DNA sequencing, there is an opportunity to take advantage of routine episodes of clinical care for biomedical and clinical research. Yet most of the data are not collected, not pooled or never connected to the explosion of molecular data."[30] But if we were serious about winning a war on cancer, a MOOM approach might be just the winning tactic and ticket.

There are also expansive ideas of how to create a MOOM from multiple sources, as shown in Figure 11.2. Not only would data come from physicians but also it would be pouring in from patients themselves, from direct-to-consumer testing companies (such as 23andMe), patient advocate foundations, online health communities (such as PatientsLikeMe), and the large number of clinical trials that are perpetually being conducted without taking full advantage of the enormous information that is generated. An oft-cited example of a highly productive collaboration between a patient advocacy organization and biotech was the development of the drug Kalydeco by Vertex Pharmaceuticals—the Cystic Fibrosis Foundation provided all their patient information, which ultimately led to a successful genomically guided treatment in five years, almost a third of the usual time span for new drug development.[30] As Patrick Soon-Shiong, the billionaire biotech founder of Abraxis, put it, "In the past, the scientific, technological and digital pieces did not exist to assemble the whole. Now they do. I like to look for patterns in science and life. It's what I do. Only

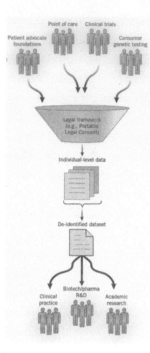

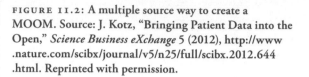

FIGURE 11.2: A multiple source way to create a MOOM. Source: J. Kotz, "Bringing Patient Data into the Open," *Science Business eXchange* 5 (2012), http://www .nature.com/scibx/journal/v5/n25/full/scibx.2012.644 .html. Reprinted with permission.

an interconnected, instantaneous, molecule-to-manufacturer managed care system can tap science and save money."[37a,37b]

Other Medical MOOMs

The same concept that drives the cancer MOOMs can be used across the board in medicine. One early application of the model has been in advancing therapeutics in rheumatoid arthritis. A single course of therapy using drugs such as Remicade, Enbrel, or Humira, which target a molecule called tumor necrosis factor, can cost $100,000. Even worse, the overall clinical response rate is only about 30 percent, yet there is little known to predict who will or will not benefit. By crowdsourcing data from large patient cohorts with integrated genetic data, treatment, and outcomes, the Rheumatoid Arthritis Responder Challenge is meant to change that.[38] The challenge will help provide better guidance and precision for patients and doctors in the future. It could even determine the biologic underpinning of poor response and set the foundation for new drug development.

Another opportunity involves medical scans. Alan Moody, the chairman of medical imaging at the University of Toronto, writes, "Many medical images are used once then filed away. This trove of clinical data should be made available to biomedical researchers." Filed away is too polite a term. That data is squandered. A population-wide image data resource could be useful in the millions of individuals who get MRIs or other scans when being evaluated for memory loss or possible Alzheimer's disease. Collecting the data, as Moody argues, could enable the weak signals emanating from subclinical disease to "rise above the background noise."[39] The potential to explore pre-disease, and early disease, at a population level via medical imaging certainly is alluring, since it is a veritable back hole in our medical knowledge base.

A similar black hole surrounds the so-called variants of unknown significance (VUS),[40] a dominant problem in cancer biology that extends to most other conditions in medicine. Patients with VUS are condemned to what has been called "genetic purgatory," and rescuing them is a task especially well suited to MOOMs. In patients with an unknown or rare disease, having all the data associated with every sequence variant in the human genome (including insertions, deletions, structural variants, polymorphisms, etc.) in an information resource, connected with detailed information on the corresponding individual's phenotype, would make such diagnoses decidedly easier.[41–43] Even genes that have been intensively studied for over twenty-five years, such as CFTR which causes cystic fibrosis, can leave many patients in genetic purgatory, as the gene has thousands of variants, many of which are VUS.[40] The best way to solve those VUS is to pool the data. Pooling can also help tackle rare or unknown diseases. Rarity may make them seem a low-priority target, but there are thirty million individuals with a rare or unknown disease in the United States alone, and their cumulative incidence approaches 7 percent of the population, while cancer's cumulative burden is under 5 percent. When you add all the rare folks together, there's a serious unsolved common problem of diagnosis. If only we could add all the medical efforts and resources together, break down the silos, and crack the cases.

One area of particular interest to me for MOOMs is the application for performing a molecular autopsy for sudden death.[44,45] Each year 1 in 100,0000 people between the ages of 1 and 35 die suddenly. Physical autopsies have been on steady decline for many years, and more than 40 percent of hospitals don't perform them at all.[46] Even when they are performed for an individual who has died suddenly, presumably from a cardiovascular cause, they are unrevealing in the majority of cases. That is, even after dissection of the human body, the medical examiner can't determine why the person died. This is especially a burdensome problem for family members, who live the rest of their lives in uncertainty, not knowing whether or when they might suffer the same fate. But there is a potential and attractive way out, which ultimately relies on the MOOM model to be informative.

The information required to solve the mystery involves three components: the DNA sequence of the deceased, the DNA sequence of the immediate family members (ideally the parents), and a worldwide MOOM repository of as many like individuals who have succumbed to sudden death and their families as possible. While there will be many families that carry rare, classic mutations in one of approximately one hundred genes that are known to potentially cause sudden death, which would be immediately informative and helpful to family members, the vast majority of the genomic variations will be uncertain. But it doesn't have to stay that way. MOOMs can enable us to demystify and definitively diagnose sudden death.

While MOOMs are a form of crowdsourcing information at a large and ideally global scale, the concept can be successfully applied on a limited basis. "Hackathons" have been popular in the tech space, and now they have made their way into medicine.[47,48] A transdisciplinary group—doctors, entrepreneurs, software developers, engineers—assembles and attacks an unmet need in medicine. An example of an outgrowth of this type of open medicine is PillPack, conceived at a medical hackathon. By supplying patients who have the challenge of a complex schedule with multiple prescription medicines, a prepackaging service labels the pills with the time to be taken to maximize adherence.[48] While it's a rather simple solution, it sets up a practical, low-cost strategy that was not previously available.

The open medicine model has also led to extensive crowdfunding, with many different flavors. Rare disease advocacy groups have used crowdfunding to cover treatment costs for individual patients in need. Consano and Watsi are examples of nonprofit foundations raising funds for medical research and care, respectively.[49,50] This can even be done at the individual level: a seven-year-old boy raised over $750,000 for his sick friend with a glycogen storage disease by selling his book called *Chocolate Bar*.[51,52] Medical device entrepreneurs are touting their innovations on the Internet to raise funds. While some of these may represent true and meaningful advances, what have been called "scampaigns" are a new prospect.[52–54]

Some companies make claims that seem too good to be true. The company Healbe pitched a wristband device called GoBe that was "the only way to automatically measure caloric intake" and raised over $1 million via Indiegogo's crowdfunding platform.[54] Similarly, Airo raised funds for a wristband that also claimed to precisely track caloric intake, but it didn't work and was abruptly withdrawn. Another example is TellSpec, which raised $400,000 for a handheld food scanner that would tell exactly the nutritional contents of any food you were eating. It remains uncertain as to whether these innovative devices are working as advertised.[52-54] So while "open" is often perceived as virtuous, there's clearly a potential flip side to the story. We'll also get into the dark side of selling data obtained through open medicine in the next chapter.

The Government and Open Medicine

We've seen the kimono opened by the US government with initiatives such as Open FDA, the release of the Medicare database, and other data resources.[26,55-62] The FDA now allows public access to information regarding four million adverse drug reactions and medication errors over the past decade.[63] After years of pressure from Dow Jones, the parent company of the *Wall Street Journal*, Medicare released a trove of medical data from 2012 on 880,000 doctors and medical providers. Any US physician who billed Medicare for a visit or procedure can be easily searched on the Internet, which provides consumers additional information in selecting a doctor. For example, it is now possible to see how many patients covered by Medicare underwent a particular operation by an individual surgeon. That's a very crude marker of quality but may serve as a first step to linking the data with other outcome measures in the future. Another new government initiative for medical researchers is PCORnet (Patient-Centered Outcomes Research Network),[64,65] which intends to gather medical records, physiologic data, and insurance claims from thirty million citizens. However, the United States is way behind other countries in such open medicine endeavors. Denmark's MedCom has a comprehensive patient data resource that tracks back to 1977, and similar efforts in Finland and Estonia are well-established health information resources.

Open Science

Open data are key to MOOMs, which as I've defined are focused on taking the medical care of patients to a new, unparalleled level. While we

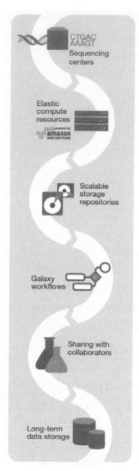

FIGURE 11.3: Sharing genomic data pipeline. Source: V. Marx, "Genomics in the Clouds," *Nature Methods* 10 (2013): 941–945. Reprinted with permission.

have not yet seen global sharing of data in medicine, some notable precedents for that have occurred in life science research. The international human genome-sequencing project set an important foundation for collaboration and openness back in the 1990s, but this has recently been taken forward more powerfully. The Global Alliance for Genomics and Health (GA4GH) was announced in 2013 with participation of seventy medical, research, and advocacy institutions from forty-one countries.[66–71] Its mission is to build a trove of data on genetic variations and medical information that would be open to all scientists, not just those who created it. By the time of the GA4GH's first meeting in 2014, there were 150 organizations represented, including Google, who joined in the effort via its new genomics branch. Early priorities in cancer and rare diseases sought to enhance understanding of genomic variations and how they connect to very specific medical conditions.[67] By being so general GA4GH is charting new ground both scientifically and legally. It requires specific patient consent for participation along with developing technical, ethical, and legal standards for the broad collaboration.

A proof of principle for how such open science can accelerate discovery was borne out in Alzheimer's disease. The gene APOε4 has long been associated with late-onset dementia but the mechanism has been elusive. By accessing all of the publicly available databases on gene expression, high-throughput genotyping and imaging of the brain, in patients with and without APOε4 carrier status, a team of researchers at Columbia University was able to elucidate the molecular pathway and other key genes involved in this type of dementia.[72,73]

In the past, publishing a paper was the standard method for sharing the data. That is completely outmoded in the era of enormous datasets, whereby sharing is enabled by the digital infrastructure, including secure cloud servers and open-source collaborative platform software such as Galaxy (Figure 11.3).[74] While the backbone for such a shared data pipeline involves some significant upfront costs, as the data resource grows there are remarkable economies of scale. With the potential of such a vast information resource, there will also likely be new ways that research grants and budgets are allocated in the future.

Open Access

While on the topic of cost and data, it's time to address the sticky problem of access to biomedical publications.[75-82] Public monies, via the National Institutes of Health or other government agencies, have funded a very large proportion of these research efforts. But when the papers are published in leading peer review journals such as *Nature, Science, Cell*, the *New England Journal of Medicine* or *JAMA*, which often charge exorbitant amounts for subscriptions and even to read single articles, the public cannot access the work that they've supported through taxes. What's more is that the price has little relationship to the actual publication costs, meaning the publishers make a hefty profit margin. For example, in a recent annual report of one of the major biomedical publishers, Elsevier, the company had a 37 percent profit margin with net revenue of over $2.5 billion.[75] In 2013, the chronic angst over this ordeal ultimately led to a boycott of the company's journals by more than twelve thousand researchers.[75] That same year the editors of the *New York Times* published, "We Paid for the Research, So Let's See It."[83] To counter the dominance of this old model, a number of open access journals have cropped up over the years, including *Public Library of Science (PLoS)*, *BioMed Central*, *PeerJ*, and *eLife*. There are also public archives where papers can be uploaded, such as *arXiv* and *bioRxiv*.

Soon after the announcement of the 2013 Nobel Prizes, the new laureate in medicine, Randy Schekman, a professor at the University of California, Berkeley, wrote a column in *The Guardian* titled "How Journals like *Nature, Cell* and *Science* are Damaging Science."[84] He wrote: "Like many successful researchers, I have published in the big brands [such as *Nature*], including the papers that won me the Nobel prize for medicine, which I will be honoured to collect tomorrow. But no longer. I have now committed my lab to avoiding luxury journals, and I encourage others to do likewise."[84,85] The article sparked remarkable controversy in the science community.[86] The disparaging term "luxury journals" was new, but the denouncement by Schekman, the editor of *eLife*, an open access journal, seemed to represent an overt conflict of interest. And the idea that once someone wins the Nobel Prize, it's OK not to publish in the luxury journals, did not escape harsh critique from young scientists, who worry that not publishing in the luxury journals would hurt their chances of finding permanent jobs.

Nevertheless, the push to open access has intensified. Two undergraduate medical students launched the Open Access Button for when someone trying to download an article hits the proverbial paywall—which typically means from $30 to over $100 per article PDF.[87] When that all too frequent problem is encountered, the button initiates a workaround plan by either finding a free author-deposited version or sending an e-mail to the author to get the PDF of the paper.[88,89] Other opportunities for peer-to-peer sharing include ResearchGate, an online social network for scientists to share papers and find collaborators, and academia.edu, which has over nine million researchers signed up to share their papers despite being slammed by takedown notices from Elsevier. Open access journals continue to grow as well.[90] The annual volume of open access articles rose from 20,702 articles in 2000 to 340,130 in 2011.[79]

The directory of open access journals (http://www.doaj.org) now lists more than eight thousand. The site codes the journals with two colors— green and gold. Green means the article is published in an open access repository, such as within a university or central resource like PubMed Central; gold denotes publishing in an open access journal. The momentum, despite considerable expense to government, universities, and to authors, who are levied fees to publish in certain open access journals, is clearly building. Ann Wolpert of MIT, in a perspective in the *New England Journal of Medicine*, wrote on the inevitability of universal open access: "There is no doubt that the public interests vested in funding agencies, universities, libraries, and authors, together with the power and reach of the Internet, have created a compelling and necessary momentum for open access. It won't be easy, and it won't be inexpensive, but it is only a matter of time."[91]

There are other related reverberations. A demand to have all references publicly accessible is resonating with Open Citations Corpus. Recent data suggest we have a long way to go here, as, of the fifty million scholarly journal articles, only about 4 percent have their bibliographic citation data accessible.[92] There's also the open patent movement, with the new database Lens that intends to cull together information for more than ninety worldwide patent jurisdictions.[93] (Although not related to medicine or life science, the recent release of all of the patents held by Tesla, the electric car manufacturer, in the "spirit of the open source movement," is noteworthy.)[94,95] And a call for open access to medications that were supported with federal funds, but not developed or made available to those in need, has also been registered. Like with research and publication that are government-funded, the premise is that taxpayers should have rights to this intellectual property.[96]

Opening Up Medical Research

When you put together open medicine, open science, open access, open source, and open data—Open[5]—all sorts of new channels of research activity become available, and existing ones become exponentially more powerful. One form is citizen medicine that is progressively enabled by having universal, free, immediate access to discoveries and innovations. It's not just about access—it's also about driving discovery and innovation. Open[5] brings into the mix all potential players, such as the Argentine car mechanic who designed new ways of delivering babies under the most difficult conditions[97] and a young American high school student, Jack Andraka, who came up with a potential low-cost, creative means of diagnosing pancreatic cancer.[98] That is also why people like Kim Goodsell (Chapter 2) are now able to make their own diagnosis of complex medical conditions. The pervasive progression toward openness is fueling a remarkable degree of activism across consumers, patient advocacy groups, research foundations, and the life science industry.

When Katherine Leon, age thirty-eight, developed an exceptionally rare heart condition known as spontaneous coronary artery dissection (SCAD), which led to a heart attack and bypass surgery, she found there was little known about the disease. She took to the Internet to find other individuals who carried the same diagnosis.[99] Partnering with the Mayo Clinic, she was able to find others who were searching Google for information on SCAD. She set up a virtual patient registry so that affected individuals could submit their medical records and scans online. Over time more than seventy individuals with SCAD were identified and now the cohort is expanding to two hundred. Sharon Hayes, the Mayo Clinic cardiologist who has worked with Leon, said, "This is not investigator-initiated research; this is patient-initiated research and to a certain extent has been patient-sustained research in the case of our study."[99]

Elena Simon, a teenager who had been diagnosed with a rare form of liver cancer at age twelve and had successful treatment and surgery, later undertook finding the genomic root cause of her cancer as a high school science project (mentioned in Chapter 1). Just before her high school graduation she published as a coauthor an article in *Science* (OK, not open access!) that revealed the mutation that caused her fibrolamellar liver tumor.[100,101] By setting up a website known as the Fibrolamellar Registry, which served as a repository of information and a means to find other affected patients, she found fourteen other patients who had developed this rare cancer, and they became part of her report, confirming the same gene with mutations as was found in sequencing her tumor. Simon said, "It's their information, it's their health, so they should have the right to do with it what they want. Perhaps the best thing patients can do is to give their data away for free to work, bit by bit, toward a cure. The open access movement has worked for software and genetics; it can work for medicine, too."[100]

By leveraging the open digital infrastructure through Internet searches and online social networks, these activist patients with rare diseases are advancing medicine, especially by enhancing our understanding of the basis for the condition. Citizen medicine can also lead to attempts at treatment. Here again open may not necessarily be considered optimal. One of the most dreaded medical conditions is amyotrophic lateral sclerosis (ALS, Lou Gehrig's disease), which is characterized by a relentless neurologic deterioration. The loss of muscle control eventually leads to severely impaired breathing and swallowing, and death two to five years from diagnosis. Although there is no treatment available or approved by the FDA, there have been reports from early, small studies that are publicly accessible. Studying them enabled one patient with ALS to conclude that the active drug in one of these early, Phase 1 studies, was sodium chlorite. Affected patients began treating themselves with this chemical, which is obtained by bleaching paper pulp. Collectively, via the social online health network PatientsLikeMe, a rapid crowdsourced clinical trial took form, albeit without controls (patients not receiving sodium chlorite) but showing no sign of efficacy. In fact, taking sodium chlorite was associated with an adverse effect.[102,103] Using clever algorithms, PatientsLikeMe can simulate a randomized trial within their database and had already demonstrated that another candidate drug for ALS, lithium bicarbonate, was ineffective using this method. That finding was subsequently validated by a traditional, expensive, and time-consuming randomized trial.

Although open is not a guarantee of good outcomes, social online networks of "ePatients" with like conditions do have real advantages over classic clinical trials. A major one is that they provide unique, real-world, relevant crowdsourcing information. The real-world setting needs emphasis, since it is altogether different from the classic clinical trial with highly select patients, often undergoing frequent and close follow-up—all in all, they are receiving care under a set of contrived, nonrepresentative conditions. For this reason, too often clinical trials are not adequately predictive of a drug's or device's true effect when commercially available. Accordingly, an electronic community that tracks individuals in their natural setting may be a particularly useful, alternative resource.

Although PatientsLikeMe, with more than 250,000 members, is the largest of the online health communities that provide this resource, there are hundreds of them that have cropped up in recent years, with cumulatively well over a million participating patients. Some are quite specialized, such as Chronology, for patients with Crohn's disease and ulcerative colitis, which was started by Sean Ahrens, age twenty-five. Patients share medications, dietary treatments, and alternative medicine on the website, and, according to Ahrens, "are recognizing that they can and need to take an active role in managing their health instead of just sitting by and going to doctor's appointments."[104]

The life science industry, and specifically the pharmaceutical companies, has clearly taken notice of this resource. In recent years PatientsLikeMe has worked with Merck and Sanofi to facilitate recruitment of patients for clinical trials. In 2014, such collaboration took a big step forward when Genentech announced a five-year contract with PatientsLikeMe—the first broad research collaboration between PatientsLikeMe and a pharmaceutical company—to work together on multiple fronts beyond simply providing access to patient recruitment.[22,105,106] Of the participating patients, the PatientsLikeMe CEO, Jamie Heywood, said, "They're not just using [the network] for personal understanding. They also understand that their data can really have greater meaning and impact the way healthcare is delivered in the United States in a much more patient-centered way."[22]

Indeed, more than 70 percent of Americans say that they would enroll in a clinical trial if recommended by their doctor.[107]ut only a tiny proportion, far less than 1 percent, ever formally participate in a clinical trial. Although it is rather difficult to navigate and comprehend, the public can access ClinicalTrials.gov, which lists more than 150,000 trials in all fifty states along with almost every country. Drug companies are increasingly tapping into online information resources to streamline clinical development of new drugs. When Sanofi and Regeneron were looking to expedite recruitment of patients with high cholesterol for their new, experimental drug alirocumab, an antibody against the PCSK9 protein, they turned to the American College of Cardiology registry.[108] Another approach, developed by researchers at Case Western Reserve University, is a software tool known as "Trial Prospector," which delves into clinical data systems to match patients with clinical trials.[109] It combines artificial intelligence and natural language processing to automate the patient screening and enrollment process, often a rate-limiting step in developing new drugs. Automated clinical trial matching programs for specific conditions, such as the Alzheimer's Association Trialmatch,[107] are proliferating. Data mining to facilitate clinical trial recruitment is offered by a number of companies, such as Blue Chip Marketing Worldwide and Acurian.[110] Ben Goldacre, the acclaimed author and one of the leading independent critics and innovators in pharma research, set up the tool "RandomiseMe," which makes it "easy to run randomized clinical trials on yourself and your friends."[111] So although clinical trial participation is remarkably rare today, there are efforts on multiple fronts to change that in the future. Wouldn't it be ideal if we learned something from each and every patient that might help the next individual who comes along?

That brings up one of the biggest reservoirs of waste and lost opportunity in medical research—the data that has been hiding within the life science industry stockades. Half of clinical trials are never published, and when they are the data presented is often quite incomplete. Only in 2013 did this long-standing chokehold of industry begin to let up, when waves of open science finally reached the shores of the life science industry. Researchers at Yale, working through a group known as Yale Open Data Access (YODA), were granted access by Medtronic to the entire patient-level data on the company's bone morphogenetic protein-2 (BMP-2) dataset.[112–114]

Back in 2011, an entire issue of *The Spine Journal* was dedicated to a takedown of BMP-2 spinal fusion, a drug and device combination used to fuse the vertebrae in patients undergoing back surgery.[112,113] The papers called out multiple serious complications that were occurring, including uncontrolled bone growth, infection, damage to the nerve supplying the bladder, infertility, and cancer. There was also the charge of conflict of interest among the researchers who were involved with BMP-2 research that led to its FDA approval nearly a decade earlier in 2002, as one of the authors had received more than $10 million in royalties and consulting payments from Medtronic. Given the controversy, it seems likely that the release of data in 2013 was not solely altruistic. But it was still noteworthy, especially given the outcome. When systematic reviews were independently performed by the Oregon Health and Science University and the University of York, coordinated by Yale, it was determined that BMP-2 had no overall efficacy, but might be useful in select patients such as when a piece of bone could not be harvested from a patient's hip.[114] The review also suggested that side effects had been understated in prior published reports. Yale's Harlan Krumholz, who leads the effort, wrote an op-ed in the *New York Times* entitled "Give the Data to the People"[115] citing YODA as "an extraordinary donation to society and a reversal of the industry's traditional tendency to treat data as an asset that would lose value if exposed to public scrutiny."[115] Representing Medtronic, Dr. Rick Kuntz said that as a result of this experience, "we will move away from the paradigm in which a single research entity, such as industry or academia, exclusively possesses and analyzes the data from a clinical study to arrive at a singular set of conclusions and interpretations about the benefits and harms of a medical intervention."[116] Certainly, if they had shared their data in 2002, they might have spared themselves a major black eye in 2011.

Following this precedent, Johnson & Johnson signed an agreement with Yale to share patient-level clinical trial data for hundreds of their drugs and other products. The worldwide chairman for Johnson & Johnson pharmaceuticals said, "To get really credible, we took the leap to set up an independent way to make sure people get access to the data."[117] The pharma march to transparency has also included GlaxoSmithKline and Roche, both making announcements of their plans to share data about products that are already on the market with qualified researchers. The National Institute of Allergy and Infectious Diseases, a division of the NIH, has made one of its data resources, which includes participant-level data open to the public, "without the need for a specific research plan or approval of the qualifications of the investigators." Highlighting the critical role of the individual-level, granular data, the European Medicine Agency (equivalent to the US FDA) has issued their policy to promote this practice.

In 2014, the Institute of Medicine published a report on clinical trial data sharing to help promote this trend.[118] Funding agencies like the Bill & Melinda Gates Foundation and the National Institutes of Health are trying to push for data sharing and transparency of clinical trials. Taking the call further, Atul Butte at Stanford wants this to be obligatory: "Mandating the release of raw, clinical trials data—with identifying details removed to preserve patient confidentiality—would enhance transparency and provide us with a better understanding of human biomedicine."[119]

This isn't the only new major trend happening to open up clinical research. Particularly stunning was the announcement between the government and a large number of pharmaceutical companies in 2014. Francis Collins, the NIH Director, announced the Accelerating Medicines Partnership, a five-year collaboration of the flagship federal research agency with ten large pharma companies concentrating on four disease states. This includes sharing of scientists, tissue and blood samples, and data.[120]

The head of research and development of one of the participating drug companies, Pfizer, summarized it as a Google Maps depiction of human disease, since the principal aim is to determine the molecular maps and biologic targets—the GIS—for each of the four diseases. As Langley and Rockoff reported in the *Wall Street Journal*, "Taking a page from the 'open-source' movement that has swept the software world, the group will share all findings with the public, for anyone to use freely to conduct their own experiments."[120] For cancer, a very large project with the National Cancer Institute,[5] pharmaceutical companies, and Foundation Medicine, a cancer sequencing company that we've discussed, was recently launched for determining optimal therapies for lung cancer.[121]

There are several crowdfunding genomic sequencing projects that recruit participants and financial donations via the Internet,[122] such as PathoMap, which collects DNA throughout New York City from subway stations, trains, parks, taxis, buses, and airports and Genome Liberty, focused on pharmacogenomic interactions.[123] The Canadian-based website Science Menu (http://sciencemenu.ca) does a great job of tracking all the crowdfunding science research projects, including genomics.

This increasingly popular form of medical research is not confined to drugs or genomics.[124–126] Likewise, substantial efforts are being advanced in the medical device industry to use open source systems. The University of Pennsylvania, with the FDA, is pursuing the Generic Infusion Pump with the goal to "print out an infusion pump using a rapid prototyping machine, download open-source software to it and have a device running within hours."[127] The University of Wisconsin has initiated the Open Source Medical Device program "to supply, at zero cost, everything necessary to build a device from scratch, including hardware specifications, source code, assembly instructions, and parts—and even recommendations on where to buy them and how much to pay."[127] There's also the Medical Device Coordination Framework from Kansas State University that is building an open source hardware platform with elements common to many devices like displays, buttons, processors, network interfaces and operating software.[127] These open medical device initiatives have the potential to propel device interoperability and the whole mobile device medical movement.

In the *Journal of Socialomics,* Limaye and Barash made the case that it is a moral imperative and professional obligation to share medical data. They wrote, "Knowledge is the basis of our ability to provide patients with high quality medical care. If healthcare organizations and professionals do not openly share knowledge, we are not living up to our professional social contract with society and not fulfilling our general human duty of beneficence."[1]

Sharing, transparency, and openness are all now fast-moving trends in medicine that have been potentiated by the digital infrastructure. It has been exhilarating to see how quickly the Open[5] movement has taken form, and yet it should still be regarded to be in its early stages. It has indeed allowed us to think big, to be imaginative about how someday the medical data from most *Homo sapiens* could potentially be culled together to promote the health of each other and future generations (recall the literal translation of *sapiens* is "wise," so MOOMs might even help promote that). We can now seize this sharing opportunity, something that was not previously possible, but has extraordinary potential, and qualifies as a moral imperative. It's democratizing medicine at a higher level, bringing together all of our GIS and treatment information to create a new path of medicine for the people. A vital issue will be tackling the analytic challenges of such enormous datasets, which we'll address subsequently. Equally important for this to be successful is dealing with big unresolved issues of privacy and security. Failure to do that could destroy the very possibilities that open medicine could realize. That's next up.

Chapter 12

Secure vs. Cure

"I do not want to live in a world where everything I do and say is recorded."

—Edward Snowden[1]

"Today's Web-enabled gadgets should come with a digital Miranda warning: Anything you say or do online, from a status update to a selfie, can and will be used as evidence against you on the Internet."

—Nick Bilton, *New York Times*[2]

In a world of Julian Assange's Wikileaks and Edward Snowden's exposé of the National Security Agency, we are progressing toward zero tolerance of governmental non-transparency.[1,3] At the same time, massive Internet security breaches are occurring or being discovered, from retailers like Target to the Heartbleed bug. Just as everything is getting digitized, making it eminently portable and accessible, we're betwixt and between. We want openness but we also want to preserve our privacy. We want a government that is transparent but that will not compromise safety and enable predators.[4,5] We want full access but we also demand complete security of our personal information. We live in a world of sophisticated hackers and "quantrepreneurs"[6] who want to sell our data to make money. To say "it's complicated" is a gross understatement.

Despite the complication, it is enormously important that we figure these issues out. We've explored the many ways that data are already being shared. A basic premise in health care these days is that big data will ultimately lead to big cures,[7,8] or at least better health. But so far there's been a lot of curating without a lot of cures. Much of that hinges upon predictive analytics, which is the topic of the next chapter. We'll explore in the next chapter the extent to which that is true, but we can't weigh the potential benefits—whether they are as incremental as a month's worth of good health or as momentous as the end of cancer—unless we have clear accounting of the downside of having individuals digitized and everybody on the net. So the weighty issues of privacy and security for digital health and medical data are where we turn next.

Our Digital Bread Crumbs and Data Brokers

We've been leaving digital bread crumbs everywhere for a few decades now, beginning with charging things on our credit cards. Things really ramped up in the past fifteen years with Google and Internet searches, Amazon and online retail purchases, Facebook likes and social network site visits, not to mention our wireless mobile devices, which provide our precise location and much more about us in real time. And then there's the National Security Agency, keeping our e-mails and cellphone calls in vast databases for warrantless searches.[9,10] The bread crumbs have become bread loaves.

Avoiding this surveillance is at best highly inconvenient. In *Dragnet Nation: A Quest for Privacy, Security, and Freedom in a World of Relentless Surveillance*,[11] Julia Angwin, a *ProPublica* investigative journalist, explains why she quit using Google search: "My searches are among the most sensitive information about me."[12] She was annoyed about Google's decision to combine information from its various services, such as search and Gmail, giving advertisers more opportunities to promote things personalized to you. So Angwin moved to DuckDuckGo, a search engine that doesn't store the user's IP address or other digital footprints.[12–14] This "small" search engine, with a billion searches a year compared to Google's one hundred billion a month, has grown quickly due to the growing interest in private searching.[15] It does post ads related to your search.

It is exceedingly difficult to protect one's privacy when tapping at a keyboard or mobile device. You can try to buy some privacy with such tools as the Blackphone, an Android smartphone costing $628,[16] which has specialized software for users to make encrypted calls and send encrypted texts, the OFF Pocket cellphone case that for $85 blocks the signal from the phone to avoid location detection.[17] The Snapchat app promises the automatic deletion of data, removing texts, photos, and videos from the recipient's device and the company's servers one to ten seconds after the data has been reviewed. (There are also Secret, Confide, Younity, Gliph, and Wickr "ephemeral" apps.)[18]

Efforts to limit data collection on a national scale have had little effect. The "Do Not Track" tool for consumers to opt out of web tracking is not at all effective, and the Consumer Privacy Bill of Rights, originally proposed by President Obama in 2012,[19-24] has not gone past the idea stage. Alexis Madrigal wrote about his experience of being tracked by 105 companies on the Web. He pointed out that "people haven't taken control of the data that's being collected and traded about them,"[25] despite President Obama's proposal, which was meant to allow users to "exercise control over what personal data companies collect from them and how they use it." Things have gone from bad to worse since.

Stephen Wolfram, the consummate informaticist, has demonstrated how much we reveal to potential hackers and e-predators when we register on Facebook.[26] Although the sharing is voluntary, it is uninformed. Few users know that even after users make privacy settings more restrictive, it's quite easy to retrieve previously entered data. Then there are the constant attempts to hack into some websites, such as online banking, by computer programs that guess the user's password. Programs like the Wireshark network analysis tool can make the danger visible,[27] revealing all the Internet data packets directed to (attacking) your computer—they are captured and filtered so you can inspect them and get even more depressed.

When you leave your insecure desktop or laptop environment, and decide to go to a store or a shopping mall, you're certainly used to tight surveillance by closed circuit TV (CCTV) cameras,[28] but that's not the half of the surveillance going on. For example, your smartphone talks to many retailers and grocery stores to let them know you have entered.[29-32] With knowledge of your profile, those companies can generate personalized promotional pitches in the form of texts or coupons. You may well have your location privacy settings on, but that doesn't matter. The pings that are emitted by a smartphone looking for a Wi-Fi antenna provide retailers rich information as customers move through a shopping mall, and so does your phone's tilt sensor.[33a] Did you know that some store shelves have hidden cameras to track your eye movements and what you pick up and examine, and that they can then algorithmically generate a coupon or other enticement to send to your smartphone? Kind of personalized, eh? There's also software that detects your mood via facial recognition to make tailored recommendations. If you are willing to give up privacy altogether, the mobile app Placed gives you coupons for providing information on what store you're in.

As you get out on the city streets and public places, there's now an unprecedented array of sensors, CCTVs, and vast wireless networks that are set up to detect your motion, sense your car, read your license plate, and capture key biometric information such as facial recognition. Then there are all the low-cost satellites from above so that "all of the Earth will be held to a mirror, in near real time, at an increasing granularity of visual infrared and other kinds of data."[33b] Wow, are we ever being watched.

Not just being watched but also identified. The NameTag app enables users of Google Glass to take a picture of a stranger and identify them in the FacialNetwork company's database, which includes occupation and social media profiles.[34] Similarly, the NEC company is developing tools to enable hotels and businesses to automatically recognize their important visitors.[35] These efforts rely on converting each person's facial data into a "faceprint" of mathematical code along with a large database to find a match. Facebook users will have a feel for faceprints, since their face-matching software, known as "Tag Suggestions," automatically suggests names of people in pictures to tag.[34-36]

While there isn't yet a faceprint database of Earth's seven billion residents, that doesn't mean there aren't companies working on it.

At the Newark International Airport, where 171 new LED light fixtures were installed in 2014, few people were aware that the fixtures were part of a new wireless sensor network that monitored all activity and movement in the terminal.[37] Such "intelligent lampposts" are now spreading across cities all over the world—from Chongqing in China, to Dubai in the United Arab Emirates, to Rio de Janeiro in Brazil. In the UK, there is one video surveillance camera for every eleven persons.[38] People and cars are thoroughly tracked in Lower Manhattan by face and object detection technology. Surveillance cameras in Boston were used to identify Dzhokhar and Tamerian Tsarnaerv, responsible for the Marathon bombings.[28,39] Subsequently, facial recognition software was shown to be capable of an immediate identification of Dzhokhar. While such software, algorithms, sensors, and full-scale surveillance are unarguably valuable in such circumstances, concerns about surveillance in "clever cities" cannot be ignored. *The Economist* wrote, "Rather than becoming paragons of democracy, they [clever cities] could turn into electronic panopticons in which everybody is constantly watched. They could be paralyzed by hackers, or by bugs in labyrinthine software."[38] Likewise, in Dave Eggers's *The Circle*,[40] a fictitious Silicon Valley company representing an evil hybrid of Facebook, Google, and Apple, pulls together personal e-mails, banking information, purchases, social networking, and a universal operating system to portray what extreme loss of privacy can induce, such as placing chips in children to prevent kidnappings.[41,42] Anthony Townsend has a more sanguine view in *Smart Cities: Big Data, Civic Hackers, and the Quest for a New Utopia*.[43] He believes the electronic surveillance is great and that we're reinventing cities with a smartphone platform.

With all the data flowing, there's big business following. The "data brokers" are the companies that collect and analyze our personal information and sell it without our knowledge.[44] Acxiom, using twenty-three thousand computer servers and processing more than fifty trillion data transactions per year, is the largest company in this multibillion dollar industry. It has more than fifteen hundred pieces of data per person on over two hundred million Americans and two hundred million mobile phone profiles.[44,45] A *New York Times* profile on these companies was entitled "Mapping, and Sharing, the Consumer Genome."[46] Acxiom and other data brokers have not only user names, income, religion, race, education level, sexual orientation, political affiliation, home valuation, vehicle ownership, how many children you have, your recent purchases, your stock portfolio, and whether you are a vegetarian, but also family medical history and medications. Companies such as Exact Data sell names of people with sexually transmitted diseases. Internet browsers and apps on mobile devices enable much of this invasion of privacy. A *60 Minutes* segment pointed out that through both Angry Birds and the Brightest Flashlight Free app, more than fifty million people, gave companies free rein to track them and sell the resulting data.[44]

Acxiom may be considered axiomatic for privacy invasion. The retailer Target combines such data with information it gathers itself to precisely target consumers. As a regulator said, "They are the unseen cyberazzi who collect information on all of us." Yes, it's as if we are all celebrities and have the paparazzi following us, just digitally.[46] The Acxiom CEO, Scott Howe, said, "Our digital reach will soon approach nearly every Internet user in the United States."[44] It's bad enough as it is now. That might well portend a digital nightmare. The creep of creepy data intensifies.

It certainly is not the case that all this data is secure. Choice Point maintained seventeen billion records on individuals and businesses.[45] They sold this data to one hundred thousand clients, which included seven thousand federal, state, and local agencies. This company was investigated for selling over 140,000 personal records to an identity theft ring. The company Court Ventures, later acquired by Experian, one of the three major credit bureau companies, sold personal records including "fullz": Social Security numbers, mothers' maiden names, and personal information necessary to secure credit cards.

Beyond selling personal data, some of these data brokers have been hacked. If there were ever a recipe for trouble, it would be hacking a massive data hoarder. A major security breach at Epsilon led to the exposure of e-mails from millions of customers at Citibank, JP Morgan Chase, Walgreens, and Target.[46] Target then fell prey to a late 2013 hacking that gave way to credit and debit card information on forty million customers.

Many seeking to defend data collection have put much weight on the distinction between data and metadata, between one's identity and the digital tags associated with us. Unfortunately, as metadata gets increasingly contextualized with more personal information, we become "metapersons."[47] Our true identity is less important but more readily established from a data collection. When the Snowden-induced NSA revelations were made, President Obama said, "There are no names, there's no content in that database."[48] Wrong. It turns out it is remarkably easy to identify an individual by one's phone number, as Stanford researchers demonstrated.[49]

This very brief overview of the predominantly nonmedical landscape is a prelude to where health care is headed. Many hospitals are using video monitoring, to observe patients who are, for example, at risk for falling or for committing suicide, as well as to be certain that doctors and nurses are washing their hands.[50] As with retail, the business implications are enormous. When I visited Stephen Colbert, I told him about the work we are doing at Scripps to embed a nanosensor in the bloodstream that would detect a heart attack days to a couple of weeks before it would otherwise occur, and relay this signal to your smartphone. Colbert quickly responded: "Now with this information I'm sure it'll come down the line that insurance companies will give you a cut if you have a monitor on you to stay healthier. But then they're going to sell your information about your present health to other people, and you'll get a ringtone that says 'Would you like 20 per cent off caskets?' Or Crestor, or something like that?" With his incomparable humor, Colbert hit on the truth. The sad part is that by having our medical selves digitized, we're making ourselves highly vulnerable, not just to marketing but so much worse.

Medical identity theft is already in high gear.[51,52] A Pew Research Institute study has shown that there is a marked increase in the United States and occurring across all age groups.[53] In 2013, according to the Identity Theft Resource Center report, 43 percent of all identity thefts in the United States were medical-related.[52] The Ponemon Institute issued a report in 2012 on medical identity theft, defined as "when one person uses another's name and personal information to fraudulently obtain medical services, prescription drugs or submits fraudulent billing," estimating that 1.84 million Americans were victims—a 20 percent increase from the previous year. The chairman of the Institute, Larry Ponemon, summed this up: "Medical identity theft is tainting the healthcare ecosystem, much like poisoning the town's water supply. Everyone will be affected."[51] Since 2009, when Health and Human Services (HHS) started keeping track, the medical records of as many as sixty-eight million Americans have been breached.[52] So when HHS requires a medical provider to notify its patients when there has been a medical record data breach of five hundred or more patients, that's just the tip of the iceberg. And what about all the breaches affecting less than five hundred patients that are not reported to the individuals? It's bad enough that a large number of medical centers in the United States, and most of the highly prestigious ones with elaborate health information systems, have suffered a breach of electronic medical records. Although some are due to hackers (in about 14 percent of cases), far more are due to a stolen laptop or USB drive (more than 50 percent of cases). Further, according to Edward Snowden, the NSA has cracked the encryption that is used to protect medical records for Americans.

With the markedly increasing use of telemedicine and virtual consults, as reviewed in Chapter 9, there must be concern about the security of these electronic exchanges. While many of the companies are using the term "secure" liberally in their promotional materials, all it will take is a full virtual visit to be widely transmitted over the Web before this type of medical encounter becomes suspect. The likelihood of cybersecurity breaches in medical clinics and hospitals is enhanced with so many visitors and employees bringing in their own wireless devices and potentially accessing the health system's "secure" inner network.

With the cost of medical care out of control, the motive for impersonators has been greatly enhanced. But that's just one dimension of the problem. Selling the information is a much bigger one, and it's gaining traction. As Sam Imandoust from the Identity Theft Resource Center said, "With a click of a few buttons, you might have access to the records of 10,000 patients. Each bit of information can be sold for $10 to $20."

Medical identity theft is a thorny issue beyond its financial consequences. You can get a new driver's license and credit cards when the victim of run of the mill identity theft. A medical theft is quite a different ordeal. As one expert put it, "It's almost impossible to clear up a medical record once medical identity theft has occurred. If someone is getting false information into your file, theirs gets laced with yours and it's impossible to segregate what information is about you and what is about them."[52]

Care.data vs. Careless.data

An enlightening and quite sobering case study of how medical data can be mishandled at scale comes from the United Kingdom's National Health Service (NHS).[54–60] The NHS is the largest public health system in the world, providing care for fifty-three million people. In August 2013, the government, seeking to build public support for sharing their medical records with scientific researchers, initiated a major campaign called Care.data. Posters were displayed in doctors' offices throughout England, and cheerleading came from the Wellcome Trust, leading charities such as Cancer Research UK, Diabetes UK, the British Heart Foundation, and key leaders like Ben Goldacre. The prime minister, David Cameron, said, "Every NHS patient should be a research participant."[57]

One of the patients in Care.data, Richard Stephens, a cancer survivor, is an exemplar of the good that was derived from this initiative. He said, "As someone who has survived two cancers, I have seen firsthand how our health records can help improve people's lives. I might not be alive today

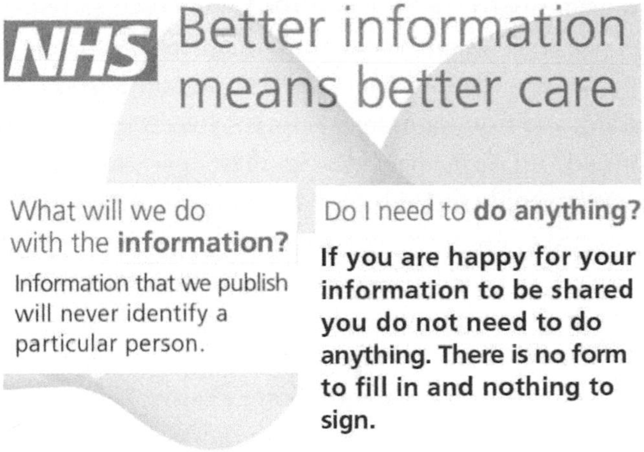

NHS Better information means better care

What will we do with the information?

Information that we publish will never identify a particular person.

Do I need to do anything?

If you are happy for your information to be shared you do not need to do anything. There is no form to fill in and nothing to sign.

FIGURE 12.1: Salient parts of the NHS leaflet for Care.data. Source: Adapted from "Better Information Means Better Care," NHS, January 14, 2014, http://www.england .nhs.uk/wp-content/uploads/2014/01/cd-leaflet-01–14.pdf.

if researchers had not been able to access the data in the health records of other cancer patients to produce the most effective treatments and the best care for me, and by making my own records available to researchers I know I am helping other patients in the future."[61]

The government sent a leaflet entitled "Better Information Means Better Care" to 26 million households (Figure 12.1).[54] Surely the NHS goal—"to achieve better health care while establishing the world's most comprehensive patient database for research"—was laudable. It would be the first time that the entire medical history of a large nation was digitized and stored in one place, a central repository at the Health and Social Care Information Centre (HSCIC).

But serious concerns about breach of privacy were voiced. A few months after the campaign began, an opposition movement, which included the British Medical Association and the Royal College of General Practitioners, went into open revolt. Unfortunately, these concerns were countered with some misconceptions. For example, Professor Liam Smeeth of the London School of Hygiene and Tropical Medicine said, "I can't guarantee there won't be a single slip, but the risk is tiny. This is not about individual people."[61] Well, it *is* precisely about individuals. Care.data consists of each person's confidential medical record with their family history, diagnoses, prescription medications, and the results of blood tests and medical scans. It only takes one person's medical identity theft to be about an individual. As with retail companies and data brokers, re-identification is altogether straightforward, and true anonymity is impossible. A more accurate term is "pseudonymized."[59] The medical identity theft of one individual's sensitive data is all that it would take to have a potentially tumultuous impact. But the worries turned out to be far greater than that. In late February 2014, a massive portion of the database, containing thirteen years of hospital data covering forty-seven million disguised patients, was sold to an insurance industry. As Ben Goldacre, outraged by the HSCIC's action, wrote, this was a violation of HSCIC's own governance charter: "They are wrong: it's like nuclear power. Medical data, rarefied and condensed, presents huge power to do good, but it also presents huge risks. When leaked, it cannot be unleaked; when lost, public trust will take decades to regain."[56] Jonathan Freedland wrote in *The Guardian,* "We now trust no one with our data—not even our doctors."[62]

Although the Care.data program was botched, it is highly instructive. It epitomizes the potentially antithetical goals of developing an immense medical information resource to help patients, but at the same time making them available to purchasers and, unfortunately, vulnerable to predators.

Medical Data and Mobile Devices

The biggest source of an individual's health data is not a MOOM or a national health repository, but a smartphone. The good news is that Internet cookies don't work well with mobile phones, so they can't follow people from a computer browser to a phone browser. The bad news is that e-advertisers, e-predators, and data brokers have found new, sophisticated ways of exploiting all of one's activities and engagement with a smartphone or tablet.[63-65] Companies like Drawbridge can match several devices to an individual user by processing the data, including websites visited, apps used, date and time stamp, and location.[32]

Privacy Rights Clearinghouse performed an in-depth study of forty-three mobile health apps that exposed "considerable" privacy risk for users.[66] Without the user's knowledge the information was apt (perhaps we should use the term *apped* here) to be unencrypted, transferred over insecure networks, and used by the app developer as well as by third parties.

Only 43 percent of the free apps posted a privacy policy.[67] A University of Colorado study showed that consumers would be willing to pay a fee to be certain their app data were kept private. I had the chance to discuss this issue with Mike Lee, the inventor and CEO of MyFitnessPal, one of the most widely used mobile apps for weight loss and promoting fitness. He strongly assured me that they do not pass on *any* individual's information to third parties. That is quite likely to be true but apparently not representative. The mobile app fitness field certainly did not get off to a good start when Fitbit, back in 2011, inadvertently exposed their users' sexual activity stats. We know too well that when mobile apps are downloaded, the user never reads the terms and conditions but just taps on "Agree."

Employers are a big part of the mobile device privacy story. While truckers have been tracked moment to moment by GPS tracking devices for location and duration of driving time for several years,[68,69] that was just the beginning of a more pervasive movement by employers to apply wearable sensors to their workers.[70,71] One example is the Hitachi Business Microscope, a device that is marketed to large employers to promote increased efficiency. It fits into the employee ID badge and includes infrared sensors, an accelerometer, a microphone sensor, and a wireless communication device. As employees interact with one another, the badges record and transmit to management "who talks to whom, how often, where, and how energetically."[70] Another wearable alternative for tracking employees is smart glasses, such as those made by Vuzix that have a microphone, GPS, accelerometer, and data display. Life-logging apps like Saga incorporate a barometer, camera, microphones, and the smartphone's location sensors to provide "a more comprehensive, automatic record of your life"[72] and know precisely where you are and what you are up to. The barometer helps distinguish exact location, along with deep acoustic and light signals for context.

But the most commonly owned wearable sensors are the wireless accelerometers like Fitbit and Jawbone.[73–75] These companies are now selling their activity trackers to thousands of employers for corporate wellness programs.[75] One large health insurer pointed out that "data collected from those gadgets may eventually impact group insurance pricing." Groups— how about individuals? Besides your employer, who may become interested in tracking you, your gym or fitness club is already on it. For so many people who buy a membership and don't use it, they might not be able to hide in the future. Life Time Fitness, with fitness clubs in twenty-four states, has a "national program manager of devices"[76] encouraging every member to allow the gym to monitor their every move. The members are reassured that they can choose which friend to share their data with, and there's always the full shield "weekend-in-Vegas" option.[76]

Medical Device Hacking

While we have yet to see wide-scale consumer use of continuous blood pressure and vital sign monitoring, enough patients have implanted medical devices to reveal many potential liabilities.[77–81] As Sadie Creese, professor of cybersecurity at the University of Oxford, put it, "If you think it's enough of a chore trying to stop thieves stealing your credit card details and hacking your Facebook, imagine trying to stop them getting into your pancreas."[82] Indeed, this has already been shown to occur with both insulin pumps and heart defibrillators, both of which have wireless connectivity to allow tracking and updating software.[83] The manufacturers have not used any security measures in these devices, but new concepts of encrypting the defibrillator with the patient's own heartbeat signal, or "salting the data" in other ways, have been proposed.[80] The databases from three of the largest medical device manufacturers in the world—Medtronic, St. Jude Medical, and Boston Scientific—were hacked, allegedly from China, and the companies were unaware until federal authorities notified them.[77] The FDA has raised awareness on the need for cybersecurity for medical devices, which are particularly vulnerable since they are interconnected to the Internet, hospital networks, smartphones, and other medical devices.[78]

The Heartbleed bug, discovered in 2014, is a major reminder of the vulnerability of popular open source, widely used software.[84–86] Called OpenSSL, we know that this code was used for encryption in a wide variety of embedded devices, making them vulnerable. Such flaws in code can certainly also happen with any closed source software, such as all of our electronic medical record systems (like EPIC, Cerner, Allscripts), which are used throughout US hospitals and health information systems.

An in-depth investigation of cybersecurity status of US hospitals and health care organizations—with interrogation of medical devices and software, including virtual private networks, firewalls, call centers, radiology imaging software, CCTVs, and routers—led to the conclusion that the state of medical cybersecurity was "appalling" and "alarming," "an illustration of how far behind the healthcare industry had fallen." The report cited inadequate current legislation, such as Health Insurance Portability and Accountability Act (HIPAA) and the Health Information Technology for Economic and Clinical Health (HITECH) Act, for setting standards of security for healthcare entities. These findings were reinforced by the results of what was described as the "healthcare industry's first cybersecurity attack simulation," conducted in 2014.[87,88a,88b] Just the fact that the first simulation took place in 2014 is telling in itself, and there were worse problems too. Participants cited the inability to coordinate across medical practices, device makers, hospital information systems, and payers.[88a,89] Jim Koenig, one of the leaders of the simulation, said he expected the exposure to attacks only to grow.[87] So, not surprisingly, hacktivist attacks on hospitals and health systems are taking off, perhaps even faster and larger than some have predicted. In April 2014, the Boston Children's Hospital's external website was hacked by the group Anonymous, making its servers nearly inoperable and forcing the hospital to temporarily shut down its e-mail communication system.[88c] Just a few months later, the 4.5 million patient, 206-hospital Community Health System was hacked by a Chinese cyberattack, with loss of personal data, names, addresses, and social security numbers.[88d] It was the largest breach of medical data yet recorded.

Your Genome

Whenever I give a public talk about genomics, the first question that I invariably get is related to the privacy issue. Currently the largest genomic data set resides at 23andMe. The company's mission is to create "the world's large, secure, private database of genotypic and phenotypic information that can be used for comparison analysis and research."[90] That mission looks good until you read in the company's terms of use about how "genetic information you share with others could be used against your interests" or about the company's potential plan for selling the anonymized data to the pharma industry.

Indeed, there are many distinct concerns surrounding privacy and security when it comes to your DNA. Let's start with getting genetic testing, which could be anything from a simple genotype to whole genome sequencing, or any of the various omics that comprise one's GIS. That decision ought to be the individual's, the owner of his or her genome, with the only exception being children, for which the parents can make the call. Unfortunately, it is very easy to undertake genetic testing without the subject's knowledge, which can be as easy as swiping a bit of your DNA from a cup, utensil, or glass you were using. That clandestine form of genetic assessment needs to be prohibited, as it represents a frank violation of privacy.

Next comes who should have access to your DNA results. Your insurer? Well, doctors are concerned, reflected by a Columbia University study that showed 5 percent of 220 internists purposefully hid or disguised the genetic data of their patients. The American Medical Association code of ethics suggests it may be necessary for doctors to maintain genetic results in a separate file, not accessible to insurers. And certainly you might be rightfully concerned about having your genome sequence results in your medical record. The electronic record could be hacked or breached, as we've reviewed. Or an insurance company could use the information to either deny coverage or demand exceptionally high premiums.[91]

After fourteen years of US Congressional dysfunctionality, the Genetics Information Nondiscrimination Act (GINA) was finally passed in 2008.[92] While that law protects individuals from having their genetic data turned over or misused by employers or health insurers, it left out life, disability, and long-term care forms of insurance. By exempting these other important types of insurance from genetic privacy and discrimination, it has engendered considerable controversy and confusion.[92]

Some experts, such as Bartha Maria Knoppers, the director of the Center of Genomics and Policy at McGill University, points out that "no study has ever clearly established the existence of systemic genetic discrimination by insurers"[93] and concludes "it is doubtful that another piece of legislation to address life, disability and long-term care insurance could really prevent discrimination."[93] Indeed, Joly and colleagues performed a systematic review of all that has been published on genetic discrimination and life insurance and concluded, "With the notable exception of studies on Huntington's disease, none of the studies reviewed here brings irrefutable evidence of a systemic problem of genetic discrimination that would yield a highly negative societal impact."[94]

Of the fifteen large life insurance companies, only one (Northwestern Mutual) currently asks potential customers in certain states about their genetic test data, if any was performed.[94] And the company points out that refusing to report the results may lead to denial or a higher rate for coverage. One life insurance broker stipulated that if an individual failed to disclose his high genetic risk for Alzheimer's dementia, such as having two copies of the apoε4 allele, that would be considered a critical omission that might invalidate a policy.[95]

Fortunately, some states have taken initiative beyond GINA to provide a more comprehensive genetics privacy law. In sixteen states there are laws for life and disability insurance genetic privacy; in ten states for long-term care insurance, and in some states, such as California and Massachusetts, there is privacy protection for all three types of insurance.[96] In the United Kingdom, insurers have thus far agreed to ignore genetic tests because hereditary conditions that would have a major impact are rare.

Nevertheless, some leading American insurance companies believe it is appropriate to have all of an applicant's health information, including their genomic data, since that is the only way to fairly and accurately assess risk. So this debate is largely unsettled. In addition, we are in a state of major flux with respect to how to interpret genomic information. Mutations that have a high probability of an individual manifesting a serious disease are predominantly rare; far more typical are the common genomic variants with uncertainty of the individual's natural history—only a probabilistic, not deterministic chance of ever developing a condition. Take apoε4 as an example. Carriers are common, at around 14 percent in the population, and have a threefold increased likelihood of developing Alzheimer's. But that still is a risk of 20 percent to 25 percent, not 100 percent. Insurance companies might want to do actuarial statistics on that, but the apoε4 story is one of the few established common alleles with some natural history defined. In the years ahead we'll learn much more about the modifier genes, which account for why some people with even two copies of apoε4 never get Alzheimer's. Only when millions of individuals with diverse medical conditions and ancestries undergo whole genome sequencing will we start to have better information on risk. Until then, we're in a zone of uncertainty and that is impeding research—almost 25 percent of individuals who are approached to enroll in genomic research studies decline because of worries about insurance issues. Yes, most people are willing to share their DNA information for research purposes, as long as it is anonymized, but there's a problem with that proviso. Several studies have shown that with extensive genomic data from an individual, it may be possible to re-identify the person. It's not easy and it's certainly not always possible,[97] but the point is that one cannot guarantee a willing participant in a genomics research study that it won't ever happen. Recent studies that have shown it is getting increasingly possible to reconstruct one's facial identity—a "genetic mugshot"—from a genome sequence add another layer of privacy concern.[98] And from facial recognition algorithms, genetic abnormalities can be identified.[99]

A few different approaches to counter this predicament have been offered. Misha Angrist from Duke University summed up the three options—better encryption, making re-identification unlawful, or just making genotype and phenotype public.[100] Having participated in the Harvard Personal Genomic Project (PGP), which is completely open, he acknowledges that most people would be uncomfortable with the last option, since your DNA could be used to frame you, among other risks like revealing nonpaternity.

Encrypting genomes is a real possibility. Cryptologists advocate the "homomorphic" methodology whereby the data are manipulated through multiplication and addition, but that does require longer computation times. And it is totally beatable: John Wilbanks, a privacy expert at Sage Bionetworks in Seattle, said, "If there's a copy of your genome out there that's heavily encrypted, it would just be better for me to shake hands with you and take some of your genetic material." We've already covered that possibility, which should be illegal. Re-identification should also be against the law, but enforcing these practices may be exceedingly difficult.

These challenges for maintaining privacy, especially concurrent with large genomic databases being assembled of millions of people, likely accounted for the view that Steven Brenner, from University of California, Berkeley, put forth in "Be Prepared for the Big Genome Leak."[101] While he made the case that big leaks are inevitable, he believes that the effects at the individual level "would probably reveal less than a typical Google search." He may be right about this today, but fast-forward to the point when genomic data becomes markedly more informative, and that may be way off the mark.

One other option has been offered up—selling your genomic sequence. A startup "Miinome" has set up a platform by which consumers get cash for selling their DNA data to marketers and researchers.[102] The CEO said, "We're the first member-controlled, portable human genomics marketplace."[102] The company gets a cut every time a purchaser accesses one of your traits. I question whether this company's business model will be at all alluring to consumers, and I think that the researchers probably do not have adequate budgets to defray the cost, but at least it begins to recognize the principles of ownership and value of one's DNA.

To sum up after reviewing these alternatives, it seems that two options are eminently doable—enhanced encryption and making re-identification illegal. While they are not perfect solutions by any means, they are both worthy in context of the heightened informativeness of genomic data in the future. Anything that will better protect the genomic privacy of an individual should be pursued.

The Path Forward

We've covered a lot of ground on privacy and security of your medical data, but there are a few critical concepts and actionable items that need attention to get this on the right track.

I've said it before but let me say it again. You have to own all your medical data. If you gathered it, such as through wearable sensors or your smartphone laboratory or imaging device, you own it. It's your body. You paid to extract the information. It has more implications for you than anyone else on the planet. Over the course of your lifetime, you may see tens of different doctors in as many different health systems and clinics, and there is no way to assure that your information will be readily available unless you have it at your immediate disposal. We're not just talking about your final reports or summaries. Raw data. Like your entire genome sequence, output from sensors, or the video loops of your ultrasound images. All of your data, at the most granular level. Even if you might not have use for it or any clue as to understanding it, having the raw medical data about yourself may prove especially helpful during a subsequent evaluation. We have a long way to go. As Lunshof and colleagues emphasized in *Science* on the vital need for raw data access: "The U.S. Presidential Commission recently reviewed thirty-two reports from the United States and worldwide on returning of findings in diverse contexts; it is striking that access to raw data by participants was not addressed in any of them."[103] A *Nature* editorial nicely articulated the charge to protect research participants: "It is a fundamental human right that people can determine how their personal medical data are used, and exceptions to specific informed consent cannot be taken for granted. Informed consent is not an obstacle to be overcome, but a principle to be respected and cherished."[55]

Next, that data set of your GIS—you, medically digitized—needs to be fully protected in your personal cloud with appropriate firewalls. It's too big a file to maintain locally. That is the only way that all your medical data from womb to tomb can be easily accessible and protected. Here the N of 1 principle is working in your favor. While you hopefully will be enthusiastic to participate in a clinical research study and share your data on an anonymized, encrypted basis in a large database, we've reviewed how these can be hacked. The larger the information resource, the more attractive it may be for such a breach. With you having a personal cloud, the chances of such data escape are diminished. The antediluvian medical information systems of today need to undergo total reconfiguration such that every bit of data about you is automatically deposited and nicely organized in your personal cloud.

We also need help from our government. Fortunately, the FDA has been unequivocal about consumer rights in genomics: "Individuals should have unfettered access to their own raw genomic data." That view, as I've previously reviewed, is not necessarily shared by medical organizations, such as the American Medical Association. But our governmental legislation is way behind across the board in digital medicine, with inadequate federal privacy and security actions. We need a new act that transcends HIPAA and HITECH, one which provides critical balance for privacy protection while at the same time promoting medical research.[89,104] The White House Consumer Privacy Bill of Rights and Do Not Track legislation desperately needs to be made law. As Stephen Fairclough, a professor at Liverpool University, correctly asserts, "Electronic devices that track our emotions, heart rate or brain waves should be regulated to protect individual privacy."[105] That circles us back to the secure vs. cure theme and title of this chapter. We clearly want to foster and harvest the remarkable opportunities of open medicine, open science, and MOOMs, while at the same time be cognizant of the risks. Curating medical information, with the right amalgam of security and openness, might someday be the foundation of curing, or at least preserving, health. I'm assuming that the right balance will eventually be struck, which certainly will not be the same for all people. With that foundation, we're ready to use the data to fulfill the dream of preventing illness—far better than a cure.

Chapter 13

Predicting and Preempting Disease

"After spending time working with leading technologists and watching one bastion of human uniqueness after another fall before the inexorable onslaught of innovation, it's becoming harder and harder to have confidence that any given task will be indefinitely resistant to automation."
— ERIK BRYNJOLFSSON AND ANDREW MCAFEE, *The Second Machine Age*[1]

"Over the next few years you are going to see predictive tech and intelligent assistants begin to appear everywhere. Not only will they be in most apps you use—they will also be in your car, in your living room, and in your office. They will also be inside the enterprise—helping doctors better treat patients."
—TIM TUTTLE, CEO, EXPECT LABS[2]

"Eventually, we won't need the doctor. Machine learning makes a better Dr. House than Dr. House."
—VINOD KHOSLA[3]

"Although doctors are devoting their lives to helping people get better, they seem to find a strange satisfaction in seeing a disease take its expected course."
—MICHAEL KINSLEY[4]

The biggest unfulfilled dream in health care is to prevent chronic illness. In the United States we spend 80 percent of the near three trillion annual health care dollars managing the burden of chronic diseases. What if there was a way to actually stop them in their tracks?

Medicine has some other big dreams, too. For over twenty years, a graph that I saw in *The Economist* (Figure 13.1) has been stuck in my mind.[5] In 1994, the magazine predicted that cancer and heart diseases would be "cured" by 2040 and the rest of most serious diseases by 2050. With that, life expectancy at birth would rise to one hundred. All of this seemed like a set of remarkably bold expectations, and many seem no closer to reality than they did in 1994. Some of their prophecies have become at least partially actualized, such as robotic surgery and an effective treatment for some types of cystic fibrosis. But not a cure—the C word—for sure. Perhaps that shouldn't be surprising. The C-word, *cure,* generally means "restore to health" or "recover from disease" or "relieve the symptoms of a disease or condition." There are remarkably few cures in medicine. Some examples are ablating an arrhythmia like atrial fibrillation (in some fortunate patients), antibiotics for pneumonia, or one of the newer treatments for hepatitis C, which has a 99 percent cure rate (for the most common genotype-1 viral subtype). Generally, once a disease strikes, it's a story of managing it. Indeed, *The Economist* prediction notwithstanding, most researchers actively pursuing cancer therapies hope to convert it to a chronic disease, as they have downgraded their ambitions for cures. Once there is congestive heart failure, chronic obstructive pulmonary disease, kidney failure, cirrhosis, dementia, or any significant organ failure, there's no real hope for a cure.

That seems a pretty grim prognosis. But medicine is morphing into a data science, now that big data, unsupervised algorithms, predictive analytics, machine learning, augmented reality, and neuromorphic computing are coming in. There's still an opportunity to change medicine for the better and at least a chance for prevention. That is, if there was a sure-fire signal before a disease had ever manifested itself in a person—and this information was highly actionable—the individual's illness might be preempted.

This dream isn't simply one of better data science, however. It is inextricably linked to the democratization of medicine. The prospect here would

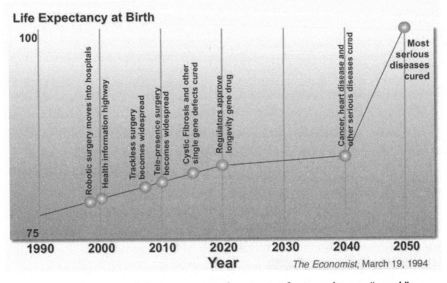

FIGURE 13.1: Increase in life expectancy and projection for most diseases "cured." Source: Adapted from "A Survey of the Future of Medicine," *The Economist*, March 19, 1994, http://www.highbeam.com/doc/1G1–15236568.html.

not be possible without exquisite tracking of individuals by themselves—recall the double entendre of the term "individualized medicine."[6] Picking up a signal long before there are any symptoms relies on one's GIS, not an annual visit with the doctor. With the little wireless devices that we carry and the Internet of Things, we're developing the capability of continuous, critical, real-time surveillance of our bodies. When that gets fully developed, as it ultimately will, *The Economist*'s predictions for the next thirty years in medicine don't seem as far-fetched.

The Economist was shooting from the hip when they made their predictions in 1994. The terms "data mining" and "predictive analytics" were certainly not in vogue and likely hadn't even been invented. But the concept of using data to predict things, like actuarial statistics for life insurance, has been around for ages. What's different now is that the data sets are digital, exponentially bigger and richer, and matched by remarkable computing power and algorithmic processing. That's what enabled Target to predict who among their customers might be pregnant,[7a] how the National Security Agency is using our phone records to spot terrorists, and for hospitals to predict which patients with congestive heart failure are going to require hospitalization.[7b,7c] And it is what will enable us to not just shoot from the hip anymore.

Predicting Things at the Population Level

Some things are pretty easy and intuitive to predict. An example is that a sick public figure drives others to search the Internet for information about their illness or treatment.[8] You could easily predict this would happen; the data mining simply provides quantification of the effect.

But what if you used the Google searches to more intelligently *predict* an illness, rather than just *quantify* the searches? That brings us to the big Google flu story, which is one of the most cited examples of prediction in health care.[9–16] Google Flu Trends (GFT), which started in 2008, has been known as the "poster child for the power of big data analysis" by tracking forty-five flu-related search terms, monitoring trends of billions of searches in twenty-nine countries,[10] and making correlations with unsupervised algorithms to predict a flu outbreak. By unsupervised, this means it is hypothesis-free, no biases—just letting the top fifty million search terms and algorithms do the work. In widely cited papers in *Nature*[12] and *Public Library of Science (PLoS) One*,[11] Google authors (Figure 13.2) claimed the ability to use web search logs to create daily estimates of influenza infection, unlike usual methods, which have built-in lags of one to two weeks. And later, in 2011: "Google Flu Trends can provide timely and accurate estimates of the influenza activity in the United States, especially during peak activity, even in the wake of a novel form of influenza."[11]

But a firestorm of controversy developed in early 2013 when it was shown that GFT grossly overestimated the flu outbreak (Figure 13.3). Later, a team of four highly respected data scientists wrote in *Science* that GFT had systematically overestimated the prevalence of flu every week since August 2011, going on to criticize "big data hubris," the "often implicit assumption that big data are a substitute for, rather than a supplement to, traditional data collection and analysis."[17] They attacked the "algorithm dynamics" of GFT, pointing out that the forty-five search terms used were never documented, key elements such as core search terms were not provided in the publications, and the original algorithm did not undergo constant adjustment and recalibration. What's more, while the GFT algorithm was static, the search engine itself underwent constant change—as many as six hundred revisions per year—which was not taken into account. Many

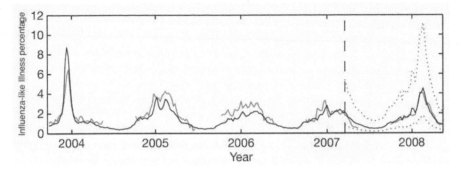

FIGURE 13.2: The CDC data (light line) compared with Google Flu Trends (dark line) for influenza outbreaks in the mid-Atlantic United States. Source: J. Ginsberg et al., "Detecting Influenza Epidemic Using Search Engine Query Data," *Nature* 457 (2009): 1012–1015. Reprinted with permission.

other editorialists opined on the matter.[13–15,18,19] Correlation rather than causation and the critical absence of context were the most prominent critique points. There was also the sampling issue as the crowdsourcing was limited to those doing searches on Google. Further, there was a major analytical problem: GFT performed so many multiple comparisons of data that they were likely to be getting spurious results. These can all be viewed as common traps when we are trying to understand the world through data.[13] As Krenchel and Madsbjerg wrote in *Wired*, "The real big data hubris is not that we have too much confidence in a set of algorithms and methods that aren't quite there yet. Rather, the issue is the blind belief that sitting behind a computer screen crunching numbers will ever be enough to understand the full extent of the world around us."[19] We want answers, not just data. Tim Harford, in the *Financial Times*, put it bluntly, "Big data has arrived, but big insights have not."[18]

Some rallied to the defense of GFT, pointing out that the data were additive to the Centers for Disease Control and Prevention (CDC) and that Google never claimed they had a magical tool. Gary Marcus and Ernest Davis expressed the most balanced perspective in their op-ed "Eight (No, Nine!) Problems With Big Data."[20] I've reviewed most of their issues already, but Marcus and Davis's point about the hype of big data and what it can (and can't) do deserve their emphasis: "BIG data is suddenly everywhere. Everyone seems to be collecting it, analyzing it, making money from it and celebrating (or fearing) its powers. . . . Big data is here to stay, as it should be. But let's be realistic: It's an important resource for anyone analyzing data, not a silver bullet."[20]

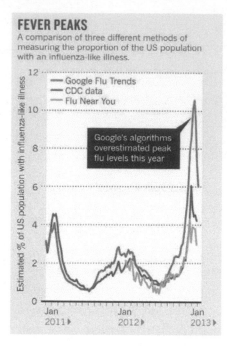

FEVER PEAKS
A comparison of three different methods of measuring the proportion of the US population with an influenza-like illness.

- Google Flu Trends
- CDC data
- Flu Near You

Google's algorithms overestimated peak flu levels this year

FIGURE 13.3: The GFT overestimate of flu. Flu Near You is another initiative launched in 2011. Source: D. Butler, "When Google Got Flu Wrong," *Nature* 494 (2013): 155–156. Reprinted with permission.

Despite the problems with GFT, this kind of effort isn't going anywhere. An alternative and more recent approach to predicting a contagious outbreak used a smaller base of individuals who were well connected on the Twitter network—so called "central nodes"—essentially exploiting these individuals as sensors.[21a] This enabled detection of viral outbreaks seven days faster than looking at the general population. Similarly, the HealthMap algorithm, which scours tens of thousands of social networks and news media, was capable of predicting the 2014 Ebola outbreak in West Africa nine days before the World Health Organization.[21b] I've delved somewhat deeply into this Google flu story and related infectious disease outbreaks because they represent the early stages of where we're headed, and how we can get off track, in using large data sets to predict things in medicine. But knowing how we got off track is important if we're ever going to stay on.

Predicting Things at the Individual Level

More powerful than data from whole populations, as with GFTs, is the combination of granular data of an individual[21c] with the granular data of the rest of the population. You've encountered this before. For example, Pandora maintains a database with the song preferences from over two hundred million registered users who have pressed collectively the like or dislike more than thirty-five billion times.[22] It knows who listens while driving or on an Android device or an iPhone, and it knows where every listener lives. As a result it can predict not just the music each listener likes but even political preferences, which it has used for political ad targeting in presidential and congressional campaigns. Eric Bieschke, Pandora's chief scientist, summed their data program up as providing "magical insights" about their users. And they can do it because they integrate two big data layers to derive these insights—your data and the data from millions of other people.[22]

Using data brokers such as Acxiom (discussed in the previous chapter), the University of Pittsburgh Medical Center performs data mining of their patients, including their shopping characteristics, to predict the likelihood of their using the emergency room facilities.[23] So does the Carolinas Health System, by mining the consumer credit card data from two million people in their region to identify high-risk patients (e.g., via purchases of fast food, cigarettes, alcohol, and drug refills).[24] The Pittsburgh predictive model showed that households using mail order and Internet shopping the most were more apt to use emergency services, something that health systems are trying to discourage. The data mining builds on itself over time, when extant patients have repeat encounters and more patients come into the system, to be better at predicting certain features. But the privacy and ethical issues are looming.

These examples can be considered a rudimentary form of artificial intelligence (AI)—machines or software exhibiting human-like intelligence. Other examples that you might have around you already include personal digital assistants such as Google Now, Future Control, Cortana,[25] and SwiftKey,[26] which cull together information from e-mails, texts, calendars, address books, search history, locations, purchases, whom you spend time with, your taste in art, and your past behavior.[27] Based on what they learn from that information, these apps pop up on your screen to tell you to leave early for your next appointment and to provide the traffic pattern for your upcoming drive or the flight status of your imminent trip. By reading your contacts' Twitter feeds, Future Control can pick up the state of mind of your contacts: "Your girlfriend is sad, get her some flowers."[28] SwiftKey even figures out how you type to compensate for consistently pecking on the wrong letter. Google Now partners with airlines and event organizers to access ticketing information and can even listen to the sound of your television to provide advance programming information.[29] As you might know, these capabilities represent far greater power than does the hunt for correlations that powers GFT, and they have great relevance to medicine.

Such predictive power relies upon machine learning, a key aspect of AI. The more data fed into the program or computer, the more it learns, the better the algorithms, and supposedly the smarter it gets.

Techniques from machine learning and artificial intelligence are what powered the triumph of the IBM Watson supercomputer over humans on *Jeopardy*. This relied upon quickly answering complex questions that would not be amenable to a Google search.[30-32] IBM Watson was taught through hundreds of thousands of questions from prior *Jeopardy* shows, armed with all the information in Wikipedia, and programmed to do predictive modeling. There's no prediction of the future here, just prediction that IBM Watson has the correct answer. Underlying its predictive capabilities was quite a portfolio of machine learning systems, including Bayesian nets, Markov chains, support vector machine algorithms, and genetic algorithms.[33] I won't go into any more depth; my brain is not smart enough to understand it all, and fortunately it's not particularly relevant to where we are going here.

Another subtype of AI and machine learning,[2,20,34-48] known as deep learning, has deep importance to medicine. Deep learning is behind Siri's ability to decode speech as well as Google Brain experiments to recognize images. Researchers at Google X extracted ten million still images from YouTube videos and fed them to the network of one thousand computers to see what the Brain, with its one million simulated neurons and one billion simulated synapses would come up with on its own.[35,36] The answer—cats. That the Internet, at least the YouTube segment (which occupies a lot of it), is chock full of cat videos. More than the cat diagnosis, this revelation exemplified the operation of cognitive, or what is also known as neuromorphic, computing.[49a] For if computers can emulate the human brain, as the theory goes, they can be taken to the next level of performance for perception, action, and cognition. Progress in neuromorphic computing is occurring at a dizzying pace. In the past year, the accuracy of computer eyesight—such as the recognition of a pedestrian, helmet, bicyclist, car—has improved from 23 to 44 percent, with a drop in error rate from 12 to less than 7 percent.[49b]

Despite the achievements of Google Brain, we clearly aren't there yet. The human brain works on low power, just about twenty watts, but the supercomputer needs millions of watts to operate.[35,49a–57] Whereas the brain doesn't need to be programmed (even though it seems that way sometimes) and loses neurons throughout one's life without much functional attrition, computers that lose a single chip can be wrecked, and they generally can't adapt to the world they're interacting with.[50] Gary Marcus, a neuroscientist at New York University, put this neuromorphic mission in perspective: "At times like these, I find it useful to remember a basic truth: the human brain is the most complicated organ in the universe, and we still have almost no idea how it works. Who said that copying its awesome power was going to be easy?"[58] Nevertheless, there has been quite a bit of progress in speech, facial, gesture, and image recognition, which are strengths of the human brain and soft spots for computers. Having attended conferences and lectured in foreign countries, with simultaneous translations, I was struck by one achievement in particular: Richard Rashid, then Microsoft's top scientist, gave a lecture in China that was not only simultaneously translated by a computer into Mandarin characters but also rendered in Rashid's own voice (as simulated) in Chinese.[36] Facebook's DeepFace program, with the world's largest photo library, can determine whether two pictures of a person's face represent the same individual at 97.25 percent accuracy.[59,60] The medical implications are already becoming manifest. Academic researchers, showing that computers can detect facial expression, like pain, more accurately than humans, have reinforced the extraordinary progress in computer facial recognition.[61-63] Stanford University computer scientists have utilized their cluster of sixteen thousand computers to train image recognition on twenty thousand different objects. More relevant to our topic, they've used these deep learning tools to determine whether a breast cancer biopsy is cancerous.[37] Harvard's Andrew Beck developed a computerized system for diagnosing breast cancer and predicting survival rates based on automatic processing of images. It turned out, with unsupervised learning, to be more accurate than pathologists, and it picked up new features that had been missed by them throughout the years.[64] And we shouldn't forget the amazing AI support that has enabled seeing and hearing devices. Orcam is a camera sensor mounted on eyeglasses for the visually impaired that sees things and transmits that information through a bone-conduction earpiece.[39] GN ReSound Linx and Starkey are two smartphone app-connected hearing aids that "give people with hearing loss the ability to outperform their normal-hearing counterparts.[65] In line with this bionic future, we have now seen wheelchairs for quadriplegics that can be controlled by thoughts.[39] So the power of AI to transform things in medicine surely can't be missed. The technology can be readily combined with robotics, or course. At the University of California, San Francisco, the hospital pharmacy is algorithmically fully automated, and the robot dispensation of medications has yet to make a mistake.

The Individual and the Internet of Medical Things

Now we're ready to tackle medicine with this accelerated intellectual capacity of our digital machines and infrastructure. Currently, the annual amount of data produced worldwide per individual is about one terabyte, or five zettabytes of data per year (or forty sextillion). But remember from Chapter 5 when we drilled down the human GIS, just the omics from an individual will add at least another five terabytes, and we haven't even gotten to real-time streaming from biosensors, which would quickly supersede sequencing for amount of data generated. That still barely gets things started when you add the other components of one's GIS, especially the data flood from the pixels of medical imaging and the coming deluge from the Internet of Medical Things.

But this is clearly not just an N of 1 story here. As reviewed in Chapter 11, although lots of data about you would be useful, the optimal condition for making the data maximally informative is to compare it to *all* the data from *every individual* on the planet (Figure 13.4). While we'll never get to all the people, the more, the better, and companies like Facebook show what can be done.

The key is that machine learning of the sort behind IBM Watson and other systems enables us to go broad (N of 7B) and deep (N of 1) not just in search of knowledge but in search of prediction and understanding. For each individual, we need to know what are the triggers and complex interrelationships at many levels—genomic, biologic, physiologic, and environmental—that account for liability to develop an illness or episode. The goal is not simply an estimate of risk during the course of one's life, but

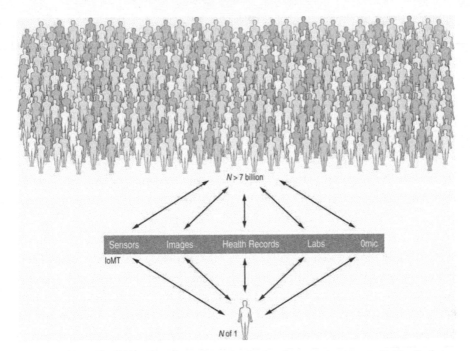

FIGURE 13.4: Really big data from the individual and comparing that individual's data with all of the Earth's population (IoMT = Internet of Medical Things). The two levels of data acquisition, comparison, and machine learning—individual and population—are critical, across all of the components of one's GIS.

at a particular time or moment. We'll also learn a great deal by examining in depth as many people as possible for their cues, enriching our understanding of what it takes for a condition to manifest or to be prevented. Only now that we can capture such panoromic data on each individual, and in populations of people, along with the ability to manage and process such enormous sets of data, are we in the enviable position of predicting illness—and maybe, just maybe, once we get good at it, even preventing diseases in some individuals from ever happening.

Predicting Disease: Who, When, How, Why, and What?

First, let's make sure we differentiate prediction from diagnosis. Online symptom checkers[66] are getting increasing electronic traffic and attention on the Internet to help people "self" (computer-assisted) diagnose, but they don't predict an illness. At best, from a cluster of symptoms that a person inputs, a differential diagnosis is offered with the right one on the list. That's useful and practical, but not predicting anything. Likewise, the Biovideo developers—who are building an app for the IBM Watson supercomputer so that "a mother with a sick child at 4 am will be able to use IBM Watson to ask what is wrong with her baby and get a 100 per cent accurate response"[67a]—may create something useful, but that something is not about prediction.

We have a very serious problem with misdiagnosis—diagnosis of a patient with the wrong disease or the correct one too late—affecting 12 million Americans per year.[67b,67c] We can look to technology and contextual computing to help alleviate this struggle. The popular TV show *House* is very instructive on this point. The central character, Dr. Gregory House, is a brilliant diagnostician who solves all the rare, mysterious cases that stump other doctors.[68–71] To accomplish this, he actually uses a Bayesian approach in which all of the information—history, physical examination, lab tests, scans—is contextualized with all previous known relevant information (what is known from Bayes's theorem as the pretest odds of a hypothesis). A yes or no answer is not obtained. Rather, there is a probability that the patient has X or Y diagnosis. That compares with the frequentist approach, yielding a yes or no based solely on probability statistics (like P <0.05). The Dr. House model is ideally suited for computer automation in medicine and it is precisely the output from IBM Watson.[70,71] The pretest probability includes all of the medical literature that has been published, up to date. When you submit to IBM Watson all the pieces of evidence about a particular patient in search of the diagnosis, you get a list of the possible ones. Attached to each is a weight or probability (likelihood ratio).

Further, the Bayesian model for computer-assisted diagnosis is quickly becoming part of clinical care and can extend to treatment recommendations. A web-based information resource known as Modernizing Medicine has collective knowledge from over fifteen million patient visits and four thousand physicians with treatments and outcomes of each patient.[72] So added to IBM Watson's differential diagnosis capability, a list of treatments with weighted assignments of probability could be generated that matches the patient at hand to all the patients in the database. (By the way, the data scientists who work in this field don't like to have their health information resources described as databases. Oops.) These exemplify the use of artificial intelligence for differential diagnoses and treatments in medicine. But again they do not represent prediction.

Then let's make sure it is clear that collecting oodles of data doesn't mean you are going to be able to predict something meaningful. At the time of Alan Turing's one-hundredth birthday, *Science* ran a number of articles, including one about "a home fully equipped with cameras and audio equipment [that] continuously recorded the life of an infant from birth to age three, amounting to ~200,000 hours of audio and video recordings, representing 85% of the child's waking experience."[73] OK, that's a triumph in data collection, but certainly not with the intent of or any likelihood of predicting illness. This is not a hypothesis-free exercise or experiment. Similarly, there are many new large-scale genome-sequencing projects of one hundred thousand people, such as the Geisenger-Regeneron, Human Longevity, Inc., Genomics England, and Institute for Systems Biology initiatives. While these programs will undoubtedly contribute to genomic science, the individuals that are being enrolled are of no specific phenotype and there is no real hypothesis. Instead, it's the idea that these endeavors are possible and worthy, and that perhaps a discovery from the data will lead to a new drug. In order to predict illness, however, specific hypotheses and very deliberate goals need to be drawn up, as we'll get into. Otherwise, we'll be blinded by a low ratio of signal to noise, lulled into thinking we have a complete picture of the data universe, and misled by spurious relationships.

Another important point is that we're trying to predict a major medical condition, not a biomarker. We're not trying to say someone will have a bad cholesterol level or an abnormal liver function test. Overall, these protein or gene markers have been particularly misleading, with a flood of candidates put out in the medical literature but very few that ever pass muster in the clinic.[74] That's because, while lab results may be useful in helping to predict the onset of a disease before it happens, they are not the endgame.

A step in the direction of big data to understand disease progression was undertaken by researchers in Denmark, who had fifteen years of data on the country's 6.2 million citizens.[75] They were able to map out many disease arcs, or as they called them, trajectories, such that one condition was apt to eventually lead to another one that was seemingly unrelated. These were temporal associations without any established cause-and-effect relationships.[75]

The fundamental goal is that we're trying to predict so we can prevent. If it's not actionable, then predicting is more of an academic exercise. For example, considerable work is going into trying to predict who will get Alzheimer's disease long before any cognitive deficit has occurred. It's unquestionably one of the most important public health issues we face, but to date, despite considerable efforts, there are no clear, validated preventive strategies.

The timing and location of a prediction is also crucial. I live in San Diego, where I see lots of surfers who ride the waves in the Pacific Ocean every day without thinking about sharks. They only kill ten people a year out of the seven billion plus inhabitants of the planet, so we can make a general prediction that the average risk of dying by shark attack in San Diego is infinitesimally small. But every now and then there is a "killer" shark sighting. On those days, it is a rarity to see any surfer go out. With predicting things, time and place are pivotal.

For predicting diseases in people, timing is everything. We can accurately tell everyone that they're going to die. If you tell someone, "You're going to die but we don't know whether that's in two weeks or two decades," it's worthless. In fact, it's worse than worthless because while it may be true, it can create emotional havoc for a patient due to lack of temporal specificity. So in an attempt to prevent a medical condition, both who and when are paramount.

A useful analogy for successful medical prediction is to think about predicting the failure of jet engines.[76,77] Companies like General Electric place their aircraft engines under continuous surveillance. They use sophisticated unsupervised algorithms, AI, and multidimensional analytics to identify predictive precursors like a hairline fracture, because there is demand for a zero probability of failure when every flight puts hundreds of passengers at risk. Most medical conditions, like a heart attack, asthma attack, stroke, autoimmune attack, are just like plane crashes happening inside the human body. We can use the same computational tools. The biggest difference is that the medical monitoring will save plane-loads of people, but only one "passenger" at a time.

Now let's go through some medical conditions that might be predicted and preempted in the future. We'll start with those that are amenable to monitoring by wearable sensors, because they provide unique, real-time, streaming data on individuals at risk, which is the best, most precise shot on goal for being informative and predictive.[78] First, I'll look at wearable sensors that are likely to be widely available soon, and then move on to conditions that would chiefly rely on bloodstream embedded sensors. Let's first turn our attention to asthma. Asthma attacks are one of the leading causes of deaths and life-threatening emergencies in children, and certainly are a major health issue in millions of adults. Each asthmatic individual has different triggers for what tips their airways to go into spasm—for some it's pollution, for others it's cold, exercise, pollen, or other allergens. If we can sense when muscles in the airway start to change in tone long before the first wheeze, we can stay in front of an attack. This might be possible by a cluster of sensors—wearables for air quality, pollen, analysis of the use of the inhaler(s) and geo-location, the breath for the presence and quantitation of nitric oxide, and measuring lung function through the microphone of the smartphone or suitable add-appter. Because immune function is tied in tightly with the gut microbiome, sampling and analysis of this omic may be useful and deserves study. Along with this, passive monitoring of respiratory rate, temperature, oxygen saturation in the blood, blood pressure, and heart rate could all be captured via a wristwatch device. Now comes the machine learning for the individual, from all these data inputs, of what characteristics are precursors to an asthma attack. That pattern, once recognized, can be used to alert the individual to take additional medication, avoid a particular exposure, or some combination of action steps. Moreover, this information becomes even more valuable once this is learned from thousands and hundreds of thousands of people with asthma—we've never before had the ability to monitor all this stuff for people "in the wild." New trigger patterns and links will inevitably be discovered. Ultimately, individuals who have never had an asthma attack but are at high risk, as determined by genome sequencing, family history, and immune system screening, will have the capability of using a sensor approach to stave off an event.

How about depression and posttraumatic stress disorder (PTSD)? Let's say a soldier has returned from Afghanistan and is being screened for PTSD. Today that is done by a questionnaire with subjective responses provided by the individual. There are many more objective ways this can be tracked, which include tone and inflection of voice, pattern of breathing, facial expression, vital signs, galvanic skin response, heart rate variability and heart rate recovery, pattern of communication, movement and activity, posture, quality and duration of sleep, and brain waves. This panel of metrics would likely diagnose susceptibility to PTSD. Similarly, depression affects over twenty million Americans, with marked impact on quality of life and functionality. If we can learn what precipitates and what alleviates depression in each individual, and for a large population, we can likely do far better in preventing depression, or at least its most severe forms. In those receiving therapy, adherence to medications can also be readily tracked to determine whether this is a precipitating factor.

The same logic train extends to congestive heart failure. Now we have ways to continuously stream heart performance beat-by-beat, fluid status, sleep quality and apneic spells, along with vital signs and daily weight. The smartphone can be used to measure labs like brain natriuretic peptide and kidney tests such as blood urea nitrogen or creatinine, which reflect both fluid status and heart muscle strength. Medication adherence can be tracked via digitized pills. In aggregate, these data should be able to identify impending heart failure before a susceptible individual has developed any shortness of breath. If imminent heart failure is detected, there are several types of medications that can be used to prevent a flooding of the lungs.

Ditto for epilepsy, which, as has been shown, may be predictable via "electrodermal" sensing in some individuals, by monitoring heart rate variability and galvanic skin response via a wristband. But supplement that with wearable EEG, sleep quality metrics, and vital sign monitoring, anticipating a seizure well before it happens could prove to be possible. And that potential is heightened when there are thousands of individuals with epilepsy who have comprehensive monitoring.

An initiative that has data on thousands of premature babies is Project Artemis, based at the University of Ontario.[79] There is a near 25 percent risk of serious infections among premies, and 10 percent of these newborns will die, but until now it has been hard to predict which baby is particularly susceptible or when this might occur. Using heart rate sensors, a significant heart rate trend marker was identified. Now neonatal units around the world can send heart rate monitor data through the cloud for minute-by-minute readings at Artemis's base to get constantly updated probability statistics. Similarly, there are programs to detect which frail, elderly individuals are likely to fall, and when.[80,81a] Using various sensors in the floor, or what has been called a "magic carpet," it appears possible to spot a trend for a person's deterioration in gait and progressive temporal risk of falling. Such falls represent one of the greatest risks for the elderly, all too frequently resulting in hip fracture and fatality. The machine learning strategy could prove especially worthwhile for preventing such events.

Now we'll pivot to some diseases that will likely require an embedded sensor (Table 13.1), because there is not an adequate way to get the critical information or insight from outside the body (at least at this point in time).[81b] By having a tiny sensor implanted in the bloodstream, such as within a miniature stent put in a vein in the wrist area, our bloodstream can be put under constant surveillance. For autoimmune diseases that include diabetes ("Type 1"), multiple sclerosis, lupus, rheumatoid and psoriatic arthritis, Crohn's disease and ulcerative colitis, the immune function—both the so-called adaptive and innate immunity pathways—could be monitored. On an individual basis, lymphocyte B cells and T cells could be sequenced along with any autoantibodies (antibodies directed to oneself) to determine modes of immune attack. Once that is accomplished in tens of thousands of individuals with immune disorders, we'll have a much broader view of the things to be monitored in the bloodstream for those at risk or who have already been diagnosed with one of these conditions. Similar to asthma, intermittent microbiome assays, particularly of the gut, will likely be helpful. If an immune attack is known to be developing, well before there are symptoms or any destruction of tissue like β-islet cells, nerve tissue, or joints (for diabetes, multiple sclerosis, and rheumatoid arthritis, respectively), there are many different therapies that can turn off the relevant portion of the immune system. That would lend itself to a far more intelligent way of preventing the toll of these diseases than our current approaches of crisis intervention or chronic therapy, even when the immune system is quiescent.

The Molecular Stethoscope and Machine Learning

As we've reviewed, the original stethoscope is quite limited with respect to the data it collects. But the concept was that it looked into the body and was an integral part of the physical exam and checkup on an individual's health. Although it didn't actually look into the body, it at least provided one's internal sounds and shaped two hundred years of medical practice.

We are at an interesting point in really looking into the body and perhaps getting information that is surprising, difficult to interpret, or just

Condition	S	Metrics	Labs	Imaging	Actionability
Heart Failure	W	Cardiac output, stroke volume, fluid status, vital signs, weight, sleep	BNP, Kidney tests	US	Fluid offload, heart unload, medication adherence
Depression	W	Voice, vital signs, breathing, communication, activity, facial expression, sleep, HRV, HRR, GSR	Neuro-hormones	EEG	Counseling, anti-depressant, medication adherence
Asthma	W	FEV_1, air quality, inhaler, GPS, allergens, vital signs	NO Microbiome	--	Preventive Rx of medications, avoidance of trigger
Epilepsy	W	HRV, GSR, sleep, activity, vital signs	--	EEG	Medication, avoidance of vulnerability
Autoimmune Diseases	E	Sequence of B and T cell repertoires in blood cells	Microbiome	--	Immunomodulation
Cancer	E	Presence of ctDNA and CTCs	Breath scan, Molecular stethoscope	--	Sequencing to determine whether/what Rx is necessary
Heart Attack	E	Presence of ceDNA or RNA	CT angiogram Molecular stethoscope	--	Anti-clotting medication

TABLE 13.1: Examples of seven diseases that may be prevented by multidimensional monitoring at both the individual and population levels. S = sensor type, W = wearable, E = embedded, HRV = heart rate variability, HRR = heart rate recovery, GSR = galvanic skin response, FEV_1 = forced expiratory volume in one second, ctDNA = circulating tumor DNA, ceDNA = circulating endothelial DNA, EEG = electroencephalogram, NO = nitric oxide, CT = computed tomography, CTC = circulating tumor cells.

too much. For example, when an expectant mother has a noninvasive prenatal test to determine whether the fetus has chromosomal abnormalities such as Down syndrome, the blood sample contains both her DNA and the baby's. Now there are many cases where tumor DNA has been found, and further evaluation of these pregnant women has confirmed that they have cancer. So a simple blood test to find out information about the fetus results in unexpected, serious molecular findings about the mother. But this represents just the tip of the iceberg, because as we move forward it is highly likely that blood samples for the cell-free DNA and RNA that is circulating in our blood will become a routine lab test—a molecular stethoscope. We'll be really looking into the body, as we've never been able to do before. When that happens, an increasing number of people will show tumor DNA. But do they have cancer?

It may well be that as part of our normal aging process, and housekeeping functions in a healthy body, a few cells here or there develop mutations that could ultimately lead to cancer. But there are defense mechanisms, such as the immune system, that see these limited number of abnormal cells and stop the process from going further. Nevertheless, the abnormal "tumor"-free DNA shows up in the blood. We really don't know what to make of it. This could lead to very extensive and expensive evaluation with scans to find out whether the individual really has cancer, and where it is located. Alternatively, we could turn to machine learning to understand the problem. Samples taken at different time points in each individual, and the same in large cohorts of individuals, with various omics, including DNA and RNA, would likely sort this conundrum out. With deep learning we should eventually be able to say to any given patient that this tumor DNA is innocent, just a sign of the healthy body doing its thing, or that it represents the earliest detection of the real deal. One might question why we should get into this over-detection mode. And the answer would be that if we are to be able to detect cancer long before it can be seen on a scan or cause symptoms, this might well be the optimal path. Especially if it is shown that catching cancer so early results in excellent outcomes.

This is just one example of many for the molecular stethoscope. In an individual who has had an organ transplant, there is always the risk for rejection, and this complication can be very difficult to detect, typically requiring a biopsy. But we don't want to do a biopsy for someone feeling perfectly fine, even though we know that rejection is far easier to treat when the process is at the earliest stage. Recent studies suggest that just looking at the blood for evidence of the organ donor's DNA might be the best way to track the rejection process. However, like with tumor DNA, if there is some low level of donor DNA in the blood, what does that mean? Again we turn to machine learning to unravel this puzzle, with as much information as possible, in large numbers of patients across all the different organ transplant types, to figure out what this signal means. The putative answer at one point in time is always subject to updating as more information is added to the learning process.

The most far-reaching component of the molecular stethoscope appears to be cell-free RNA, which can potentially be used to monitor any organ of the body.[82] Previously that was unthinkable in a healthy person. How could one possibly conceive of doing a brain or liver biopsy in someone as part of a normal checkup? Using high-throughput sequencing of cell-free RNA in the blood, and sophisticated bioinformatic methods to analyze this data, Stephen Quake and his colleagues at Stanford were able to show it is possible to follow the gene expression from each of the body's organs from a simple blood sample. And that is changing all the time in each of us. This is an ideal case for deep learning to determine what these dynamic genomic signatures mean, to determine what can be done to change the natural history of a disease in the making, and to develop the path for prevention. Furthermore, besides a blood test that could be looked at from time to time, this molecular stethoscope could potentially be made into an embedded sensor. But whether this promising window to the molecular operations of the body will pan out or wind up like most of the 150,000 biomarkers that go nowhere remains to be seen.[74] We hardly have to be reminded of how complex human biology is, and that comprehending all the interdependent interactions—systems medicine—for each individual will likely prove to be a tough nut to crack.

These are strategies that represent novel, yet to be validated means of preempting critical illnesses. It's easy to be imaginative when extraordinary patient-generated data comes to smartphones connected to and processed by artificial intelligence. And when we can use these same data capture and predictive analytics at both the individual and population levels, as medicine becomes a data science, we all may even start to look halfway intelligent.

Chapter 14

Flattening the Earth

"It has been clear to me that one of the biggest obstacles to improving the lives of the world's poorest people is the ability to accurately measure in real time the burden of ill-health. Because if we can't measure it, how can we do anything about it?"
—SETH BERKLEY, CEO OF GAVI ALLIANCE[1]

"We believe that digital health technology can serve as a powerful equalizer for improving health education and access to care among minority and low-income communities by reaching people where they are spending time—at school, at church, in their neighborhoods and on-the-go with real time solutions that easily fit into their daily lives."
—GARTH GRAHAM, PRESIDENT OF THE AETNA FOUNDATION[2]

When you hear or read about Murray and López, you are probably thinking of Andy Murray and Feliciano López, playing a big tennis match. But whenever I see the names Murray and Lopez, I think of the Global Burden of Disease.[3,4] Launched in 1991 by the World Health Organization and the World Bank, the project is an extraordinary source of worldwide medical data, providing longitudinal perspective on what is going on in the health of the world's population.

In Figure 14.1, you'll see the world's leading causes of death and disability.

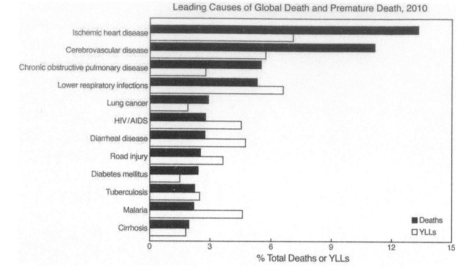

FIGURE 14.1: Global Burden of Disease: leading causes of death and years of life lost due to premature death (YLLs), 2010. Source: Adapted from C. Murray et al., "The Global Burden of Disease: Generating Evidence, Guiding Policy," Institute for Health Metrics and Evaluation, July 23, 2013, http://www.healthdata.org/sites/default/files/files/policy_report/2013/GBD_GeneratingEvidence/IHME_GBD_GeneratingEvidence_FullReport.pdf.

But when we are thinking about the burden of disease, it's not just about death. Even greater is the toll of disability. Table 14.1 shows the cost of disease as measured in disability adjusted life years (DALYs), a unit combining the effects of premature death and living with debilitating disease, with the 95 percent confidence intervals around these estimates.[3]

You can see that there is considerable overlap of the causes of death and disability, but there have also been pronounced changes over the past two decades in the developing world, with an uprising of non-communicable diseases like diabetes, cancer, and heart disease (Figure 14.2). While communicable, infectious diseases have markedly decreased—lower respiratory tract infections, diarrhea, tuberculosis, and meningitis have been reduced by 20 percent to 50 percent—there are two notable exceptions: HIV/AIDS has increased by 350 percent and malaria has increased by over 20 percent.[4]

That is, the leading causes of death in the developed world are now becoming important causes of death in the developing world attributable to increasingly pervasive risk factors such as obesity, hypertension, and the

Cause	Rank	2010 DALYs (95% UI) *in thousands*
Ischemic heart disease	1	129,795 (119,218–137,398)
Lower respiratory tract infections	2	115,227 (102,255–126,972)
Stroke	3	102,239 (90,472–108,003)
Diarrhea	4	89,524 (77,595–99,193)
HIV–AIDS	5	81,549 (74,698–88,371)
Malaria	6	82,689 (63,465–109,846)
Low back pain	7	80,667 (56,066–108,723)
Preterm birth complications	8	76,980 (66,210–88,132)
Chronic obstructive pulmonary disease	9	76,779 (66,000–89,147)
Road-traffic injury	10	75,487 (61,555–94,777)
Major depressive disorder	11	63,239 (47,894–80,784)
Neonatal encephalopathy	12	50,163 (40,351–59,810)
Tuberculosis	13	49,399 (40,027–56,009)
Diabetes mellitus	14	46,857 (40,212–55,252)
Iron-deficiency anemia	15	45,350 (31,046–64,616)
Sepsis and other infectious disorders in newborns	16	44,236 (27,349–72,418)
Congenital anomalies	17	38,890 (31,891–45,739)
Self-harm	18	36,655 (26,894–44,652)
Falls	19	35,406 (28,583–44,052)
Protein-energy malnutrition	20	34,874 (27,957–41,662)

TABLE 14.1: Global Causes of Disability. Source: Adapted from C. Murray and A. López, "Measuring the Global Burden of Disease," *New England Journal of Medicine* 369 (2013): 448–457.

increase in cigarette smoking.[4] The next figures show which risk factors and conditions are associated with the most deaths and disabilities (Figures 14.2 and 14.3).[5] The deaths due to non-communicable disease exceed infections and maternal, neonatal, and nutritional diseases by a 3 to 1 ratio (Figure 14.3).

Again, we see problems formerly found specifically in the developed world: note the surges in high blood pressure, body mass index, and fasting glucose. The impact of smoking, a diet low in fruit or high in sodium, and physical inactivity are particularly remarkable.

The changing landscape of risk factors and disease in the developing world are important, not just because they represent critical public health issues, but because this trend toward uniformity lends itself to more homogenous approaches for prevention and treatment. Economic development

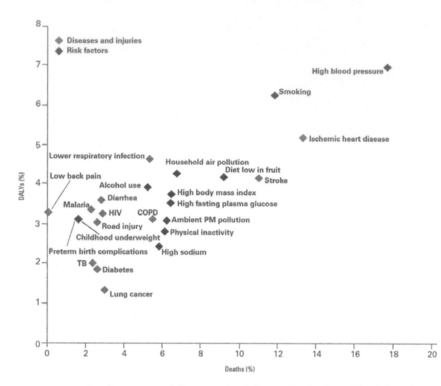

FIGURE 14.2: Leading causes of disease and risk factors for death and disability. Source: C. Murray et al., "The Global Burden of Disease: Generating Evidence, Guiding Policy," Institute for Health Metrics and Evaluation, July 23, 2013, http://www.healthdata.org/ sites/default/files/files/policy_report/2013/GBD_GeneratingEvidence/IHME_GBD _GeneratingEvidence_FullReport.pdf.

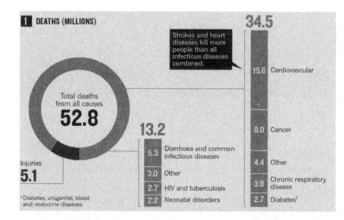

FIGURE 14.3: Deadly and Neglected. Non-communicable diseases (NCDs) such as cancer and diabetes caused more deaths and disabilities in 2010 than did infectious ones, but received disproportionately low investment. Source: L. O. Gostin, "Healthy Living Needs Global Governance," *Nature* 511 (2014): 147–149. Reprinted with permission.

can flatten the Earth in the future. Although that might mean new health risks, it also means new health opportunities. Indeed, it means a chance to fully democratize medicine, making it available not only to wealthy Westerners but truly to all people.

Communicable Diseases

Chronic diseases are becoming big problems, but infectious diseases remain important. They still represent the #2 (pneumonia), #4 (diarrhea), #5 (HIV), and #6 (malaria) causes of disability in the world.[3,4] Twice as many children under fifteen years old contract tuberculosis as previously thought—roughly one million per year worldwide.[6] And there are several other infectious diseases in the top twenty medical conditions. For a large part of the developing world, such as in Africa, infections still account for the leading cause of death and disability; non-malarial febrile illness is the leading cause of childhood mortality in low-income countries. Of the 196 countries in the world, 22 (11 percent) have very high rates of tuberculosis, a combined result of poor distribution of antibiotics and the emergence of multidrug antibiotic-resistant strains.[7] The world at large is not blind to the problem, and, in 2014, the United States along with twenty-six other countries formed the Global Health Security Agenda to deal with infectious disease outbreaks, albeit with an emphasis on preventing pandemics that might reach industrialized countries.[7] This is quite a formidable goal because there is a global mismatch—medical technology is characteristically set up for high-resource settings with plenty of infrastructure, but most of the world's health care is needed in low-resource settings with donated equipment that usually doesn't work.

Tackling infectious disease is going to demand new tools. Enter the cellphone. As of 2013, there were over 630 million cellphone subscribers in Africa, with 93 million of them using smartphones. And these numbers, especially the individuals connected to mobile Internet, are rising quickly. For example, in Nigeria in 2000 there were only 30,000 cellphone subscribers but now there are over 140 million.[1] Just having cellphones so widely distributed enables education. Project Masiluleke in South Africa, for example, sends a million text messages each day to prompt people to be tested and treated for HIV/AIDS.[8] Throughout rural malaria-endemic areas, mobile phone texting provides surveillance and promotes medication adherence. Cellphones enable parents to readily register the birth of a child, allowing governments to plan vaccination schedules. Educational initiatives via texting have been utilized for tuberculosis, malaria, and sexually transmitted diseases. Such programs are beginning to show good results: an educational program called Helping Babies Breathe, developed by the American Academy of Pediatrics, has reduced early neonatal mortality in Tanzania by 47 percent.[9] Mobile phone data from fifteen million people in Kenya were used to map the geo-temporal patterns and human carrier travel dynamics to understand the spread of malaria.[10] Seth Berkley, the CEO of GAVI Alliance, pointed out that "even if cell phone data were to improve upon existing models by just 1 percent, that would translate into the prevention of the deaths of 69,000 children under age five a year."[1]

Recent efforts are making the cellphone more than just a medium of communication. Converting the mobile phone into a high-powered microscope can be readily accomplished through an attachment, and it has been shown to reliably diagnose malaria-infected red blood cells using simple light microscopy and tuberculosis via fluorescent microscopy.[11a] With a laser diode attachment for the smartphone camera, Aydogan Ozcan and his team at UCLA have been able to image a single human cytomegalovirus (CMV) virus, which is 150–300 nanometers (nm), and things that are 1,000 times slimmer than a human hair (100,000 nm).[1] Engineers at Caltech have taken the smartphone-based microscope a step further, eliminating the need for a dedicated light source.[11b]

Microfluidic devices, known as lab-on-a-chip or miniature total analysis systems (µTASs),[12] have been highly successful in facilitating infectious disease diagnoses. Cornell University engineers have used such a chemically based system for a smartphone-assisted diagnosis of the herpes virus that causes Kaposi's sarcoma.[13] A cheap photodetector for an optical readout was used in Rwanda to diagnose HIV in seventy patients (only missing one) within twenty minutes, with sensitivity and specificity that are comparable to the classic ELISA (enzyme-linked immunoabsorbent assay antibody) test.[12] Very low-cost, high-performance diagnostics using paper-based analytic devices, known as µPADs,[12] wick bodily fluids such as blood or urine, with rapid results for both infectious and non-communicable diseases.[14]

But the innovative use of paper has transcended microfluidics, and moved into microscopy. The "origami" microscope, invented by Manu Prakash at Stanford University, is a remarkable, frugal innovation (Figure

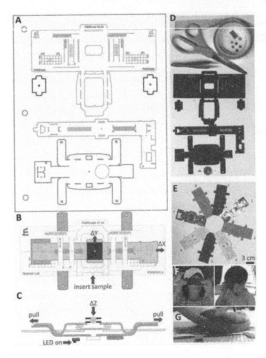

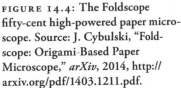

FIGURE 14.4: The Foldscope fifty-cent high-powered paper microscope. Source: J. Cybulski, "Foldscope: Origami-Based Paper Microscope," *arXiv*, 2014, http://arxiv.org/pdf/1403.1211.pdf.

14.4).[15–20] Assembled from a flat sheet of paper within ten minutes, the "Foldscope" fits in the pocket, requires no external power, weighs less than two nickels, and can magnify an object by more than two thousand times. It requires a tiny lens that costs fifty-six cents and a three volt button battery that costs six cents, an LED that costs twenty-one cents, along with some tape and a switch—a cumulative cost of under $1. It has been demonstrated to image Leishmania donovani, Trypanosoma cruzi, E. coli, Schistosoma haematobium, Giardia lamblia, and many other bacteria and parasites.[19]

New ways to rapidly diagnose malaria, which kills approximately six hundred thousand people each year, are indicative of the general trend toward very inexpensive, handheld diagnostic tools.[10,21–23] Malaria parasites produce hemozoin iron crystals when they digest hemoglobin.[24] The crystals can be detected via nanobubbles that form and pop when infected cells are subjected to near-infrared laser energy. The characteristic sound enables detection of malaria (Figure 14.5) "in the same way a destroyer detects a submarine."[24] Not only does this skin test give instant results, detecting malaria at any point in its life cycle, without reagents or drawing

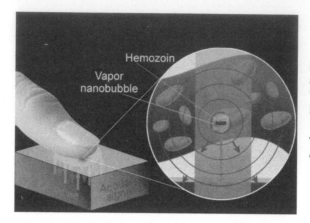

FIGURE 14.5: Nanobubble skin test for malaria. Source: "In This Issue: Transdermal Detection of Malaria," *PNAS* 111 (2013): 877–878, http://www.pnas.org/content/111/3/877.full.pdf+html.

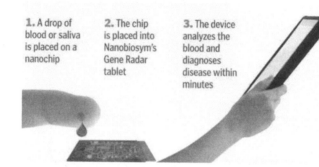

FIGURE 14.6: Gene Radar nanotechnology to diagnose tuberculosis, malaria, and HIV via a mobile device. Source: M. Farrell, "Blood Tests in Minutes, Not Days or Weeks," *Boston Globe*, September 29, 2013, http://www.bostonglobe.com/business/2013/09/29/rapid-blood-test-device-could-game-changer/ZEQQzCzwfNoFATUIW2Le3M/story.html.

blood, but remarkably the sensitivity is at a level of detecting a single infected red blood cell out of eight hundred, without false positives. It takes twenty seconds and costs fifty cents. While first validated in mice, it is now well into clinical trials. Another malaria detection device is worn on the wrist and detects the malaria-induced hemozoin through a reusable, combined magnetic and optical sensor.[25] There are several other novel malaria diagnostics using a quantitative polymerase chain reaction (qPCR) of a pinprick of blood, such as the startup Amplino. Particularly attractive is incorporating qPCR into a handheld mobile device such as Nanobiosym's "Gene Radar,"[26] QuantuMDx, and Biomeme (Figures 14.6 and 14.7).[27–30] The point-of-care sequencing capability expands the potential to do handheld DNA sequencing for a variety of pathogens, including gonorrhea and

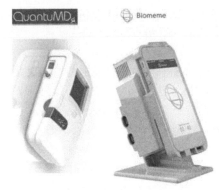

FIGURE 14.7: QuantuMDx and Biomeme handheld qPCR devices.
Sources: http://www.quantumdx.com and http://bio-meme.com.

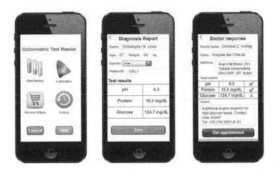

FIGURE 14.8: The Colorimetrix app from University of Cambridge. Source: A. Yetisen,
"A Smartphone Algorithm with Inter-Phone Repeatability for the Analysis of Colorimetric Tests," *Sensors and Actuators B: Chemical* 196 (2014): 156–160. Reprinted with
permission.

other sexually transmitted diseases, West Nile virus, dengue, and tuberculosis. An even simpler method using a colorimetric assay for tuberculosis,
malaria, or HIV, performed directly with a test strip and a smartphone
camera, was developed by the University of Cambridge (Figure 14.8).[31,32]

Other tools are becoming available in low-infrastructure environments.
The precipitous drop in the cost and time required for genome sequencing provides the newfound capability to diagnose antimicrobial resistance
by sequencing the pathogen from culture, and even more quickly from a
sample such as sputum. While body fluids are a great source for molecular
diagnostics, so is breath.[33] Mass spectrometry analysis of breath has been
used to diagnose tuberculosis and was shown to have concordance with
traditional sputum smear microscopy.[33] The latter is not especially a gold
standard, as it missed the diagnosis in 40 percent to 60 percent of cases.

Although breath analysis has not been subject to large-scale testing, a specific point-of-care test known as Xpert, which uses DNA amplification to pick up tuberculosis along with rifampin resistance, was assessed in a randomized trial in South Africa, Zimbabwe, Zambia, and Tanzania in over fifteen hundred individuals.[34] While it did not improve overall morbidity (the primary endpoint), the Xpert test resulted in higher rates of initiating treatment, lower rates of dropout, and was easily accomplished with non-specialized personnel.[34]

The pathogen (bug) is not the only point deserving attention. Indeed, there is vital evidence that has mounted on the importance of the host (person). Malnutrition is exceptionally important in the developing world both because it predisposes individuals to infection, and because the cause of many infections is highly influenced by the gut microbiome.[35–39] More than twenty million children worldwide suffer from severe malnutrition, and fatality rates for hospitalized children with kwashiorkor—a protein-deficient form of malnutrition—is as high as 50 percent. A randomized trial in rural Malawi, representative of sub-Saharan Africa, tested two different antibiotics and matching placebo in 2,767 children, ages six months to five years (Figure 14.9). There was a significant reduction in fatalities with antibiotics, but it is clear the number of deaths is still exceedingly high on treatment.[40,41] But in another study of 317 twin pairs from Malawi, with only one of the twins suffering from acute malnutrition, the gut microbiome showed that the imbalance in bacterial populations could be restored with fortified peanut butter.[37] That represents a significant change from the typical Malawian diet, which is very high in starch. When the less diverse gut microbiome from children with kwashiorkor was transplanted (via fecal samples) to mice, the animals reacquired their lost weight when fed enriched peanut butter. These two impressive studies demonstrated the interrelationship between diet, the microbiome, and the host for acute, severe malnutrition, along with critical salutary intervention with diet and antibiotics. But in another sense they can be seen as just the first step now that the underlying culprit has been identified. In the future, cheap, point-of-care sequencing tools (Figures 14.5, 14.6, 14.7 and 14.8) may be able to precisely and rapidly define the causative bacterial species and imbalance and lead to tailored use of specific probiotics.[42,43]

A perhaps even more amazing application of mobile technology will come when it is paired with the upcoming ability to send a vaccine over

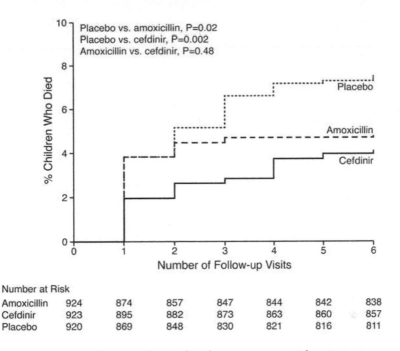

FIGURE 14.9: Antibiotic randomized trial in severe, acute malnutrition management. Source: I. Trehan, "Antibiotics as Part of the Management of Severe Acute Malnutrition," *New England Journal of Medicine* 368 (2013): 425–435.

the Internet. Venter and colleagues have already demonstrated the capability to rapidly create synthetic influenza vaccine matched for the causative strain (Figure 14.10), the code that can, at least theoretically, be electronically dispersed in real time anywhere on the planet for a primary pandemic response system.[44] Of course, influenza is just representative of a large number of microorganisms that could be similarly approached with this strategy. This certainly represents one of the most exciting near-term opportunities of synthetic biology, and exemplifies the fusion of the digital and biological information domains to improve medicine.

Non-Communicable Diseases

Not only is there an increased toll of non-communicable diseases in the developing world, but also cancer alone causes more deaths than the combination of HIV, tuberculosis, and malaria. Of the fourteen million people

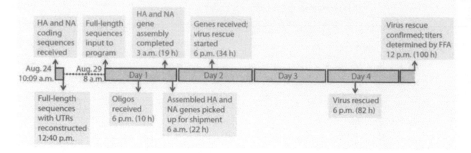

FIGURE 14.10: Influenza virus strain quickly sequenced and vaccine produced, ready for Internet transfer. Source: P. R. Dormitzer et al., "Synthetic Generation of Influenza Vaccine Viruses for Rapid Response to Pandemics," *Science Translational Medicine* 5, no. 185 (2013): 1–13. Reprinted with permission.

diagnosed with cancer each year, 57 percent are individuals from low- and middle-income countries, and they account for approximately 70 percent of the deaths attributable to cancer (and 80 percent of avoidable deaths) worldwide.[45] Such is the case for breast cancer, now clearly a global disease: of the twenty million cases projected to occur in the upcoming decade, more than half will be in low- and middle-income countries.[46] Not only are oncologists and health care professionals of any kind desperately lacking in many of those countries, but so are the treatment centers and infrastructure to effectively diagnose and treat cancer in the developing world. But like the paper-based analytics for infectious diseases, similar innovations are appearing for cancer.[47–49] Engineers at MIT have developed a rapid, low-cost urine test that relies on nanoparticles interacting with tumor proteins for detection.[50] Sangeeta Bhatia, the senior author of the publication said, "For the developing world, we thought it would be exciting to adapt it instead to a paper test that could be performed on unprocessed samples in a rural setting, without the need for any specialized equipment. The simple readout could even be transmitted to a remote caregiver by a picture on a mobile phone."[50] So patients would receive an injection of the nanoparticles and urinate on a paper test strip coated with antibodies that detect the nanoparticles bound to abnormal cancer proteins. In practice, once validated, it would function a lot like a home pregnancy test.[47] The researchers are even gearing up for long-term, as opposed to one-off, measurements, with a nanoparticle formulation that would be implanted under the skin.

Another creative means of detecting cancer uses a smartphone, sunlight, and a tiny DNA sample. Instead of the usual way a PCR is performed, requiring electricity, a primer, and precision electronics to heat and cool the sample, this Cornell-developed method simply taps into sunlight via a lens and disc to drive the PCR.[49] Besides application in cancer testing, another paper-based device, with a per-test cost of ten cents as compared to the usual $4 per test, has been developed to measure liver function tests. A drop of blood flows within the paper that has patterned hydrophobic barriers embedded in it. The results are analyzed and transmitted with a cellphone camera.[51]

The digitizing, GIS approach that has been developed earlier in the book involving sensors, imaging, and omics fully applies to individuals with non-communicable diseases in the developing world. But getting this technology requires more than a mobile phone signal, and a number of crowdfunding projects have been launched to get the sensors—such as The Sensor Project[52]—and the imaging devices—such as Imaging the World[53]—necessary for medical GIS to work. One impressive example of handheld, high-resolution ultrasound imaging has been demonstrated for reducing perinatal mortality. By giving the device to a group of nurse midwives along with just one day of education on recognizing the top five imaging risk factors for pregnancy, such as placenta previa or breech fetal position, there was a greater than 70 percent reduction in fatal events in Ghana and rural India. Newborn health has been addressed via mobile devices in many ways throughout remote parts of Africa and India, with programs such as texting expectant mother gestational age-timed information and getting women with signs of obstetric complications to have facility-based deliveries.[54] And preeclampsia, a condition that affects 10 percent of pregnant women and markedly increases their risk of complications, can be detected early with a low-cost smartphone device for measuring oxygen in the blood.[55] The Sensor Project is raising funds to provide this sensor for eighty thousand women in India, Pakistan, Nigeria, and Mozambique.[52]

The theme of frugal technology, connected to smartphones, is central to the democratization of digital medicine to the developing world. There are even more tools—including a $50 endoscope that can do an entire exam of the ears, nose, and throat, which has been field-tested in the rural mountain area of Taiwan,[56] or a Stanford-developed smartphone ophthalmology kit that for $90 performs the same testing—including the conjunctiva, lens, cornea, and iris—as the standard devices that cost $20,000–$30,000, without a slit lamp.[57] It has been dubbed the "eye phone," and one of its researchers called it "The Instagram for the Eye."[57,58] Using a 3-D printer, the Australian National University creates a tiny microscope lens for one cent, which when attached to a smartphone achieves equivalent functionality to a dermascope that costs $300.[59a] Harvard engineers invented a "universal mobile electrochemical detector," which, for a cost of approximately $25 to manufacture, with a 3.7 V lithium battery, can go for months or even years assaying most routine chemistries like glucose or sodium. This handheld device relies on a smartphone-to-cloud connection to perform real-time, off-site analysis of the sample.[59b,59c] The MIT media lab designed Eye Netra, a $2 reusable attachment to the smartphone that refracts eyes and has restored useful visual acuity to thousands of people in the developing world. But even these relatively low prices could be too high, and so as each of the new tools are developed, from vital sign monitoring to genome sequencing, it is imperative to consider how the cost can be brought down to *de minimis* so that the worldwide opportunity for improved health care can be maximized.

Lack of Health Professionals

Technology at extreme low cost alone is not enough: there still is the critical need for enough health care professionals. This is a profound global problem, as shown in Figure 14.11, with all of the darkened areas representing critically low numbers of doctors, nurses, and midwives.

The mismatch has been described previously, with the areas of lowest health professionals having the highest burden of chronic disease, as measured by DALYs. The World Health Organization estimates there is already a global shortage of well over four million doctors and nurses.[60] As a result of the scarcity of health professionals, innovations are occurring. For example, Mozambique nurses have had added training to perform cesarean sections (to become known as *técnicos do cirurgia*) and achieved equivalent outcomes as physicians.[60] Overall, there has been a major increase and reliance upon community health workers and paraprofessionals in the developing world. Telemedicine is also an attractive strategy and has been getting legs.[61] One of the companies, VSee, has set up a telemedicine field kit with multiple medical devices that enable remote diagnosis. Using eHealth Opinion software, the Virtual Doctor Project connects

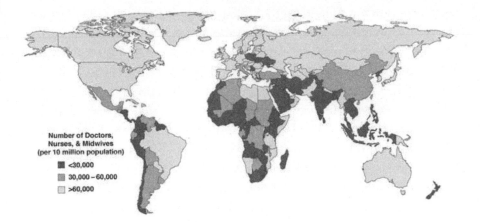

Number of Doctors, Nurses, & Midwives (per 10 million population)
■ <30,000
▨ 30,000 – 60,000
□ >60,000

FIGURE 14.11: Doctors, nurses, and midwives per ten million people, 2011. Source: N. Crisp and L. Chen, "Global Supply of Health Professionals," *New England Journal of Medicine* 370 (2014): 950–957.

rural patients with physician experts in the United States and China. It was initiated in Zambia and has expanded in many parts of the developing world.[62] These pioneering efforts are just the beginning of how patients and health care professionals can be connected, and hopefully someday will effectively deal with the otherwise insurmountable problem of inadequate professional personnel.

Will Flattening Increase or Decrease Health Disparities?

Nicole Ellison, an associate professor in the School of Information at the University of Michigan, predicted, "As more of the global population comes online, there will be increased awareness of the massive disparities in access to health care, clean water, education, food, and human rights."[63] There are two divergent effects of relying on digital tools to improve health care throughout the world. On the one hand, it can, as we've seen through many examples, provide state-of-the-art medicine anywhere there is a mobile signal, and especially with a smartphone with Internet connectivity. That proviso emphasizes the importance of the digital divide, which is surely not just a problem outside the United States. Although the Obama administration put more than \$7 billion into expanding broadband Internet reach throughout America, millions have been left by the e-wayside.[64] Still about 20 percent of adults in the United States do not use the Internet via any means, including a mobile device. It isn't just about lack of computer literacy—access is expensive and seemingly grows ever more so. The underrepresented, minority populations are especially overrepresented in the nonaccess group. Some will be surprised that the United States ranks seventh among the top twenty global economies for Internet adoption.[65] Simply pouring more money into this does not appear to be enough: Joseph Morris, director of Internet policy at the US Commerce Department, calls the digital divide "a complex, multi-faceted challenge with no simple, one-size-fits-all solution."[64] This makes it all the more important to start investigating multiple responses.

Despite this very significant challenge of democratizing broadband access and assuring universal adoption, there are signs that the current infrastructure is helping people we might not have expected it to help. As it turns out, in at least one study, more than 70 percent of homeless individuals getting health care through emergency departments owned cellphones and were eager to receive texts and calls.[66] The authors of the study concluded: "Smartphones can meet their Internet and application needs as they relate to health care when stable housing with landlines, desktops, laptops, and Wi-Fi access are not available."[66] Interestingly, homeless individuals in this study were more receptive to getting health information through texting and calls than their stably housed counterparts.

But there's no question that much more needs to be done to bridge the digital divide, which is a global phenomenon. Virtually every time a mobile health strategy is tested, the evidence mounts that patient care can be improved. A study of diabetics in rural Honduras among individuals with only five years of education and an annual income of \$2,500 showed marked improvement in glucose regulation with just six weeks of Internet-based phone calls.[67] In a poor urban area in Brazil, one hundred elderly patients with multiple chronic illnesses had remote monitoring and showed evidence of less hospitalizations and marked reduction in cost of care.[68]

The head of that project made a point with relevance far beyond his own study: "At a time when the global urban population is aging rapidly and going through a shift from communicable to chronic diseases, our project shows the great potential benefits that [mHealth] technology can bring to urban healthcare globally. We should not wait for this kind of innovation to slowly trickle down to the bottom of the pyramid. This study shows that we can and should start where better access to healthcare is needed most and we should do so using the best available technology."[68]

Whether with regard to rural or urban, the developed or developing world, there's mounting evidence that digital medical tools can democratize medicine. That means that, even as the cost of add-on medical devices drops, so too must the cost of phones. Indeed, smartphone costs are plummeting and projected to get well below $50 in the next few years (Figure 14.12).[69,70] Free Wi-Fi is starting to emerge in the rural developing world, connecting Africa's unconnected through such initiatives as Internet.org and free mobile service plans.[71,72] One simple strategy appears to be helping to some degree—recycling.[73,74] Daniel Fletcher, an engineer researcher at University of California, Berkeley, wrote an op-ed titled "Why Your iPhone Upgrade Is Good for the Poor."[73] The reason for this odd coupling between affluent smartphone purchasers and the poor is simple: "The enormous capabilities of smartphones are being repurposed and redirected for use in the developing world. Seven years ago, when one-megapixel cameras started appearing on phones, I began working with a group of students in my lab at the University of California at Berkeley to see if those cameras could capture images of human cells similar to those captured on our $150,000 research microscope. By attaching a simple set of lenses to a Nokia phone borrowed from my sister, we were able to image blood cells, malaria parasites and the bacteria that cause tuberculosis."[73] Now Fletcher

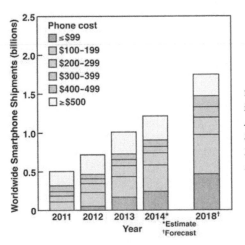

FIGURE 14.12: The relentless reduction in the cost of smartphones. Source: Adapted from "The Rise of the Cheap Smartphone," *The Economist*, April 3, 2014, http://www.economist.com/node /21600134.

and his team are recycling smartphone cameras to detect parasitic worms in Cameroon, retinal diseases in Thailand, and oral cancer in India. Other teams have transformed the recycled smartphones into a portable ultrasound system for imaging.

This kind of innovation is just another example of what it will take for smartphone medicine to reach all corners of the globe. It takes the Gates Foundation, Vodafone Foundation, Verizon Foundation, the World Health Organization, and countless others to make it happen. And unwittingly, even those with "affluenza" are helping the cause when they get the latest smartphone upgrade. Back to Gutenberg's press, smartphones are markedly promoting literacy—we're in the midst of a "reading revolution" in poor countries.[75] This will further improve the uptake of health education initiatives. Over time, we'll asymptotically approach the end goal of making digital medicine available to all people. We can't afford to leave any folks behind.

Chapter 15

The Emancipated Consumer

"It's not the owner of a stage coach who builds railways."
—Joseph Schumpeter[1]

"The relationship between doctors and patients will surely be much more equal; indeed, health will be the business primarily of patients, with doctors as advisers, guides, and facilitators. Much of medical practice will be conducted online, with online consultations routine."
—Richard Smith, editor, *British Medical Journal*[2]

"We can only see a short distance ahead, but we can see plenty there that needs to be done."
—Alan Turing[3]

Profound change has not ever gone over well in the medical community. When Dr. Ignaz Semmelweis published findings in 1848 that hand washing could markedly reduce mortality, it was summarily dismissed by doctors who were offended at the suggestion they should wash their hands and saw no scientific explanation for the claim.[4] Likewise, in 1990, there was strong opposition to the use of ultrasound during pregnancy. In the *American Journal of Obstetrics & Gynecology* (the leading medical journal of the specialty), in response to an article touting its use, Ewigman and colleagues wrote: "These authors' ethical argument that patient autonomy justifies offering ultrasonography routinely would lead to unrealistic expectations of physicians and the health care system, cause an inappropriate legal liability, and may be harmful to patients."[5] Even the stethoscope, invented by Rene Laennec in 1816, was not received well by doctors, to put it mildly. There was an intense rebellion against the new device for interfering with the traditional physical examination. It took twenty years for the stethoscope to be generally accepted, with the proclamation in 1838 that "Auscultation has withstood the most violent assaults that have ever stormed any science."[6] Today, we're in a similar predicament. We are at the cusp of something far more impactful than a stethoscope.

My patient, Kim Goodsell (see Chapter 2), who has been called "The Patient of the Future," wrote me in a recent e-mail about the changes medicine is undergoing, and the challenges that patients and physicians each are facing. "Novel challenges," she wrote, "will undoubtedly continue to arise as patients have unlimited access to information, become engaged and better educated." Nevertheless, she saw that "the compass heading is pointing towards a future collaborative patient/physician dynamic. Thank you again for affording me the opportunity to participate in 'co-production of medical intelligence.'"

These few sentences capture, from the perspective of a patient, the essence of emancipation, the ultimate form of democratization. With medicine that is digitized and unplugged, we move from the flip phone to flipping the entire health care model. We now have the formula for freedom, for relative autonomy from the canonical medical community that forced patients to be subservient and dependent.[7-18] No longer.

As medicine radically upgrades from a heterogeneous admixture of art and science to become a real data science—one with the individual's GIS and predictive analytics—the world of health care is irrevocably transformed. Where once patients could not even access their data, today they can actually generate and own it.[19-24] Where once there were profound access issues, today there is medicine on demand. Today patients can rapidly diagnose their skin lesion or child's ear infection without a doctor. That's just the beginning. We've seen how your smartphone will become central to labs, physical exams, and even medical imaging; and how you can have ICU-like monitoring in the safety, reduced expense, and convenience of your home. How a supercomputer will process hundreds of millions of articles in seconds about your symptoms and data from the complete, fully updated medical literature, and how, when a medical evaluation is necessary, you can now immediately "see" the doctor, with pricing information and ratings of doctors and hospitals instantly accessible via your mobile device. In short, we're seeing an unprecedented shake-up in a paternalistic profession that has never been seriously challenged since the era of Hippocrates, 400 BC. As in every other sector in our lives, when data becomes eminently portable and granular, when there's so much more of it and it's free flowing, fully transparent, and there's seemingly unlimited computing power to process it, historic change takes place. Just think of the impact of Google or Amazon. But searching and purchasing anywhere, anytime is old stuff. The ability to share data and contextually compute it led the nonmedical world to progress many could not have even imagined, leading to advances like driverless cars. The shake-up of medicine will be just as strong.

Driverless Cars and Doctorless Patients?

When I'm driving in back of a big truck and can't see anything in front of me except the truck, I feel vulnerable because I'm lacking critical information about the traffic and road conditions. The parallels to health care are irresistible. The big truck is our doctor, out in front, dominating the road, and unwittingly obscuring our vision. With our medical GIS in place, there are no trucks obscuring our view of the road. Instead of one-off measurements in the contrived setting of a doctor's office, we can now capture our own data in real time, in the real world. Suddenly, we patients are the ones driving in front of the big truck.

Of course, that's not the only way to avoid the big truck problem. We could just leave the driving to Google. The Google driverless car is now electric without brakes, an accelerator, or a steering wheel.[25–31] It has a 360-degree field of view—eliminating any blind spots—with hundreds of laser and radar sensors. It can now recognize pedestrians and bicyclists, along with their hand gestures, better than human beings can, and has a sterling safety record that surpasses driving by humans. And it can be summoned by a smartphone. If we can build self-driving cars with this sensor and computing technology, are we ready to develop doctorless patients?

I think the answer is much more autonomous patients, yes, without question, but truly doctorless, no. Much of the practice of medicine will reboot and bypass the current deeply engrained, sacrosanct doctor-dependent operations.[32-34] Just as you can do your electrocardiogram by your smartphone today and get an immediate computer algorithm inter-pretation, so it will be the case for many diagnostics in the future, such as whether you have sleep apnea or hypertension—anything with simple quantitative data to record, process, and quickly return to you. If you're just interested in checking symptoms, it will be straightforward to enter them into your little device, connect to a supercomputer, and get a top five list with likelihood rankings of what condition you have. And, of course, a comprehensive list of references if you're so inclined to look them up.

Diagnostics extend to labs. The home pregnancy test alone was a big deal when it appeared in drugstores in 1977, but very soon you won't have to go too far to get any routine lab test, from determining whether you have an infection and what bug it is, to organ function and much more.

But the doctorless autonomy isn't restricted to just making a diagnosis. There's the monitoring dimension, which represents a sweet spot for tech-nology. Close, quantitative, real-time assessment of mood for depression, heart performance parameters (like cardiac output, stroke volume, and fluid status) for heart failure, lung and respiratory function for asthma and chronic obstructive pulmonary disease, and muscle movements and tremor for Parkinson's are some examples. There's hardly a chronic condition that isn't amenable to sensor, lab, and smartphone monitoring. Once the data are captured, it's just about having validated algorithms that provide con-tinuous feedback to the patient.

I've already seen the impact of going doctorless with the most elemental monitoring task—monitoring blood pressure—in so many of my patients with hypertension. Once the goal parameters are set, such as 130 systolic and 80 diastolic, the patient takes over. With frequent readings and nice data visualization on the smartphone screen, the patient now diagnoses whether control has been achieved and if not, why not. Having the context of one's life experiences provides an immense advantage for pinpointing the reasons and remedies for abnormal blood pressures.

Of course there are limits as to how far one can go doctorless. It's not going to ever extend to most treatments, such as surgeries or proce-dures. (We may have robots to vacuum the house and assist surgeons, but they're not going to be developed for one's own heart bypass.) Although likely not for many prescriptions, I do believe that once we fully accept

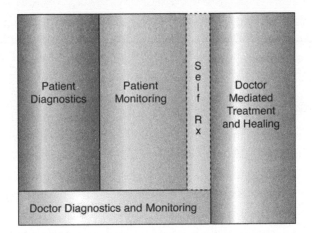

FIGURE 15.1: The doctorless patient model: Diagnostics and monitoring largely become the domain of the patient.

patient-generated data and algorithmic interpretation, the movement to self-prescription for certain conditions will take hold (Figure 15.1, dotted line). For instance, when a parent has objective proof that a child has strep throat, along with a record of allergies and all prior drug exposures, why is a doctor necessary to get an antibiotic prescription? To many health care policy aficionados, "doctorless" might denote transfer of responsibility to nurses, pharmacists, and other medical personnel. Patients having so much of their information will indeed make that transfer of authority possible, but the big shift will be the diminished dependence on all health care professionals in favor of patients' relative autonomy.

It's only when we get to healing that the line for autonomy is drawn (Figure 15.1). Now we're talking about providing the paramount human definitive treatment combined with healing touch. This really builds on the differentiating capabilities of doctors—having an exceptional base of knowledge and judgment to contextualize the patient's information, while at the same time providing empathy, inspiration, and support for the individual to stay or get healthy. As Abraham Verghese nicely put it in his 2014 Stanford medical school commencement address, "You can heal even when you cannot cure by that simple act of being at the bedside—your presence."[35] To that end, it's hard to improve upon the words of the sixteenth century physician Paracelsus (his full name was Philippus Aureolus Theophrastus Bombastus von Hohenheim!), "This is my vow: to love the sick, each and all of them, more than if my own body were at stake."[35] There will never be algorithms, supercomputers, avatars, or robots to pull that off. The Turing test for medicine won't be passed, and Kurzweil's "singularity" will remain a plurality.

A New Wisdom of the Body

While some people connect "wisdom of the body" with the notion that infants can innately self-select their diet for proper nutrition[36] or that food cravings during pregnancy are for critically needed nutrients,[37] the term goes back to Walter Cannon's *The Wisdom of the Body* book published in 1932.[38] Cannon, an eminent Harvard physiologist and medical researcher, developed the concept of homeostasis—that our body tightly regulates itself, with steady-state levels of blood glucose, electrolytes, pH, body temperature, and many other components. Each of these has feedback loops to promote auto-correction and equilibrium, such as sweating or shivering to maintain the body temperature in a narrow range, and thirst or concentrating the urine to preserve fluid status. Cannon even got into the concept of social homeostasis, understanding the human organism's complex interactions with the environment and one another. These breakthrough ideas reshaped our understanding of human physiology.

Now we are ready to move to a new dimension of human homeostasis, because each individual can have direct feedback loops with their medical data. This represents an external rather than intrinsic mechanism of achieving a steady state. Going back to the example of blood pressure, our body often does not do well in maintaining the ideal range. But now that information can be continually fed back to the individual, who can take corrective steps, be it determining one's salt sensitivity, interactions with diet, and the quantitative effects of weight loss, exercise, and sleep, and, if needed, the right medications and doses. It's not just an individual's sensor, lab, or image data; it's also data sharing among peers that can provide yet another feedback loop for the person. While not part of Cannon's original theories about homeostasis, it's not hard to envision a new path toward an improved equilibrium of key health metrics that goes beyond what a doctor could ever provide. Unlike many of the body's functions, this external system of autoregulation is not automatic. It involves active participation of the individual, and can be facilitated by computer processing of one's data with algorithm-derived recommendations for action. These added feedback loops, propelled by having data that was previously unattainable, have the potential to supplement and enhance Cannon's inherent wisdom of our bodies.

Ownership of Your Body's Data

Throughout the book I've stressed the importance of ownership of your data. Clearly, the value of one's data in a data-driven economy has markedly increased. You just have to consider the valuation of Amazon, Facebook, and Twitter to appreciate how much personal data is worth now, not to mention the imminent flood of individualized health and medical data. To highlight one individual's take on the importance of ownership of data, let's turn to Jennifer Lyn Morone.[39] She has created both a software platform for personal data management and a company (JLM Inc.)—an incorporated person—for explicit ownership and control of her data. Using a multisensor device that she wears most of the time (Figure 15.2) and software called DOME (database of me), the platform can be used to package and sell her "biological, physical and mental services" data. This will likely be an N of 1 experiment, but it does reflect the newfound regard for how valuable—and how important ownership of—your data has become.

The ownership of property is central to emancipation. It's unquestionably appropriate, a self-evident truth, that each individual is entitled to own all of his or her medical data. This is not about the intellectual property of patents; it's about the body property of patients. We're not there yet, but just as the value of patient engagement was rather precipitously realized, so will we reach an inflection point that sees right of ownership vigorously pursued. We'll have to get beyond medical paternalism, have the data eminently portable, develop innovative technology for patients to generate their own data, and have the digital infrastructure for sharing it.

It's not as simple a concept as it seems. Ownership is not zero or one. You think you own your cellphone data, but companies like Verizon or AT&T have control over your account access, your data storage, and what third parties may get to see of your information (like the National Security Agency). We've seen a good model of ownership of genomic data at the Coriell Institute for Medical Research, whereby a person's genome is stored in their computers and can only be selectively accessed by one's providers once owner-approved. But ownership, once achieved, is not enough. It has

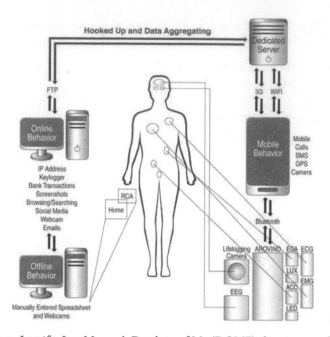

FIGURE 15.2: Jennifer Lyn Morone's Database of Me (DOME) that stores and manages all the data she generates. Source: Adapted from Jennifer Lyn Morone, Inc., accessed August 12, 2014, http://jenniferlynmorone.com/.

to be protected. One's data cannot be used, sold, or disseminated without the willingness and consent of the individual. And that cannot be by an app that prompts (forces) you to tap "I Agree." As we've reviewed, most people are willing to have their data used for research if their identity is protected. Some, like Jennifer Lyn Morone, might even be happy to sell their data and give up anonymity. With the very worrisome rise in personal data and smartphone theft, new methods for maximizing security of one's medical information are desperately needed. The onus of minimizing vulnerability to e-theft extends to the individual. Fortunately, new methods for personal data ownership with protection are being developed.[40,41] Eventually, each individual will not only own their data, but it will be secured in a personal cloud or system, with the owner granting rights for others to access. Now that's a flip.

Rebooting the Employer-Employee Relationship

The antiquated American health system is employer-based, unique in the industrialized world, yet has been largely embraced by the Affordable Care

Act.[42] To achieve real emancipation, we would need to put an end to employees' dependence on their employers for health insurance, an idea that has been revitalized in the wake of the recent Supreme Court decision (*Burwell vs. Hobby Lobby*, in favor of employers for what coverage, such as for contraception, they are willing to provide).[43] While we should continue to strive for employer-based emancipation, it appears that we may well be stuck with this illogical, inefficient, and outdated platform for some time.[43,44] Nevertheless, there is at least one part that can be addressed— corporate wellness programs. They are a big business of over $6 billion a year, with more than half of companies with over fifty employees having a wellness initiative that costs an average of $600 per employee.[45-47] The goals include less consumption of medical resources, reduced absenteeism, durable changes in healthy lifestyle, or improved productivity. But they have been largely unsuccessful; indeed many would say a blatant failure, when one looks at them for a return on investment.[48-50] These programs typically offer screens for hypertension and cholesterol, performance of a health-risk assessment, antismoking and weight reduction efforts, and health education. Some provide financial incentives for reaching particular goals. In general, however, they simply scratch the surface of what health is, and in some ways—as when they require annual checkups as most do—these wellness programs may well make things worse.[51-54] Now that employees will own their data, can wellness programs be rebooted and made successful?[53,55-58] While no one could rightfully question the importance of lifestyle for impacting health, durable behavioral change is exceptionally difficult to achieve. However, we've not previously had the tools to get granular data on each individual's pattern, no less their relevant and panoromic medical information. And now that we can, there are data suggesting that when good behavior, such as exercise, is fun and "gamified," it's particularly well received and motivating.[59] Having participated in some employer-managed competition groups for lifestyle improvement (detailed in the postscript of *The Creative Destruction of Medicine*),[60a] it's hard for me to think that harnessing such competitive juices would not be influential. British Petroleum and Autodesk are large companies that have incorporated wearable sensors for their employee base, initially tracking exercise and sleep.[60b] Appirio, with 1,000 employees, claims a savings of five percent of their health care bill with the use of wearable activity tracking sensors.[60c] With the imminent commercial availability of much broader medical sensor capabilities, such programs could markedly expand. An important caveat to come back to is the employee ownership of the data, his or her decision whether to share it, and, if affirmative, that such information would not be used in any way without the individual's knowledge and consent. These programs would be better known as employee—not employer—health and wellness initiatives, denoting the power of the information holder and generator.

Taking Down Walls

Freeing the people from traditional medical shackles entails freeing the data, and there are signs this is beginning to take off. One such indication is the joint venture of Philips, a major supplier of medical sensors, with Salesforce, a pioneer in cloud computing, to create an "open cloud-based health care platform" for software developers, providers, medical device producers, and insurance companies.[61,62] Open medicine initiatives build on the Power of One. If you've never seen that one-minute video, and are looking to be inspired by individuals who've impacted the world, it's worth a look: https://www.youtube.com/watch?v=GOXOImxK0NA. When the data and information of each individual become part of a platform that can benefit all people, that's another dimension of emancipation. I like to think of it as "reverse epidemiology." Today's epidemiology is the study of populations, a top-down approach, analyzing patterns, causes, and effects of health and disease conditions. By its nature, it is average-oriented, because it is looking at data from large numbers of people without high definition of any particular person. In contrast, reverse epidemiology, now with the unprecedented capability of having each individual's GIS, is bottom-up. Loaded with the power of many, we can now fully acknowledge that average is over, and understand much more precisely what drives health and disease. Until now, however, too may initiatives have centered on data collection, going from big data to bigger data, overlooking the critical goal of deep analytics and learning. Today less than 5 percent of such data are analyzed. It's time to move from data hoarding to knowledge transforming.[63] We are at a unique time in medicine where transdisciplinary efforts will be required to not only free and amass the data, but also to maximize its value. The lack of boundaries between academia, the life science industry, and the information technology sectors is just what is needed to tap into

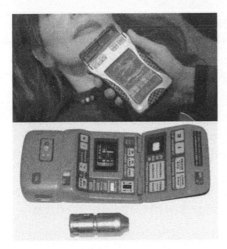

FIGURE 15.3: The tricorder device with detachable high-resolution scanner. Sources: (top) io9, accessed August 12, 2014, http://io9.com/meet-the-teams-who-are-building-the-worlds-first-medic-1543000639; and (bottom) Starbase 484, accessed August 12, 2014, http://sb484.kersare.net/nova/index.php/wiki/view/page/24.

the boundless potential. To say "it takes a village" would be an extreme understatement. But when accomplished, this will get us to the wisdom of the population.

The Road to Emancipation

One of my intellectual and visionary heroes is Marshall McLuhan, the original media guru, whom you will note has been widely quoted in this book. Back in 1962, he published *The Gutenberg Galaxy: The Making of Typographic Man.*[64] He provided remarkable insights on the impact of the printing press and subsequent forms of mass communication. This led him to propose, way ahead of their time, the concepts of a "global village" and "surfing" related to the accumulated body of recorded works of human art and knowledge. Even though it would be many decades before the Web existed, he foresaw the ability to rapidly and mutidirectionally move from one document to another in the electric age. He realized that it wasn't about the technology *per se,* but that the people and their culture were reinvented by books and printed materials. McLuhan probably understood the impact of mass media better than and before anyone else, and realized that without the printing press there would not ever have been media and the world as he knew it and as it has further evolved today.

In a similar vein, there would not be democratized medicine without smartphones, along with the entire digital infrastructure that supports them. The culture stands to change dramatically once the tricorder comes online. In *Star Trek*'s vision of the twenty-third century, Dr. Leonard "Bones" McCoy used the handheld device to immediately diagnose disease with three input recording functions—GEO (geographical), MET (meteorological) and BIO (biological) (Figure 15.3).[65–67] In 2015, just before *Star Trek*'s fiftieth anniversary, Qualcomm is awarding a $10 million X-Prize to the team that produces the best version of a modern tricorder.[68] There's a big difference, however: this device isn't meant to be used by Bones or a doctor, but rather a device that is fully operated by the patient.

Moving From Autocratic to Semi-Autonomous Medicine

We know the road to medical emancipation is within our reach. The technology to digitize human beings has required innovation; it's here and continuing to rapidly evolve. But that's relatively easy compared with its implementation and achieving the democratization of health care. So I propose the iMedicine Galaxy (Figure 15.4) as a model to bring the requisite interdependent forces together and achieve transformation. Let me briefly review what we need from each of them.

The Large Employers

The biggest companies have hundreds of thousands of employees and are paying billions of dollars a year on health care. Rather than having these companies leave the United States to reduce their tax burden to be able to pay employee health care costs (such as Abbvie or Medtronic) or go bankrupt (like General Motors), this book provides a far more attractive option. Lead the charge; buck the system. If they promote democratized medicine for all their employees, it would strip down the costs of care for office visits, hospitalizations, lab tests, imaging, and other diagnostic procedures. Why should these companies pay for an elaborate ultrasound study, with charges averaging $800–$1,000, when in most cases the necessary imaging can be done as part of a mobile-technology-driven physical exam, and essentially for free? Why are patients kept in the hospital or even admitted, at the $4,500 per day average fee, when they could have remote monitoring? Why pay for sleep studies in a hospital laboratory that cost at least $3,500 when they could be performed for free, at least a screening exam, in the patient's home? Why haven't such employers enforced all of the hundreds of Choosing Wisely's modest but clear-cut recommendations of unnecessary tests and procedures?[69] These are but some of the ways large

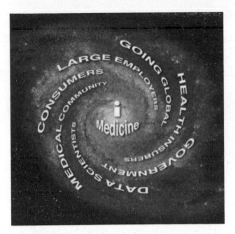

FIGURE 15.4: The iMedicine Galaxy. Source: Adapted from the Whirlpool Galaxy (Spiral Galaxy M51, NGC 5194) imaged by NASA and ESA using the Hubble Space Telescope.

employers can exercise their massive muscle to reduce costs and catalyze bottom-up medicine. They also can have marked influence over the big health insurance companies they hire, like United Health, Wellpoint, and Aetna, but no big company has moved to use it yet. If just one becomes a first mover, and challenges the status quo along with the baseless charges of "rationing," this could take off.

Consumers

It may be harder to mobilize the consumer base even though they are at peak frustration and have picked up a considerably higher burden of their health care costs in the form of "co-pays." We know they want their data, want better engagement and interaction with their doctors, and are the prey for countless unnecessary tests and procedures every year. There hasn't yet been the one big thing or the public figure with overpowering clout to rally the public. But that doesn't mean it won't happen. A large international survey of adult smartphone users in fourteen countries, including the United States, has shown that 80 percent of consumers want to interact with their doctors on mobile devices, and nearly 70 percent would prefer to get medical advice on their mobile devices instead of going to the doctor's office.[70,71] The social network is in place; there are multiple precedents for a grassroots revolution. When Apple debuted their 2014 new software campaign that included the Health and Healthkit apps, it was called "You're More Powerful Than You Think."[72a] They sure got that one right. Collectively, more like a sleeping giant waiting to erupt. The power of people indeed seems palpable when you see that parents of kids with muscular dystrophy are the key drivers in writing the regulatory guidance documents for new drug approvals[72b] or the magnificent spike in research fundraising for the Amyotrophic Lateral Sclerosis Association driven by social media and the "Ice Bucket Challenge."[72c]

Government

Although tremendous political capital was used to get the Affordable Care Act passed, and access has improved as a result, nothing has been done to truly democratize American medicine. We have an outmoded Center for Medicare and Medicaid Services (CMS) with 140,000 codes for describing needed care, even nine for different injuries caused by turkeys. Estimates of fraud run as high as $272 billion per year, giving rise to the notion that the only people who love America's health care system are its thieves. Tackling even a fraction of that fraud could free up the $40 billion investment needed to drive the use of interoperable electronic medical records that include each individual's GIS. So too would doing something about CMS reimbursement, which needs a complete overhaul with proper information systems in place, and a simplified, rational system that fosters rather than suppresses consumer empowerment. Why does CMS reimburse $300 for a simple drug interaction genotype when it costs pennies to perform? And why doesn't CMS negotiate pricing of drugs, devices, and diagnostics like every other country in the developed world? If you ask health policy wonks or legal eagles "why?" the answer is "that's the law." Well, it's time to change the law.

Patient ownership of data also demands changes to the law. The White House continues to publish white papers on the "Consumer's Privacy Bill of Rights" without any follow-up action. Protected ownership can only be asserted with new legislation. The Federal Trade Commission needs to be charged with proscribing the selling of an individual's medical data without their unconditional consent.[73] If we cannot provide the absolute maximal assurance of privacy and security for each individual's medical data, or if the government decides to effectively tolerate hacking, medical emancipation will never get started. New technologies to achieve this critical goal, such as quantum cryptography,[74a] deserve careful consideration.

The Food and Drug Administration, while paying lip service to innovation, has done little to alter its regulatory approval processes to catalyze the ways that each individual can assume a greater role in their medical care. That's why your smartphone isn't as smart as it could be[74b] in an ambiguous regulatory landscape.[74c] It will be a hard and slow slog to new medicine without marked changes in the way innovation is recognized and encouraged, such as by faster reviews, conditional approval, and tight post-market electronic surveillance.

Surely, even if lack of progressive reimbursement and regulatory procedures in the United States means that democratized medicine does not take hold here, these frugal—and better—technologies will find homes in the rest of the world, where there are virtually no perverse incentives and immediate opportunities for nonlinear, leapfrog change. This has already been seen with multiple devices, including the modern handheld ultrasound stethoscope. The most far-reaching opportunity that lies ahead for governments around the world is the support and promotion of massive online open medicine (MOOM)—the planetary database of everyone's de-identified GIS that enables matching and the best-known treatment and outcomes for all human beings.

Doctors and the Medical Community

With disinclination to change embedded in the medical community, reflected by the average time gap of seventeen years from innovation to adoption in medical practice, we need a cultural change. While digital native doctors just coming out of medical school or finishing residency training understand the sea change that is unfolding, there are millions of practicing physicians around the world who do not. We don't have time to wait for a new generation of doctors and health care professionals to take hold. Cultural change is exceedingly difficult, but given the other forces in the iMedicine galaxy, especially the health care economic crisis that has engendered desperation, it may be possible to accomplish. An aggressive commitment to the education and training of practicing physicians to foster their use of the new tools would not only empower their patients, but also themselves. Eliminating the enormous burden of electronic charting or use of scribes by an all-out effort for natural language processing of voice during a visit would indeed be liberating. It's long overdue for physicians and health professionals to be constantly cognizant of actual costs, eliminate unnecessary tests and procedures,[75a] and engage in exquisite electronic communication, which includes e-mail, and sharing notes and all data. If financial incentives are needed, they may be well worth the investment.

Data Scientists

Government and recalcitrant doctors are major potential impediments, but the biggest bottleneck to advancing the field is unquestionably dealing with data. Here is the paradox: there is no shortage of data to capture and aggregate, yet we have a profound shortage of the people who can write algorithms, separate signals from noise, and actualize the full potential of computers to perform deep learning. While there are a relatively small number of such professionals in a world inundated with data challenges in every sector, health care has not been able to attract enough gifted individuals proportional to the size and importance of this field. The irony now is that data scientists are the ones being referred to as the "high priests."[75b]

The iMedicine Galaxy

Patients, companies, employers, doctors, government, data scientists: these major forces are like stars gravitationally bound in a galaxy, the movement of any one of them affecting all the others. What I have tried to convey here is that we have a new galaxy in the making. Just as the printing press was the great object around which modern culture has orbited, the smartphone and iMedicine are forcing a comparable transformation. There is a time ahead when every human being has the potential for the same access to medical care, provided they have a mobile signal, when medicine is no longer paternalistic and autocratic, when a reformation and a renaissance of medicine can take hold. Only then can we move from an era in which Desmore asserted, "medicine is not a science, [but] empiricism founded on a network of blunders" to a new medicine as a real data science with each individual capable of calling the shots, making the choices.

As with any model, particularly one that is going after a new, emancipated form of medicine, there will be no shortage of naysayers. They'll say that it's ill founded, underdeveloped, impossible, or even irrational. Yet technology to achieve this is accelerating; we have what were envisioned as futuristic, twenty-third century capabilities now. I consider it inevitable; the biggest question is the matter of timing. For centuries medicine's galaxy has orbited the doctor. If just one of those major forces exerts itself, these changes could happen very quickly. Maybe Angelina Jolie will tip the scales and change medicine's orbit. Or maybe it will be you.

ACKNOWLEDGMENTS

Once the digitization of medicine got legs, it became increasingly clear that democratization would be the next phase. It took a deep dive in research and writing to try and capture this movement, and predict where it would be going, and I'm especially grateful to many individuals who facilitated this endeavor.

First and foremost is my editor, Thomas—TJ—Kelleher, editorial director, sciences, at Basic Books, whom I've had the real privilege to work with on both *The Creative Destruction of Medicine* and this book. He has been exceptional in helping me sharpen the message, providing remarkably insightful critique and inspiration. Next is my family my wife, Susan, and our adult kids, Sarah and Evan—who have tolerated my long periods of hibernation in order to get this project accomplished. I'm especially thankful to my colleagues at Scripps, including Michelle Miller, who helped me get the over 1,250 references and 80 figures ready for publication (which numbered over 120 before cutting proved to be necessary); Steven Steinhubl, who reviewed the manuscript and provided great feedback and emotional support; and Janet Hightower, who worked on the graphics. Our Scripps Translational Science Institute (STSI) grant from the National Institutes of Health (NIH/NCATS 8 UL1 TR001114) has been critical for energizing all of us to be innovative in thinking about the future of medicine and how human health can be improved. My literary agent, Katinka Matson, president at Brockman Inc., has been a great resource at many points along the way.

I want to acknowledge my bias and potential conflict of interests. Clearly, I have a bias that technology will radically transform and improve health care. I've tried to calibrate that bias throughout the book, by harping on the issues that are critical to address, such as preserving privacy, security, human touch, and the need for rigorous validation. You are likely in touch with my techno-optimistic predisposition and hopefully will see the balance. I am an advisor to various companies for which I help develop their digital medicine strategy. The consumer related ones are AT&T, Google, and Walgreens. The digital sensor companies are Dexcom (I'm on the board of directors), Sotera Wireless, Quanttus, and Perminova. I also work with the genomics companies Illumina, Edico Genome, Genapsys, and Cypher to help get sequencing technology integrated into medical care. Cypher Genomics, in particular, was cofounded by three STSI colleagues and me to automate interpretation of whole genome sequences. At STSI, we were fortunate to receive a grant from the Qualcomm Foundation to advance our research efforts in digital and genomic medicine. Working with these diverse consumer, life science, and information technology companies has given me enhanced perspective about the opportunities and challenges for democratizing medicine. I have zero interest in promoting any of these companies or their products in this book, and have done everything possible to prevent that from occurring. Nevertheless, the relationships are important for you to know about.

I'd like to express my appreciation to all of you who read this book and actively contribute to the democratization of medicine. It'll take a galaxy, not a village, to get this achieved. But when it happens, we'll all be in for better health. What could be more important and far-reaching?

NOTES

Chapter 1

1. E. Hill, "Smart Patients," *The Lancet* 15 (2014): 140–141.

2. D. M. Cutler, "Why Medicine Will Be More Like Walmart," in *MIT Technology Review*. September 20, 2013, http://www.technologyreview.com/news/518906/why-medicine-will-be-more-like -walmart/.

3. E. Brynjolfsson and A. McAfee, *The Second Machine Age* (New York, NY: W.W. Norton & Company, 2014), p. 96.

4. "Essay: The Playboy Interview: Marshall McLuhan," *Playboy*, March 1969, accessed August 12, 2014, Next Nature, http://www.nextnature.net/2009/12/the-playboy-interview-marshall-mcluhan/.

5. "The Package" *(Seinfeld)*, in *Wikipedia*, accessed August 12, 2014, http://en.wikipedia.org/wiki/ The_Package_(Seinfeld).

6. D. L. Frosch et al., "Authoritarian Physicians and Patients' Fear of Being Labeled 'Difficult' Among Key Obstacles to Shared Decision Making," *Health Affairs* 31, no. 5 (2012): 1030–1038.

7. L. Landro, "How Doctors Rate Patients," *Wall Street Journal*, March 31, 2014, http://online.wsj .com/news/articles/SB10001424052702304432604579473301109907412.

8. B. Greene, "Doctor, LOOK at Me," *CNN Opinion*, March 9, 2014, http://edition.cnn.com/2014 /03/09/opinion/greene-doctor-patient-computers/index.html.

9. L. Landro, "Health-Care Providers Want Patients to Read Medical Records, Spot Errors," *Wall Street Journal*, June 9, 2014, http://online.wsj.com/articles/health-care-providers-want-patients-to-read -medical-records-spot-errors-1402354902.

10. "Uberification of the US Service Economy," *Schlaf's Notes*, April 4, 2014, http://schlaf.me/post /81679927670.

11. A. Srivastava, "2 Billion Smartphone Users by 2015 : 83% of Internet Usage from Mobiles," Daze Info, January 23, 2014, http://www.dazeinfo.com/2014/01/23/smartphone-users-growth-mobile-internet -2014-2017/.

12. M. Zuckerberg, "Mark Zuckerberg on a Future Where the Internet Is Available to All," *Wall Street Journal*, July 7, 2014, http://online.wsj.com/articles/mark-zuckerberg-on-a-future-where-the -internet-is-available-to-all-1404762276.

13. "The Rise of the Cheap Smartphone," *The Economist*, April 5, 2014, http://www.economist.com /node/21600134/print.

14. M. Honan, "Don't Diss Cheap Smartphones. They're About to Change Everything," *Wired*, May 16, 2014, http://www.wired.com/2014/05/cheap-smartphones.

15. A. Kessler, "The Cheap-Smartphone Revolution," *Wall Street Journal*, May 12, 2014, http:// online.wsj.com/news/articles/SB10001424052702304101504579546393363686978.

16. R. Snow, C. Humphrey, and J. Sandall, "What Happens When Patients Know More Than Their Doctors? Experiences of Health Interactions After Diabetes Patient Education: A Qualitative Patient-Led Study," *British Medical Journal* 3 (2013): e003583.

17. T. Shenfield, "Collaborating with Patients in the Digital Information Age," HealthWorks Collective, April 23, 2014, http://healthworkscollective.com/talishenfield/160421/collaborating-patients -digital-information-age.

18. U. Wijayawardhana, "Smart Patients," Island Online, April 23, 2014, http://www.island.lk/index .php?code_title=100181&page=article-details&page_cat=article-details.

19. J. Erdmann and H. Schunkert, "Forty-five Years to Diagnosis," *Neuromuscular Disorders* 23 (2013): 503–505.

20. J. N. Honeyman et al., "Detection of a Recurrent DNAJB1-PRKACA Chimeric Transcript in Fibrolamellar Hepatocellular Carcinoma," *Science* 343 (2014): 1010–1014.

21. R. Winslow, "Teen Helped Research Her Own Disease," *Wall Street Journal,* February 27, 2014, http://online.wsj.com/news/articles/SB10001424052702304071004579409260544992476.

22. L. Neergaard, "Teen Helps Scientists Study Her Own Rare Disease," Associated Press, February 27, 2014, http://bigstory.ap.org/article/teen-helps-scientists-study-her-own-rare-disease.

23. S. Naggiar, "Teen Makes Genetic Discovery of Her Own Rare Cancer," *NBC News,* April 16, 2014, http://www.nbcnews.com/health/cancer/teen-makes-genetic-discovery-her-own-rare-cancer -n75991.

24. G. Marcus, "Open-Sourcing a Treatment for Cancer," *New Yorker,* February 27, 2014, http:// www.newyorker.com/online/blogs/elements/2014/02/open-sourcing-cancer.html?printable =true&currentPage=all.

25. J. Wilson, "Kids Who Don't Cry: New Genetic Disorder Discovered," in *CNN Health,* March 20, 2014, http://www.cnn.com/2014/03/20/health/ngly1-genetic-disorder/.

26a. M. Might and M. Wilsey, "The Shifting Model in Clinical Diagnostics: How Next-Generation Sequencing and Families Are Altering the Way Rare Diseases Are Discovered, Studied, and Treated," *Genetics in Medicine,* 2014, http://www.nature.com/gim/journal/vaop/ncurrent/full/gim201423a.html.

26b. S. Mnookin, "One of a Kind," *The New Yorker,* July 21, 2014, http://www.newyorker.com/ magazine/2014/07/21/one-of-a-kind-2.

27. G. M. Enns et al., "Mutations in NGLY1 Cause an Inherited Disorder of the Endoplasmic Reticulum-Associated Degradation Pathway," *Genetics in Medicine,* 2014, http://www.nature.com/gim/ journal/vaop/ncurrent/full/gim201422a.html.

28. A. Regalado, "Business Adapts to a New Style of Computer," *MIT Technology Review,* May 20, 2014, http://www.technologyreview.com/news/527356/business-adapts-to-a-new-style-of-computer/.

29. E. Topol, *The Creative Destruction of Medicine* (New York, NY: Basic Books, 2012).

30. W. Ghonim, *Revolution 2.0: The Power of the People Is Greater Than the People in Power* (New York, NY: Houghton Mifflin Harcourt, 2012).

Chapter 2

1a. M. Specter, "The Operator," *New Yorker,* February 4, 2013, http://www.newyorker.com/ reporting/2013/02/04/130204fa_fact_specter?currentPage=all.

1b. H. Brubach, "Dislocation, Italian Style," *New York Times,* July 18, 2014, http://www.nytimes .com/2014/07/19/opinion/sunday/dislocation-italian-style.html?ref=opinion.

2. J. Aw, "Patients Who Question Their Doctors Are Changing the Face of Medicine—and Physicians Are Embracing the Shift," *National Post,* March 11, 2014, http://life.nationalpost.com/2014/03/11 /patients-who-question-their-doctors-are-changing-the-face-of-medicine-and-physicians-are-embracing -the-shift/.

3. B. J. Fikes, "The Patient from the Future, Here Today," *San Diego Union Tribune,* March 5, 2014, http://www.utsandiego.com/news/2014/Mar/05/kim-goodsell-genomic-medicine-topol/.

4. K. Goodsell, "Profile on Kim Goodsell," Wireless Life-Sciences Alliance, accessed August 13, 2014, http://wirelesslifesciences.org/summit-speakers/#Kim%20Goodsell.

5a. J. J. Liang et al., "LMNA-Mediated Arrhythmogenic Right Ventricular Cardiomyopathy and Charcot-Marie-Tooth Type 2B1: a Patient-Discovered Unifying Diagnosis," *Heart Rhythm Society* abstract update, 2014, http://ondemand.hrsonline.org/common/presentation-detail.aspx/15/23/1386/9568.

5b. E. Yong, "DIY Diagnosis: How an Extreme Athlete Uncovered Her Genetic Flaw Mosaic," Mosaic Science, August 19, 2014, http://mosaicscience.com/story/diy-diagnosis-how-extreme-athlete-uncovered-her-genetic-flaw.

6. "Imhotep," *Wikipedia,* accessed August 13, 2014, http://en.wikipedia.org/wiki/Imhotep.

7. T. Koch, *Thieves of Virtue* (Cambridge, MA: The MIT Press, 2012), 23.

8. R. M. Veatch, *Patient, Heal Thyself* (New York, NY: Oxford University Press, 2009).

9. J. Katz, *The Silent World of Doctor and Patient* (Baltimore, MD: Johns Hopkins University Press, 1983).

10. L. B. McCullough, "Was Bioethics Founded on Historical and Conceptual Mistakes about Medical Paternalism?" *Bioethics* 25, no. 2 (2011): 66–74.

11. T. Koch, *Thieves of Virtue.*

12. S. F. Kurtz, "The Law of Informed Consent: From 'Doctor Is Right' to 'Patient Has Rights,'" *Syracuse Law Review* 50, no. 4 (2000): 1243–1260.

13. "Oath of Hippocrates," *in* J. Chadwick and W. Mann, *Hippocratic Writings* (Harmondsworth, UK: Penguin Books, 1950), accessed from National Institutes of Health, August 13, 2014, http://history.nih.gov/research/downloads/hippocratic.pdf.

14. S. B. Nuland, "Autonomy Amuck," New Republic Online, June 5, 2009, http://www.powells.com/review/2009_06_25.

15. L. Lasagna, "Hippocratic Oath," 1964, *in* P. Tyson, "The Hippocratic Oath Today," NOVA, March 27, 2001, http://www.pbs.org/wgbh/nova/body/hippocratic-oath-today.html.

16. Katz, *The Silent World of Doctor and Patient,* p. 4–8.

17. Ibid., 8.

18. Ibid., 7.

19. Veatch, *Patient, Heal Thyself,* p. 45.

20. Katz, *The Silent World of Doctor and Patient,* p. 9.

21. Ibid., 17–20.

22. Ibid., 13.

23. M. Siegler, "The Progression of Medicine From Physician Paternalism to Patient Autonomy to Bureaucratic Parsimony," *Archives of Internal Medicine* 145 (1985): 713–715.

24. Koch, *Thieves of Virtue,* 31–33.

25. American Medical Association, accessed August 13, 2014, http://www.ama-assn.org/ama.

26. R. Collier, "American Medical Association Membership Woes Continue," *Canadian Medical Association Journal* 183, no. 11 (2011): E713–E714.

27. R. Winslow, "The Wireless Revolution Hits Medicine," *Wall Street Journal,* February 14, 2013, http://online.wsj.com/news/articles/SB10001424052702303404704577311421888663472.

28. American Medical Association, *Code of Medical Ethics,* 1847, http://www.ama-assn.org/ama/pub/about-ama/our-history/history-ama-ethics.page.

29. American Medical Association, *Principles of Medical Ethics,* 1903, http://www.ama-assn.org/ama/pub/about-ama/our-history/history-ama-ethics.page.

30. Veatch, *Patient, Heal Thyself,* p. 33.

31. American Medical Association, *Principles of Medical Ethics,* 1958, http://www.ama-assn.org/ama/pub/about-ama/our-history/history-ama-ethics.page.

32. American Medical Association, *Principles of Medical Ethics,* 1980, http://www.ama-assn.org/ama/pub/about-ama/our-history/history-ama-ethics.page.

33. D. Oken, "What to Tell Cancer Patients: A Study of Medical Attitudes," *Journal of the American Medical Association* 175, no. 13 (1961): 1120–1128.

34. S. Mukherjee, *The Emperor of All Maladies* (New York, NY: Scribner, 2010).

35. Veatch, *Patient, Heal Thyself,* 17.

36. Ibid., 34.

37. L. Keslar, "Lucian Leape: Rooting Out Disrespect," *Proto,* Fall 2013, http://protomag.com/assets/interview-lucian-leape-rooting-out-disrespect.

38. L. L. Leape et al., "Perspective: A Culture of Respect, Part 2: Creating a Culture of Respect," *Academic Medicine* 87, no. 7 (2012): 853–858.

39. J. E. Brody, "Medical Radiation Soars, with Risks Often Overlooked," *New York Times,* August 20, 2012, http://well.blogs.nytimes.com/2012/08/20/medical-radiation-soars-with-risks-often -overlooked/.

40. E. Topol, *The Creative Destruction of Medicine* (New York, NY: Basic Books, 2012), 126–127.

41. R. F. Redberg and R. Smith-Bindman, "We Are Giving Ourselves Cancer," *New York Times,* January 31, 2014, http://www.nytimes.com/2014/01/31/opinion/we-are-giving-ourselves-cancer.html.

42. L. Landro, "Where Do You Keep All Those Images?," *Wall Street Journal,* April 8, 2013, http:// online.wsj.com/news/articles/SB10001424127887323419104578374420820705296.

43. L. Landro, "New Tracking of a Patient's Radiation Exposure," *Wall Street Journal,* May 21, 2013, http://online.wsj.com/news/articles/SB10001424127887324767004578489413973896412.

44. Veatch, *Patient, Heal Thyself,* 69.

45. K. S. Sibert, "Today's 'Evidence-Based Medicine' May Be Tomorrow's Malpractice," *aPenned-Point,* February 13, 2014, http://apennedpoint.com/todays-evidence-based-medicine-may-be-tomorrows -malpractice/.

46. E. Oster, "Patients Can Face Grave Risks When Doctors Stick to the Rules Too Much," FiveThir-tyEight Science, June 13, 2014, http://fivethirtyeight.com/features/patients-can-face-grave-risks-when -doctors-stick-to-the-rules-too-much/.

47. M. J. Pencina et al., "Application of New Cholesterol Guidelines to a Population-Based Sample," *New England Journal of Medicine* 370 (2014): 1422–1431.

48. J. D. Abramson and R. F. Redberg, "Don't Give More Patients Statins," *New York Times,* November 14, 2013, http://www.nytimes.com/2013/11/14/opinion/dont-give-more-patients-statins.html.

49. J. Karlawish, "Statins by Numbers," *New York Times,* November 30, 2013, http://www.nytimes .com/2013/11/30/opinion/statins-by-numbers.html.

50. J. P. A. Ioannidis, "More Than a Billion People Taking Statins?" *Journal of the American Medical Association* 311, no. 5 (2014): 463–464.

51. H. Moses et al., "The Anatomy of Health Care in the United States," *Journal of the American Medical Association* 310, no. 18 (2013): 1947–1963.

52. G. Kolata, "Bumps in the Road to New Cholesterol Guidelines," *New York Times,* November 26, 2013, http://www.nytimes.com/2013/11/26/health/heart-and-stroke-study-hit-by-a-wave-of-criticism .html.

53. Veatch, *Patient, Heal Thyself,* 220.

54. B. McFadden, "Cholesterol Overhaul," *New York Times,* July 8, 2013, http://www.nytimes.com /slideshow/2012/07/08/opinion/sunday/the-strip.html.

55. H. E. Bloomfield et al., "Screening Pelvic Examinations in Asymptomatic, Average-Risk Adult Women: An Evidence Report for a Clinical Practice Guideline from the American College of Physicians," *Annals of Internal Medicine* 161 (2014): 46–53.

56. L. T. Krogsbøll et al., "General Health Checks in Adults for Reducing Morbidity and Mortality from Disease: Cochrane Systematic Review and Meta-Analysis," *British Medical Journal* 345 (2012): e7191.

57. C. Lane, "The NIMH Withdraws Support for DSM-5," *Psychology Today,* May 4, 2013, http:// www.psychologytoday.com/blog/side-effects/201305/the-nimh-withdraws-support-dsm-5.

58. D. W. Bianchi et al., "DNA Sequencing versus Standard Prenatal Aneuploidy Screening," *New England Journal of Medicine* 370, no. 9 (2014): 799–808.

59. N. Biller-Andorno and P. Jüni, "Abolishing Mammography Screening Programs? A View from the Swiss Medical Board," *New England Journal of Medicine* 370 (2014): 1965–1967.

60. T. M. Burton, "FDA Approves HPV Test That Could Be Used Instead of Pap Smear," *Wall Street Journal,* April 24, 2014, http://online.wsj.com/news/articles/SB10001424052702304788404579522182353831794.

61. A. Pollack, "Looser Guidelines Issued on Prostate Screening," *New York Times,* May 4, 2013, http://www.nytimes.com/2013/05/04/business/prostate-screening-guidelines-are-loosened.html.

62. American Urological Association, "AUA Releases New Clinical Guideline on Prostate Cancer Screening," news release, May 3, 2013, https://www.auanet.org/advnews/press releases/article.cfm ?articleNo=290.

63. B. Goldacre, "Statins Are a Mess: We Need Better Data, and Shared Decision Making," *British Medical Journal* 348 (2014): g3306.

64. Katz, *The Silent World of Doctor and Patient*, 39.

Chapter 3

1. E. L. Eisenstein, *The Printing Press as an Agent of Change* (New York, NY: Cambridge University Press, 1979), 243.

2. M. McLuhan, *The Gutenberg Galaxy* (Toronto, Canada: University of Toronto Press, 1962).

3. H. Blodget and T. Danova, "Future of Digital: 2013," Business Insider, November 12, 2013, http://www.businessinsider.com/the-future-of-digital-2013-2013-11.

4. J. Matthew, "The World's Most Expensive Book Just Sold For Over $14 Million," Business Insider, November 26, 2013, http://www.businessinsider.com/worlds-most-expensive-book-sells-for-14 -million-2013-11.

5. Eisenstein, *The Printing Press as an Agent of Change*, 152.

6. Ibid., 159.

7. N. Silver, *The Signal and the Noise* (New York, NY: Penguin, 2012), 2.

8. N. Carr, *The Shallows: What the Internet Is Doing to Our Brains* (New York, NY: W.W. Norton, 2010), 69.

9. Silver, *The Signal and the Noise*, 12.

10. Eisenstein, *The Printing Press as an Agent of Change*, 41.

11. McLuhan, *The Gutenberg Galaxy*, 124.

12. Silver, *The Signal and the Noise*, 7.

13. Ibid., 3.

14. Carr, *The Shallows: What the Internet Is Doing to Our Brains*, 71.

15. "The Book of Jobs: Hope, Hype, and Apple's iPad," *The Economist*, January 30–February 5, 2010.

16. Eisenstein, *The Printing Press as an Agent of Change*, 75.

17. Ibid., 119.

18. McLuhan, *The Gutenberg Galaxy*, 206.

19. S. Turkle, *Alone Together* (New York, NY: Basic Books, 2011), 166.

20. Eisenstein, *The Printing Press as an Agent of Change*, 132.

21. T. Standage, "Social Networking in the 1600s," *New York Times*, June 23, 2013, http://www .nytimes.com/2013/06/23/opinion/sunday/social-networking-in-the-1600s.html?pagewanted=all.

22. Eisenstein, *The Printing Press as an Agent of Change*, 53.

23. V. Goel, "Our Daily Cup of Facebook," *New York Times*, August 13, 2013, http://bits.blogs .nytimes.com/2013/08/13/our-daily-cup-of-facebook/?ref=technology&_r=0&pagewanted=print.

24. N. Silver, *The Signal and the Noise*, 2.

25. "The March of Protest," *The Economist*, June 29, 2013, http://www.economist.com/printedition /2013-06-29.

26. W. Ghonim, *Revolution 2.0: The Power of the People Is Greater Than the People in Power* (New York: Houghton Mifflin Harcourt, 2012).

27. Eisenstein, *The Printing Press as an Agent of Change*, 129.

28. M. B. Hall, *The Scientific Renaissance 1450–1630* (New York, NY: Harper & Brothers, 1962), 130.

29. Eisenstein, *The Printing Press as an Agent of Change*, 268.

30. N. Schmidle, "A Very Rare Book," *New Yorker*, December 16, 2013, http://www.newyorker.com /reporting/2013/12/16/131216fa_fact_schmidle.

31. I. Cohen, "Review of The Mathematical Papers of Isaac Newton," *Scientific American* 1 (1968): 139–144.

32. Eisenstein, *The Printing Press as an Agent of Change*, 245.

33. Ibid., 179.

34. Carr, *The Shallows: What the Internet Is Doing to Our Brains*, 74.

35. Ericsson, "On The Pulse of the Networked Society," *Ericsson Mobility Report*, June 2014, http://www.ericsson.com/res/docs/2014/ericsson-mobility-report-june-2014.pdf.

36. A. Toor, "Cellphones Ignite a 'Reading Revolution' in Poor Countries," *The Verge*, April 23, 2014, http://www.theverge.com/2014/4/23/5643058/mobile-phone-reading-illiteracy-developing-countries-unesco.

37. Eisenstein, *The Printing Press as an Agent of Change*, 113.

38. Ibid., 250.

39. J. Rifkin, *Third Industrial Revolution* (New York, NY: Palgrave MacMillan, 2011), 18.

40. E. L.Eisenstein, *The Printing Press as an Agent of Change* (Cambridge, United Kingdom: Cambridge University Press, 2009), 32.

41. "The Ninety-Five Theses," *Wikipedia*, accessed August 13, 2014, http://en.wikipedia.org/wiki/The_Ninety-Five_Theses.

42. J. Katz, *The Silent World of Doctor and Patient* (Baltimore, MD: Johns Hopkins University Press, 1984), 7–8.

43. American Medical Association, *Code of Medical Ethics*, 1847, http://www.ama-assn.org/ama/pub/about-ama/our-history/history-ama-ethics.page.

44. Eisenstein, *The Printing Press as an Agent of Change*, 303.

45. "Sacrosanctum Concilium," *Wikipedia*, accessed August 13, 2014, http://en.wikipedia.org/wiki/Sacrosanctum_Concilium.

46. "Ad Orientem," *Wikipedia*, accessed August 13, 2013, http://en.wikipedia.org/wiki/Ad_orientem.

47. J. Schuessler, "Wired: Putting a Writer and Readers to a Test," *New York Times*, November 30, 2013, http://www.nytimes.com/2013/11/30/books/arnon-grunberg-is-writing-while-connected-to-electrodes.html.

48. "MIT Researchers Create Wearable Books," *PressTV*, January 30, 2014, http://www.presstv.ir/detail/2014/01/30/348428/mit-researchers-create-wearable-books/.

Chapter 4

1. A. Jolie, "My Medical Choice," *New York Times*, May 14, 2013, http://www.nytimes.com/2013/05/14/opinion/my-medical-choice.html.

2. "23andMe and the FDA: A Regulator Brings a Genetic Company to a Halt," *The Economist*, November 30, 2013, http://www.economist.com/news/business/21590941-regulator-brings-genetics-company-halt-and-fda/print.

3. M. Dowd, "Cascading Confessions," *New York Times*, May 15, 2013, http://www.nytimes.com/2013/05/15/opinion/dowd-cascading-confessions.html.

4. "Angelina Jolie," *Wikipedia*, accessed August 13, 2014, http://en.wikipedia.org/wiki/Angelina_Jolie.

5. K. Blake, "Angelina Jolie Effect: Breast Cancer Awareness vs. Knowledge," Health News from Health Canal, December 20, 2013, http://www.healthcanal.com/cancers/breast-cancer/46121-angelina-jolie-effect-breast-cancer-awareness-vs-knowledge.html.

6. A. L. Caplan, "The Actress, the Court, and What Needs to Be Done to Guarantee the Future of Clinical Genomics," *PLoS Biology* 11, no. 9 (2013): e1001663.

7. T. E. Board, "Angelina Jolie's Disclosure," *New York Times*, May 18, 2013, http://www.nytimes.com/2013/05/18/opinion/angelina-jolies-disclosure.html.

8. D. L. G. Borzekowski et al., "The Angelina Effect: Immediate Reach, Grasp, and Impact of Going Public," *Genetics in Medicine*, December 19, 2013, http://www.nature.com/gim/journal/vaop/ncurrent/pdf/gim2013181a.pdf.

9. A. Breznican, "Angelina Jolie Recounts 'All the Kindness' That Helped Her Through Her Health Scare," *Entertainment Weekly*, March 5, 2014, http://insidemovies.ew.com/2014/03/05/angelina-jolie-health-exclusive/.

10. E. Christakis, "Angelina's Mastectomy: Altered Bodies Are Already the Norm," *TIME,* May 15, 2013, http://ideas.time.com/2013/05/15/angelinas-surgery-altered-body-parts-are-already-the-norm/print/.

11. L. Rothman, "Angelina Jolie's Public-Image Turnaround," *TIME,* May 14, 2013, http://entertainment.time.com/2013/05/14/angelina-jolies-public-image-turnaround/print/.

12. J. Kluger and A. Park, "The Angelina Effect," *TIME,* May 27, 2013, http://content.time.com/time/subscriber/printout/0,8816,2143559,00.html.

13. D. Kotz, "Increase in Breast Cancer Gene Screening: The Angelina Jolie Effect," *Boston Globe,* December 3, 2013, http://www.boston.com/lifestyle/health/blogs/daily-dose/2013/12/03/increase-breast-cancer-gene-screening-the-angelina-jolie-effect/2HsXjeZh6MdTE5B8T3nGMI/blog.html.

14. L. Corner, "Why Are More Women Having Mastectomies?," *The Independent,* December 1, 2013, http://www.independent.co.uk/life-style/health-and-families/features/why-are-more-women-having-mastectomies-8969889.html.

15. P. Orenstein, "Reacting to Angelina Jolie's Breast Cancer News," *6th Floor,* May 15, 2013, http://6thfloor.blogs.nytimes.com/2013/05/15/reacting-to-angelina-jolies-breast-cancer-news/.

16. K. Pickert, "Lessons from Angelina: The Tricky Calculus of Cancer Testing," *TIME,* May 15, 2013, http://nation.time.com/2013/05/15/lessons-from-angelina-the-tricky-calculus-of-cancer-testing/print/.

17. P. B. Bach, "A Pioneering Force," *Town & Country,* October 2013, http://www.townandcountrymag.com/print-this/dr-kristi-funk-pink-lotus?page=all.

18. K. Funk, "A Patient's Journey: Angelina Jolie," Breast Cancer 101, May 14, 2013, http://pinklotusbreastcenter.com/breast-cancer-101/2013/05/a-patients-journey-angelina-jolie/.

19. A. W. Kepler, "Angelina Jolie's Aunt Dies of Breast Cancer," *New York Times,* May 27, 2013, http://artsbeat.blogs.nytimes.com/2013/05/27/angelina-jolies-aunt-dies-of-breast-cancer/.

20. M. Melton, "Dr. Kristi Funk," *Los Angeles Magazine,* September 10, 2013, http://www.lamag.com/lawoman/article/2013/09/10/dr-kristi-funk.

21. R. C. Rabin, "No Easy Choices on Breast Reconstruction," *New York Times,* May 20, 2013, http://well.blogs.nytimes.com/2013/05/20/no-easy-choices-on-breast-reconstruction/.

22. D. Grady, T. Parker-Pope, and P. Belluck, "Jolie's Disclosure of Preventive Mastectomy Highlights Dilemma," *New York Times,* May 15, 2013, http://www.nytimes.com/2013/05/15/health/angelina-jolies-disclosure-highlights-a-breast-cancer-dilemma.html.

23. H. D. Nelson et al., "Risk Assessment, Genetic Counseling, and Genetic Testing for BRCA-Related Cancer in Women: A Systematic Review to Update the US Preventive Services Task Force Recommendation," *Annals of Internal Medicine* 160 (2014): 255–266.

24. G. Rennert et al., "Clinical Outcomes of Breast Cancer in Carriers of BRCA1 and BRCA2 Mutations," *New England Journal of Medicine* 357, no. 2 (2007): 115–123.

25. R. Winslow, "Early Ovary Removal Reduces Long-Term Cancer Risk: Study," *Wall Street Journal,* February 24, 2013, http://online.wsj.com/news/article_email/SB10001424052702304834704579403421175065210-lMyQjAxMTA0MDIwNTEyNDUyWj.

26. A. P. Finch et al., "Impact of Oophorectomy on Cancer Incidence and Mortality in Women with a BRCA1 or BRCA2 Mutation," *Journal of Clinical Oncology* 32, no. 15 (2014): 1549–1554.

27. N. D. Kauff et al., "Risk-Reducing Salpingo-oophorectomy in Women with a BRCA1 or BRCA2 Mutation," *New England Journal of Medicine* 346, no. 21 (2002): 1609–1615.

28. S. J. Hoffman and C. Tan, "Following Celebrities' Medical Advice: Meta-Narrative Analysis," *British Medical Journal* 347 (2013): f7151.

29. J. Bulluz and S. J. Hoffman, "Katie Couric and the Celebrity Medicine Syndrome," *Los Angeles Times,* December 18, 2013, http://www.latimes.com/opinion/commentary/la-oe-hoffman-celebrities-health-advice-20131218,0,3861833.story.

30. K. Kamenova, A. Reshef, and T. Caulfield, "Angelina Jolie's Faulty Gene: Newspaper Coverage of a Celebrity's Preventive Bilateral Mastectomy in Canada, the United States, and the United Kingdom," *Genetics in Medicine* 16, no. 7 (2013): 522–528, http://www.nature.com/gim/journal/vaop/ncurrent/full/gim2013199a.html.

31. "Myriad Genetics Q1 Revenues Shoot up 52 Percent; Angelina Jolie Effect Cited," *GenomeWeb*, November 6, 2013, http://www.genomeweb.com/clinical-genomics/myriad-genetics-q1-revenues-shoot -52-percent-angelina-jolie-effect-cited.

32. R. C. Rabin, "In Israel, a Push to Screen for Cancer Gene Leaves Many Conflicted," *New York Times,* November 27, 2013, http://www.nytimes.com/2013/11/27/health/in-israel-a-push-to-screen-for -cancer-gene-leaves-many-conflicted.html.

33. E. Murphy, "Inside 23andMe Founder Anne Wojcicki's $99 DNA Revolution," *Fast Company,* October 14, 2013: http://www.fastcompany.com/3018598/for-99-this-ceo-can-tell-you-what-might-kill -you-inside-23andme-founder-anne-wojcickis-dna-r.

34. FDA, "Inspections, Compliance, Enforcement, and Criminal Investigations: Warning Letter to Ann Wojcicki," November 22, 2013, http://www.fda.gov/ICECI/EnforcementActions/WarningLetters /2013/ucm376296.htm.

35. A. Pollack, "FDA Orders Genetic Testing Firm to Stop Selling DNA Analysis Service," *New York Times,* November 26, 2013, http://www.nytimes.com/2013/11/26/business/fda-demands-a-halt-to-a-dna -test-kits-marketing.html.

36. A. Pollack, "Genetic Tester to Stop Providing Data on Health Risks," *New York Times,* December 6, 2013, http://www.nytimes.com/2013/12/06/business/genetic-tester-to-stop-providing-data-on-health -risks.html.

37. F. Polli, "Why 23andMe Deserves a Second Chance," *Forbes,* January 14, 2014, http://www .forbes.com/sites/fridapolli/2014/01/14/why-23andme-deserves-a-second-chance/.

38. T. Ray, "Facing FDA Warning Letter and Lawsuit, Can 23andMe Stay True to Its DTC Credo in 15 Days?," *GenomeWeb,* December 4, 2013, http://www.genomeweb.com/print/1319176?utm_source =SilverpopMai%C9 PGx Uncertainty.

39. R. Rekhi, "A Government Ban on 23andMe's Genetic Testing Services Ignores Reality," *The Guardian,* December 4, 2013, http://www.theguardian.com/commentisfree/2013/dec/04/23andme -consumer-genomics-fda-ban-regulation/print.

40. R. Khan, "The FDA's Battle With 23andMe Won't Mean Anything in the Long Run," *Slate,* November 25, 2013, http://www.slate.com/blogs/future_tense/2013/11/25/fda_letter_to_23andme _won_t_mean_anything_in_the_long_run.html.

41. R. Khan and D. Mittelman, "Rumors of the Death of Consumer Genomics Are Greatly Exaggerated," *Genome Biology* 14 (2013): 139, http://genomebiology.com/2013/14/11/139.

42. C. J. Janssens, "It Is Game Over for 23andMe, and Rightly So," *The Conversation,* November 26, 2013, http://theconversation.com/it-is-game-over-for-23andme-and-rightly-so-20744.

43. L. Jamal, "What Do We Gain or Lose by Regulating 23andMe?," *Berman Institute of Bioethics Bulletin*, November 27, 2013, http://bioethicsbulletin.org/archive/what-do-we-gain-or-lose-by-regulating -23andme/print/.

44. T. Hay, "23andMe Flap With FDA Just a Bump in the Road, One Genetics-Testing Investor Says," *Wall Street Journal*, December 16, 2013, http://blogs.wsj.com/venturecapital/2013/12/16/23andme -flap-with-fda-just-a-bump-in-the-road-one-genetics-testing-investor-says/tab/print/.

45. H. Greely, "The FDA Drops an Anvil on 23andMe—Now What?," *Law and Biosciences Blog,* November 25, 2013, https://blogs.law.stanford.edu/lawandbiosciences/2013/11/25/the-fda-drops-an -anvil-on-23andme-now-what/.

46. M. F. Murray, "Why We Should Care About What We Get for 'Only $99' From a Personal Genomic Service," *Annals of Internal Medicine* 160, no. 7 (2014): 507–508.

47. G. Neff, "In the Battle Over Personal Health Data, 23andMe and the FDA Are Both Wrong," *Slate,* December 13, 2013, http://www.slate.com/blogs/future_tense/2013/12/13/_23andme_vs_the_fda _both_are_wrong.html.

48. R. Bailey, "Let My Genes Go! And Leave 23andMe Alone," Reason.com, November 29, 2013, http://reason.com/archives/2013/11/29/why-the-fda-should-leave-23andme-alone/print.

49. S. Usdin, "The Sky Isn't Falling," *BioCentury,* June 17, 2013, http://www.biocentury.com/biotech -pharma-news/politics/2013-06-17/scotus-myriad-protects-biotech-patenting-but-leaves-important-gray -areas-a13.

50. E. Vayena, "Direct-to-Consumer Genomics on the Scales of Autonomy," *Journal of Medical Ethics,* May 5, 2014, http://jme.bmj.com/content/early/2014/05/05/medethics-2014-102026.full.

51. J. K. Wagner, "The Sky Is Falling for Personal Genomics! Oh, Nevermind. It's Just a Cease & Desist Letter from the FDA to 23andMe," *Genomics Law Report,* December 3, 2013, http://www .genomicslawreport.com/index.php/2013/12/03/the-sky-is-falling-for-personal-genomics-oh-nevermind -its-just-a-cease-desist-letter-from-the-fda-to-23andme/.

52. "Doing the Genomic Revolution Right," *Huffington Post,* December 20, 2013, http://www .huffingtonpost.com/tricia-page/doing-the-genomic-revolution-right_b_4480887.html?view =print&comm_ref=false.

53. A. J. Burke, "23andMe's FDA Battle Provokes Furious Debate," Techonomy, December 2, 2013, http://techonomy.com/2013/12/just-tip-iceberg-23andme-medicine/.

54. "Multiple Testing an Issue for 23andMe," *Bits of DNA,* November 30, 2013, http://liorpachter .wordpress.com/2013/11/30/23andme-genotypes-are-all-wrong/.

55. "23andMe: State of Debate," *Bio-IT World,* November 27, 2013, http://www.bio-itworld.com /2013/11/27/23andme-state-of-debate.html.

56. M. Hiltzik, "23andMe's Genetic Tests Are More Misleading Than Helpful," *Los Angeles Times,* December 15, 2013, http://www.latimes.com/business/la-fi-hiltzik-20131215,0,1359952.column.

57. K. Hill, "The FDA Just Ruined Your Plans to Buy 23andMe's DNA Test as a Christmas Present," *Forbes,* November 25, 2013, http://www.forbes.com/sites/kashmirhill/2013/11/25/fda-23andme/.

58. L. Kish, "The Social Conquest of Medicine: The 23andMe and Conflict," *HL7 Standards,* January 7, 2014, http://www.hl7standards.com/blog/2014/01/07/23andme/.

59. J. Kiss, "23andMe Admits FDA Order 'Significantly Slowed Up' New Customers," *The Guardian,* March 9, 2014, http://www.theguardian.com/technology/2014/mar/09/google-23andme-anne -wojcicki-genetics-healthcare-dna/print.

60. A. Krol, "Show, Don't Tell: 23andMe Pursues Health Research in the Shadow of the FDA," *Bio-IT World,* March 24, 2014, http://www.bio-itworld.com/2014/3/24/show-dont-tell-23andme -pursues-health-research-shadow-fda.html.

61. D. Kroll, "Why The FDA Can't Be Flexible With 23andMe," *Forbes,* November 28, 2013, http:// www.forbes.com/sites/davidkroll/2013/11/28/why-the-fda-cant-be-flexible-with-23andme-by-law/.

62. P. Loftus, "23andMe Stops Genetic Test Marketing," *Wall Street Journal,* December 2, 2013, http://online.wsj.com/news/articles/SB10001424052702304579404579234503409624522.

63. P. Loftus, "Genetic Test Service 23andMe Ordered to Halt Marketing by FDA," *Wall Street Journal,* November 25, 2013: http://online.wsj.com/news/articles/SB1000142405270230428100457921 9893863966448.

64. P. Loftus and R. Winslow, "23andMe CEO Responds to FDA Warning Letter," *Wall Street Journal,* November 27, 2013, http://online.wsj.com/news/articles/SB1000142405270230333290457922 4093983156448.

65. G. Lyon, "Stopping 23andMe Will Only Delay the Revolution Medicine Needs," *The Conversation,* November 25, 2013, http://theconversation.com/stopping-23andme-will-only-delay-the-revolution -medicine-needs-20743.

66. V. Hughes, "23 and You," *Medium,* December 4, 2013, https://medium.com/matter /66e87553d22c.

67. "The FDA vs. 23andMe: A Lesson for Health Care Entrepreneurs," *Knowledge at Wharton (K@W),* December 18, 2013, http://knowledge.wharton.upenn.edu/article/fda-vs-23andme-lesson-health -care-entrepreneurs/.

68. R. Bailey, "Leave 23andMe Alone," Reason.com, February 25, 2014, http://reason.com/archives /2014/02/25/leave-23andme-alone/print.

69. H. Binswanger, "FDA Says, 'No Gene Test for You: You Can't Handle the Truth,'" *Forbes,* November 26, 2013, http://www.forbes.com/sites/harrybinswanger/2013/11/26/fda-says-no-gene-test-for -you-you-cant-handle-the-truth/.

70. M. Allison, "Direct-to-Consumer Genomics Reinvents Itself," *Nature Biotechnology* 30, no. 11 (2012): 1027–1029.

71. G. J. Annas and S. Elias, "23andMe and the FDA," *New England Journal of Medicine* 370 (2014): 985–988.

72. M. White, "The FDA is Not Anti-Genetics," *Pacific Standard,* January 17, 2014: http://www .psmag.com/navigation/nature-and-technology/fda-anti-genetics-72987/.

73. C. Wood, "Does the FDA Think You're Stupid?," Casey Research, December 5, 2013, http://www.caseyresearch.com/cdd/does-the-fda-think-youre-stupid.

74. C. Farr, "23andMe Remains Optimistic Despite FDA Issues: 'We Are Not Going Anywhere' (Exclusive)," *Venture Beat,* December 7, 2013, http://venturebeat.com/2013/12/07/23andme-remains-defiant-despite-fda-issues-we-are-not-going-anywhere-exclusive/2/.

75. L. Downes and P. Nunes, "Regulating 23andMe to Death Won't Stop the New Age of Genetic Testing," *Wired,* January 1, 2014, http://www.wired.com/opinion/2014/01/the-fda-may-win-the-battle-this-holiday-season-but-23andme-will-win-the-war/.

76. N. S. Downing and J. S. Ross, "Innovation, Risk, and Patient Empowerment The FDA-Mandated Withdrawal of 23andMe's Personal Genome Service," *Journal of the American Medical Association* 311, no. 8 (2014): 793–794.

77. "Irresistible Force Meets Immoveable Object," *Nature Biotechnology* 32, no. 1 (2014): 1.

78. D. Dobbs, "The F.D.A. vs. Personal Genetic Testing," *New Yorker,* November 27, 2013, http://www.newyorker.com/online/blogs/elements/2013/11/the-fda-vs-personal-genetic-testing.html?printable=true&currentPage=all.

79. G. Marchant, "The FDA Could Set Personal Genetics Rights Back Decades," *Slate,* November 26, 2013, http://www.slate.com/articles/technology/future_tense/2013/11/_23andme_fda_letter_premarket_approval_requirement_could_kill_at_home_genetic.html.

80. U. Francke et al., "Dealing with the Unexpected: Consumer Responses to Direct-Access BRCA Mutation Testing," *PeerJ,* February 12, 2013, https://peerj.com/articles/8/.

81. R. Epstein, "The FDA Strikes Again: Its Ban on Home Testing Kits Is, as Usual, Likely to Do More Harm Than Good," *Point of Law,* November 27, 2013: http://www.pointoflaw.com/archives/2013/11/t.php.

82. A. Wolfe, "Anne Wojcicki's Quest for Better Health Care," *Wall Street Journal,* June 27, 2014, http://online.wsj.com/articles/anne-wojcickis-quest-for-better-health-care-1403892088.

83. C. Bloss, N. Schork, and E. Topol, "Effect of Direct-to-Consumer Genomewide Profiling to Assess Disease Risk," *New England Journal of Medicine* 364, no. 6 (2011): 524–534.

84. R. C. Green and N. A. Farahany, "The FDA Is Overcautious on Consumer Genomics," *Nature* 505 (2014): 2.

85. R. Leuty, "23andMe's Andy Page Gets Disruptive with the Masses," *San Francisco Business Times,* October 22, 2013, http://www.bizjournals.com/sanfrancisco/blog/biotech/2013/10/23andme-andy-page-anne-wojcicki.html?page=all.

86. N. Fliesler, "Direct-to-Consumer Genetic Testing: A Case of Potential Harm," *Boston Children's Hospital science and clinical innovation blog,* May 5, 2014, http://vectorblog.org/2014/05/direct-to-consumer-genetic-testing-a-case-of-potential-harm/.

87. S. Pasha, "23andMe Revealed a Condition It Took My Doctors Six Years to Diagnose," *Quartz,* November 28, 2013, http://qz.com/151817/23andme-revealed-a-condition-it-took-my-doctors-six-years-to-diagnose/.

88. "The FDA and Thee," *Wall Street Journal,* November 25, 2013: http://online.wsj.com/news/articles/SB10001424052702304465604579220003539640102.

89. M. A. Hamburg, "FDA Supports Development of Innovative Genetic Tests," *Wall Street Journal,* December 3, 2013: http://online.wsj.com/news/articles/SB1000142405270230401130457922111609444156.

90. F. S. Collins and M. A. Hamburg, "First FDA Authorization for Next-Generation Sequencer," *New England Journal of Medicine* 369 (2013): 2369–2371.

91. "Regulation of Laboratory Developed Tests (LDTs)," American Society for Clinical Pathology, 2010, http://www.ascp.org/PDF/Advocacy/Regulation-of-laboratory-developed-tests-LDTs.aspx.

92. P. Offit, *Do You Believe in Magic?* (New York, NY: HarperCollins, 2013).

93. A. O'Connor, "Spike in Harm to Liver Is Tied to Dietary Aids," *New York Times,* December 22, 2013, http://www.nytimes.com/2013/12/22/us/spike-in-harm-to-liver-is-tied-to-dietary-aids.html.

94. J. Pickrell, "Should the FDA Regulate the Interpretation of Traditional Epidemiology?," Genomes Unzipped, February 12, 2013, http://www.genomesunzipped.org/2013/12/should-the-fda-regulate-the-interpretation-of-traditional-epidemiology.php.

95. D. Dobbs, "Is the National Cancer Institute Telling Me to Remove My Breasts?," *Neuron Culture,* December 2, 2013, http://daviddobbs.net/smoothpebbles/is-the-national-cancer-institute-telling-me-to -remove-my-breasts/.

96. M. Eisen, "FDA vs. 23andMe: How Do We Want Genetic Testing to Be Regulated?," *it is NOT junk,* November 26, 2013, http://www.michaeleisen.org/blog/?p=1480.

97. "The FDA and me," *Nature* 504 (2013): 7–8.

98. C. Seife, "23andMe Is Terrifying, but Not for the Reasons the FDA Thinks," *Scientific American,* November 27, 2013, http://www.scientificamerican.com/article.cfm?id=23andme-is-terrifying-but-not -for-reasons-fda.

99. A. R. Venkitaraman, "Cancer Suppression by the Chromosome Custodians, BRCA1 and BRCA2," *Science* 343 (2014): 1470–1475.

100. D. B. Agus, "The Outrageous Cost of a Gene Test," *New York Times,* May 21, 2013, http://www .nytimes.com/2013/05/21/opinion/the-outrageous-cost-of-a-gene-test.html.

101. Supreme Court of the United States, "Association for Molecular Pathology et al. versus Myriad Genetics, Inc., et al." SCOTUS, 2013, http://www.supremecourt.gov/opinions/12pdf/12-398_1b7d.pdf.

102. M. Specter, "Can We Patent Life?," *New Yorker,* April 1, 2013, http://www.newyorker.com/online /blogs/elements/2013/04/myriad-genetics-patent-genes.html.

103. E. Marshall, "Supreme Court Rules Out Patents on 'Natural' Genes," *Science* 340 (2013): 1387–1388.

104. N. Feldman, "The Supreme Court's Bad Science on Gene Patents," *Bloomberg View,* June 13, 2013, http://www.bloombergview.com/articles/2013-06-13/the-supreme-court-s-bad-science-on-gene -patents.

105. R. Cook-Deegan, "Are Human Genes Patentable?" *Annals of Internal Medicine* 159, no. 4 (2013): 298–299.

106. N. Totenberg, "Supreme Court Asks: Can Human Genes Be Patented?," *NPR Shots,* April 15, 2013, http://www.npr.org/blogs/health/2013/04/15/177035299/supreme-court-asks-can-human-genes -be-patented.

107. E. J. Topol, "DNA & Supreme Court: Nature Cannot Be Patented," *Union-Tribune San Diego,* April 27, 2013, http://www.utsandiego.com/news/2013/apr/27/dna-supreme-court-nature-cannot-be -patented/.

108. J. Guo, "The Supreme Court Reveals Its Ignorance of Genetics," *New Republic,* June 13, 2013, http://www.newrepublic.com//article/113476/supreme-court-genetics-ruling-reveals-judges-ignorance.

109. D. J. Kevles, "Can They Patent Your Genes?," *New York Review of Books,* March 7, 2013, http:// www.nybooks.com/articles/archives/2013/mar/07/can-they-patent-your-genes/.

110. C. Y. Johnson, "Eric Lander Weighs In on Gene Patenting Case," *Boston Globe,* February 26, 2013, http://www.bostonglobe.com/lifestyle/health-wellness/2013/02/26/eric-lander-human-genome -project-leader-weighs-supreme-court-gene-patenting-case/EjRae5IRYwUYRVLg6NXTZL/story.html.

111. L. O. Gostin, "Who Owns Human Genes? Is DNA Patentable?," *Journal of the American Medical Association* 310, no. 8 (2013): 791–792.

112. G. Mohan, "Researchers Hail Supreme Court Decision on Gene Patent," *Los Angeles Times,* June 13, 2013,: http://www.latimes.com/news/science/sciencenow/la-sci-sn-gene-patent-reaction-20130613,0, 6362625,print.story.

113. H. Ledford, "Myriad Ruling Causes Confusion," *Nature* 498 (2013): 281–282.

114. S. Reardon, "I Discovered the BRCA Genes," *Slate,* June 15, 2013, http://www.slate.com/articles /health_and_science/new_scientist/2013/06/brca_gene_discovery_mary_claire_king_says_the_supreme _court_is_right_not.html.

115. J. Carlson, "Myriad Stock Falls as Competitors Offer Lower Prices for Gene Testing," *Modern Healthcare,* June 13, 2013, http://www.modernhealthcare.com/article/20130613/NEWS/306139947/.

116. J. Walker, "Reimbursement for Breast-Cancer Risk Test to Be Cut," *Wall Street Journal,* December 29, 2013, http://online.wsj.com/news/article_email/SB10001424052702304361604579288591617575358-lMyQjAxMTA0MDIwOTEyNDkyWj.

117. C. Gunter, "SCOTUS Ruling Means Cheaper Genetic Testing," *Double X Science,* June 14, 2013, http://www.doublexscience.org/myriad-genetics-ruling/.

118. J. Carlson, "'The Cost Will Drop,'" *Modern Healthcare,* June 15, 2013, http://www.modernhealthcare.com/article/20130615/MAGAZINE/306159974/.

119. M. Scudellari, "Myriad Sues Developers of Competing Breast Cancer Tests," *Nature Medicine* 19, no. 8 (2013): 948.

120. R. Nussbaum, "Free Our Genetic Data," *MIT Technology Review,* July 25, 2013, http://www.technologyreview.com/view/517526/free-our-genetic-data/.

121. "Life on Mars? Discover Magazine Announces the Top 100 Stories of 2013," *Discover,* Jan–Feb 2014, http://discovermagazine.com/2014/jan-feb.

Chapter 5

1. A. Pentland, "How Big Data Can Transform Society for the Better," *Scientific American,* October 1, 2014, http://www.scientificamerican.com/article/how-big-data-can-transform-society-for-the-better/.

2. S. Lohr, "Sizing Up Big Data, Broadening Beyond the Internet," *New York Times,* June 19, 2013, http://bits.blogs.nytimes.com/2013/06/19/sizing-up-big-data-broadening-beyond-the-internet/.

3. "Epidemiology," *Wikipedia,* accessed August 13, 2014, 2014, http://en.wikipedia.org/wiki/Epidemiology.

4. J. L. Gardy et al., "Whole-Genome Sequencing and Social-Network Analysis of a Tuberculosis Outbreak," *The New England Journal of Medicine* 364 (2011): 730–739.

5. E. Topol, "Individualized Medicine from Prewomb to Tomb," *Cell* 157 (2014): 241–253.

6. T. Simonite, "Life's Trajectory Seen Through Facebook Data," *MIT Technology Review,* April 24, 2013, http://www.technologyreview.com/view/514186/lifes-trajectory-seen-through-facebook-data/.

7. A. Regalado, "Stephen Wolfram on Personal Analytics," *MIT Technology Review,* May 8, 2013, http://www.technologyreview.com/news/514356/stephen-wolfram-on-personal-analytics/.

8. N. A. Christakis and J. H. Fowler, *Connected* (New York, NY: Little, Brown and Co., 2009).

9. "Phenotype," *Wikipedia,* accessed August 13, 2014, http://en.wikipedia.org/wiki/Phenotype.

10. "Microphones as Sensors: Teaching Old Microphones New Tricks," *The Economist,* June 1, 2013, http://www.economist.com/news/technology-quarterly/21578518-sensor-technology-microphones-are-designed-capture-sound-they-turn-out.

11. G. Slabodkin, "Study: iPhone App for Speech Laterality Just as Reliable as Lab Brain Tests," *FierceMobileHealthcare,* February 12, 2013, http://www.fiercemobilehealthcare.com/story/study-iphone-app-speech-laterality-just-reliable-lab-brain-tests/2013-02-12.

12. I. Ezkurdia et al., "Multiple Evidence Strands Suggest That There May Be as Few as 19,000 Human Protein-Coding Genes," *Human Molecular Genetics,* June 16, 2014, http://www.ncbi.nlm.nih.gov/pubmed/24939910.

13. A. Butte, "Should Healthy People Have Their Genomes Sequenced at This Time?," *Wall Street Journal,* February 15, 2013, http://online.wsj.com/news/articles/SB10000872396390443884104577645783975993656.

14. E. C. Hayden, "Non-Invasive Method Devised to Sequence DNA of Human Eggs," *Nature News & Comment,* December 19, 2013, http://www.nature.com/news/non-invasive-method-devised-to-sequence-dna-of-human-eggs-1.14412.

15. R. W. Taylor et al., "Use of Whole-Exome Sequencing to Determine the Genetic Basis of Multiple Mitochondrial Respiratory Chain Complex Deficiencies," *Journal of the American Medical Association* 312, no. 1 (2014): 68–77.

16. J. Lupski, "Genetics. Genome Mosaicism—One Human, Multiple Genomes," *Science* 341 (2013): 358–359.

17. M. J. McConnell et al., "Mosaic Copy Number Variation in Human Neurons," *Science* 342 (2013): 632.

18. I. Cho and M. Blaser, "The Human Microbiome: At the Interface of Health and Disease," *Nature Reviews Genetics* 13 (2012): 260–270.

19. R. Chen et al., "Personal Omics Profiling Reveals Dynamic Molecular and Medical Phenotypes," *Cell* 148 (2012): 1293–1307.

20. E. Aiden and J.-B. Michel, "The Predictive Power of Big Data," *Newsweek,* December 25, 2013, http://www.newsweek.com/predictive-power-big-data-225125.

21. R. Almeling, "The Unregulated Sperm Industry," *New York Times*, December 1, 2013, http://www.nytimes.com/2013/12/01/opinion/sunday/the-unregulated-sperm-industry.html .

22. M. Allyse and M. Michie, "You Can't Predict Destiny by Designing Your Baby's Genome," *Wall Street Journal*, November 8, 2013, http://online.wsj.com/news/articles/SB10001424052702304448204579182353852538422.

23. G. Naik, "'Designer Babies:' Patented Process Could Lead to Selection of Genes for Specific Traits," *Wall Street Journal*, October 3, 2013, http://online.wsj.com/article/SB10001424052702303492504579113293429460678.html.

24. S. Morain, M. Greene, and M. Mello, "A New Era of Noninvasive Prenatal Testing," *New England Journal of Medicine* 369 (2013): 499–501.

25. A. Agarwal et al., "Commercial Landscape of Noninvasive Prenatal Testing in the United States," *Prenatal Diagnosis* 33 (2013): 521–531.

26. Illumina, "Verinata Health's verifi® Prenatal Test Available Through the California Prenatal Screening Program," Illumina Investor Relations News Release, November 1, 2013, http://investor.illumina.com/phoenix.zhtml?c=121127&p=irol-newsArticle&ID=1871236&highlight=.

27. A. Schaffer, "Too Much Information," *MIT Technology Review*, December 17, 2013, http://www.technologyreview.com/review/522661/too-much-information/.

28. A. D. Marcus, "Genetic Testing Leaves More Patients Living in Limbo," *Wall Street Journal*, November 20, 2013, http://online.wsj.com/news/articles/SB10001424052702303755504579206000052566432.

29. B. Wilcken, "Newborn Screening: Gaps in the Evidence," *Science* 342 (2013): 197–198.

30. E. Gabler, "Delays at Hospitals Across the Country Undermine Newborn Screening Programs, Putting Babies at Risk of Disability and Death," *Journal Sentinel*, November 16, 2013, http://www.jsonline.com/watchdog/watchdogreports/Deadly-Delays-Watchdog-Report-Delays-at-hospitals-across-the-country-undermine-newborn-screening-programs-putting-babies-at-risk-of-disability-and-death-228832111.html.

31. R. Greenfield, "Tracked Since Birth: The Rise of Extreme Baby Monitoring," *Fast Company*, November 15, 2013, http://www.fastcompany.com/3021601/innovation-agents/tracked-since-birth-the-pros-and-cons-of-extreme-baby-monitoring.

32. D. Epstein, *The Sports Gene* (New York, NY: Penguin, 2013), 256.

33. W. Koh et al., "Noninvasive In Vivo Monitoring of Tissue-Specific Global Gene Expression in Humans," *PNAS Early Edition*, May 2, 2014, http://www.pnas.org/content/early/2014/03/02/1403328111.

34. A. R. McLean, "Coming to an Airport Near You," *Science* 342 (2013): 1330–1331.

35. M. R. Wilson et al., "Actionable Diagnosis of Neuroleptospirosis by Next-Generation Sequencing," *New England Journal of Medicine*, June 19, 2014, http://www.nejm.org/doi/full/10.1056/NEJMoa1401268.

36. J. N. Weinstein et al., "The Cancer Genome Atlas Pan-Cancer Analysis Project," *Nature Genetics* 45, no. 10 (2013): 1113–1120.

37. G. Frampton et al., "Development and Validation of a Clinical Cancer Genomic Profiling Test Based on Massively Parallel DNA Sequencing," *Nature Biotechnology* 31 (2013): 1023–1031.

38. J. Couzin-Frankel, "Cancer Immunotherapy," *Science* 342 (2013): 1432–1433.

39. A. L. Williams et al., "Sequence Variants in SLC16A11 Are a Common Risk Factor for Type 2 Diabetes in Mexico," *Nature* 506 (2014): 97–101.

40. J. C. Florez et al., "Association of a Low-Frequency Variant in HNF1A With Type 2 Diabetes in a Latino Population," *Journal of the American Medical Association* 311, no. 22 (2014): 2305–2314.

41. I. Moltke et al., "A Common Greenlandic TBC1D4 Variant Confers Muscle Insulin Resistance and Type 2 Diabetes," *Nature*, June 18, 2014, http://www.nature.com/nature/journal/vaop/ncurrent/full/nature13425.html.

42. A. R. Harper and E. J. Topol, "Pharmacogenomics in Clinical Practice and Drug Development," *Nature Biotechnology* 30, no. 11 (2012): 1117–1124.

43. C.-H. Chen et al., "Variant GADL1 and Response to Lithium Therapy in Bipolar I Disorder," *New England Journal of Medicine* 370 (2013): 119–128.

44. A. B. Jorgensen et al., "Loss-of-Function Mutations in APOC3 and Risk of Ischemic Vascular Disease," *New England Journal of Medicine,* July 3, 2014, http://www.nejm.org/doi/full/10.1056/NEJMoa 1308027.

45. A. K. Pandey et al., "Functionally Enigmatic Genes: A Case Study of the Brain Ignorome," *PLoS One* 9, no. 2 (2014): 1–11.

46. M. M. Newman, "Sudden Cardiac Arrest: A Healthcare Crisis," Sudden Cardiac Arrest Foundation, 2013, accessed August 18, 2014 http://www.sca-aware.org/about-sca.

Chapter 6

1. A. Sabar, "Inside the Technology That Can Turn Your Smartphone into a Personal Doctor," *Smithsonian,* May 2014, http://www.smithsonianmag.com/innovation/inside-technology-can-turn-your -smartphone-personal-doctor-180951177/?no-ist.

2. R. Parloff, "This CEO Is Out for Blood," *Fortune,* June 12, 2014, http://fortune.com/2014/06/12 /theranos-blood-holmes/.

3. D. Goldhill, "'Catastrophic Care': An Exchange," *New York Review of Books,* October 24, 2013, http://www.nybooks.com/articles/archives/2013/oct/24/catastrophic-care-exchange/.

4. D. Sipress, "It's a simple stress test—I do your blood work, send it to the lab, and never get back to you with the results," *New Yorker,* accessed August 18, 2014, http://www.condenaststore.com/-sp/It -s-a-simple-stress-test-I-do-your-blood-work-send-it-to-the-lab-and-n-Prints_i9373568_.html.

5. J. Rago, "Elizabeth Holmes: The Breakthrough of Instant Diagnosis," *Wall Street Journal,* September 8, 2013, http://online.wsj.com/article/SB10001424127887324123004579055003869574012 .html - printMode.

6. D. Hernandez, "What Health Care Needs Is a Real-Time Snapshot of You," *Wired Science,* November 6, 2013, http://www.wired.com/wiredscience/2013/11/wired-data-life-theranos.

7. L. H. Bernstein, "Stanford Dropout Is Already Drawing Comparisons with Steve Jobs," *Pharmaceutical Magazine,* November 26, 2013, http://pharmaceuticalintelligence.com/2013/11/26/stanford -dropout-is-already-drawing-comparisons-with-steve-jobs/.

8. Theranos, "Welcome to a Revolution in Lab Testing," accessed August 13, 2014, http://www .theranos.com.

9. E. J. Topol and E. Holmes, "Creative Disruption? She's 29 and Set to Reboot Lab Medicine," *Medscape,* November 18, 2013, http://www.medscape.com/viewarticle/814233_print.

10. F. N. Pelzman, "Patients Must Be Given the Results of Their Tests," *KevinMD,* November 28, 2013, http://www.kevinmd.com/blog/2013/11/patients-results-tests.html.

11. T. D. Giardina and H. Singh, "Should Patients Get Direct Access to Their Laboratory Test Results?," *Journal of the American Medical Association* 306, no. 22 (2011): 2502.

12. K. Christensen, "Viewing Laboratory Test Results Online: Patients' Actions and Reactions," *Journal of Participatory Medicine,* October 3, 2013, http://www.jopm.org/evidence/research/2013/10/03 /viewing-laboratory-test-results-online-patients-actions-and-reactions/.

13. B. Snow, "Online Blood Work: No Doctor's Visit Required," *Fox News,* April 5, 2014, http://www .foxnews.com/health/2014/04/05/online-blood-work-no-doctors-visit-required/.

14. M. Cohen, "HHS Says Labs Must Give Patients Access to Test Results. So, What Does That Really Mean?," *MedCity News,* February 12, 2014, http://medcitynews.com/2014/02/hhs-says-labs-must -give-patients-access-test-results-really-mean/.

15. M. Beck, "New Rule Grants Patients Direct Access to Lab Results," *Wall Street Journal,* February 3, 2014, http://online.wsj.com/news/articles/SB10001424052702303442704579360901817015152.

16. D. Harlow, "Patients to Have Right to Access Lab Test Result Data—Finally!," *e-Patients,* February 4, 2014, http://e-patients.net/archives/2014/02/patients-to-have-right-to-access-lab-test-result-data.html.

17. J. Conn, "HHS Issues Rule Granting Patients Direct Access to Lab Test Results," *Modern Healthcare,* February 3, 2014, http://www.modernhealthcare.com/article/20140203/NEWS/302039958 /h%C9rce=articlelink&utm_medium=website&utm_campaign=Todays.

18. R. Pear, "Medical Boards Draft Plan to Ease Path to Out-of-State and Online Treatment," *New York Times,* June 30, 2014, http://www.nytimes.com/2014/06/30/us/medical-boards-draft-plan-to-ease -path-to-out-of-state-and-online-treatment.html.

19a. K. Sebelius, "HHS Strengthens Patients' Right to Access Lab Test Reports," HHS.gov, February 3, 2014, http://www.hhs.gov/news/press/2014pres/02/20140203a.html.

19b. M. J. Young, E. Scheinberg, and H. Bursztajn, "Direct-to-Patient Laboratory Test Reporting: Balancing Access with Effective Clinical Communication," *Journal of the American Medical Association* 312, no. 2 (2014): 127–128.

20. A. Jha, "The Incredible Shrinking Laboratory or 'Lab-on-a-Chip,'" *The Guardian,* November 28, 2011, http://www.theguardian.com/science/2011/nov/28/incredible-shrinking-laboratory-lab-chip.

21. R. Komatireddy and E. J. Topol, "Medicine Unplugged: The Future of Laboratory Medicine," *Clinical Chemistry* 58, no. 12 (2012): 1644–1647.

22. M. Kim, "Imagine a Smartphone Medical Lab," *philly.com,* January 6, 2014, http://www.philly.com/philly/health/20140105_Imagine_a_smartphone_medical_lab.html.

23. "Spit on Your iPhone to Diagnose Diseases," *Lab Test Consult,* December 2, 2011, http://www.labtestconsult.com/spit-on-your-iphone-to-diagnose-diseases/.

24. J. Hewitt, "Turning the Smartphone from a Telephone into a Tricorder," *ExtremeTech,* November 3, 2012, http://www.extremetech.com/extreme/138658-turning-the-smartphone-from-a-telephone-into-a-tricorder?

25. E. Schwartz, "Can Smartphones Really Cut It as Diagnostic Tools?," *mHealthNews,* January 2, 2014, http://www.mhealthnews.com/news/can-smartphones-really-cut-it-diagnostic-tools-mhealth-mobile.

26. "Acoustic Microfluidics: What a Sound Idea," *The Economist,* June 2, 2012, http://www.economist.com/node/21556091/print.

27. B. Tansey, "Genia Aims to Build the iPhone of Gene Sequencing," *Xconomy,* October 16, 2013, http://www.xconomy.com/san-francisco/2013/10/16/genia-aims-build-iphone-gene-sequencing/2/.

28. "Cradle Turns Smartphone into Handheld Biosensor," *Science Daily,* May 23, 2013, http://www.sciencedaily.com/releases/2013/05/130523162250.htm.

29. G. Slabodkin, "Malaria Detection Device to Be Field Tested a Year Ahead of Schedule," *FierceMobileHealthcare,* April 29, 2013, http://www.fiercemobilehealthcare.com/story/malaria-detection-device-be-field-tested-year-ahead-schedule/2013-04-29.

30. K. Struck, "Heart Failure: Is There a Breath Test?," *MedPage Today,* March 25, 2013, http://www.medpagetoday.com/CriticalCare/CHF/38076?utm_content=.

31. D. Aksr, "A Virus on the Camera Roll," *Wall Street Journal,* September 27, 2013, http://online.wsj.com/article/SB10001424052702304213904579095460624936226.html.

32. N. N. Watkins et al., "Microfluidic CD4+ and CD8+ T Lymphocyte Counters for Point-of-Care HIV Diagnostics Using Whole Blood," *Science Translational Medicine* 5, no. 214 (2013): 1–12.

33. "Detecting Disease with a Smartphone Accessory," *Science Daily,* June 4, 2013, http://www.sciencedaily.com/releases/2013/06/130604113959.htm.

34. B. Ouyang, "New Mobile Technology Allows Users to Track Cholesterol Levels with a Smartphone (VIDEO)," *MedGadget,* December 17, 2013, http://www.medgadget.com/2013/12/new-mobile-technology-allows-users-to-track-cholesterol-levels-with-a-smartphone-video.html.

35. I. I. Bogoch et al., "Mobile Phone Microscopy for the Diagnosis of Soil-Transmitted Helminth Infections: A Proof-of-Concept Study," *American Journal of Tropical Medicine and Hygiene,* March 11, 2013, http://www.ajtmh.org/content/early/2013/03/07/ajtmh.12-0742.abstract.

36. D. N. Breslauer et al., "Mobile Phone Based Clinical Microscopy for Global Health Applications," *PLoS One* 4, no. 7 (2009): e6320.

37. M. Colombo, "Mobile Devices Not Just for Facebook, They Are Poised to Revolutionize Healthcare," *Healthcare Blog,* October 4, 2013, http://info.calgaryscientific.com/blog/bid/339938/Mobile-devices-n%C9Mc3VWFlKrPfKbt-qzZXfCtJMa3-C1RYVYbc5LegsLEZ6LJDH2A&_hsmi=10496393.

38. G. Corley, "Paper-Based Microfluidic Technology May Let You Print Your Own Health Tests," *MedGadget,* February 20, 2012, http://medgadget.com/2012/02/paper-based-microfluidic-technology-may-let-you-print-your-own-health-tests.html.

39. A. F. Coskun et al., "Albumin Testing in Urine Using a Smart-Phone," *Lab on a Chip* 13, no. 21 (2013): 4231–4238.

40. T. M. Andrews, "Breathalyzers of the Future Today," *Atlantic*, June 2013, http://www.theatlantic.com/health/print/2013/06/breathalyzers-of-the-future-today/277249/.

41. R. Ferris, "These Amazing Dogs Can Smell Cancer," *Business Insider,* August 15, 2013, http://www.businessinsider.com/working-dog-center-dogs-can-smell-cancer-2013-8.

42. V. Greenwood, "What Does Cancer Smell Like?," *New York Times*, November 14, 2013, http://www.nytimes.com/2013/11/24/magazine/what-does-cancer-smell-like.html.

43. N. Savage, "Spotting the First Signs," *Nature* 471 (2011): S14–S15.

44. D. G. McNeil, "Dogs Excel on Smell Test to Find Cancer," *New York Times*, January 17, 2006, http://www.nytimes.com/2006/01/17/health/17dog.html.

45. W. Kremer, "Sniffing Out Cancer with Electronic Noses," *BBC News Magazine*, March 8, 2014, http://www.bbc.com/news/magazine-26472225.

46. H. Williams and A. Pembroke, "Sniffer Dogs in the Melanoma Clinic?," *The Lancet* 1 (1989): 734.

47. B. Palmer, "Roll Over! Shake! Smell This Mole!," *Slate*, May 27, 2014, http://www.slate.com/articles/health_and_science/medical_examiner/2014/05/cancer_sniffing_dogs_can_dogs_detect_and_screen_for_disease.html.

48. "Electronic Nose Sniffs Out Prostate Cancer Using Urine Samples," *eHealth News*, May 13, 2014, http://www.ehealthnews.eu/research/3929-electronic-nose-sniffs-out-prostate-cancer-using-urine-samples.

49. A. Zimm, "Canines' Cancer-Sniffing Snouts Showing 90%-Plus Accuracy," Bloomberg, May 18, 2014, http://www.bloomberg.com/news/2014-05-18/canines-cancer-sniffing-snouts-offer-new-testing-option.html.

50. A. Roine et al., "Detection of Prostate Cancer by an Electronic Nose: A Proof of Principle Study," *Journal of Urology* 192, no. 1 (2014): 230–235.

51. V. Combs, "Physicist Building Nanotech Sensor to Track Your Health Through Your Breath," *MedCity News,* September 10, 2013, http://medcitynews.com/2013/09/physicist-building-nanotech-sensor-to-track-your-health-through-your-breath/print/.

52. K. Bourzac, "Cancer Breath Test Enters Clinical Trials," *MIT Technology Review*, February 14, 2012, http://www.technologyreview.com/news/426894/cancer-breath-test-enters-clinical-trials/.

53. W. Jia et al., "Electrochemical Tattoo Biosensors for Real-Time Noninvasive Lactate Monitoring in Human Perspiration," *Analytical Chemistry* 85 (2013): 6553–6560.

54. K. Belson, "New Tests for Brain Trauma Create Hope, and Skepticism," *New York Times*, December 26, 2013, http://www.nytimes.com/2013/12/26/sports/football/new-tests-for-brain-trauma-create-hope-and-skepticism.html.

55. G. Poste, "Bring on the Biomarkers," *Nature* 469 (2011): 156–157.

56. T. T. Ruckh and H. A. Clark, "Implantable Nanosensors: Toward Continuous Physiologic Monitoring," *Analytical Chemistry* 86, no. 3 (2013): 1314–1323.

57. S. Johnson, "Someday Electronic Devices Could Be On or Inside People," *Seattle Times*, December 24, 2013, http://seattletimes.com/html/nationworld/2022524089_implanttechxml.html.

58. B. S. Ferguson et al., "Real-Time, Aptamer-Based Tracking of Circulating Therapeutic Agents in Living Animals," *Science Translational Medicine* 5, no. 213 (2013): 213ra165.

59. Y. Ling et al., "Implantable Magnetic Relaxation Sensors Measure Cumulative Exposure to Cardiac Biomarkers," *Nature Biotechnology* 29 (2011): 273–272.

60. T.-I. Kim et al., "Injectable, Cellular-Scale Optoelectronics with Applications for Wireless Optogenetics," *Science* 340 (2013): 211–216.

61. "Nanotube-Based Sensors Can Be Implanted Under the Skin for a Year," Nanowerk, November 3, 2013, http://www.nanowerk.com/news2/newsid=33040.php.

62. A. Myers, "Swimming Through the Blood Stream: Stanford Engineers Create Wireless, Self-Propelled Medical Device," *Stanford University News,* February 22, 2012, http://news.stanford.edu/news/2012/february/micro-device-implant-022212.html.

63. R. Smith-Bindman et al., "Use of Diagnostic Imaging Studies and Associated Radiation Exposure for Patients Enrolled in Large Integrated Health Care Systems, 1996–2010," *Journal of the American Medical Association* 302, no. 22 (2012): 2400–2409.

64. B. Owens, "Enhanced Medical Vision," *Nature* 502 (2013): S82–S83.

65. D. L. Miglioretti et al., "The Use of Computed Tomography in Pediatrics and the Associated Radiation Exposure and Estimated Cancer Risk," *JAMA Pediatrics* 167, no. 8 (2013): 700–707.

66. R. F. Redberg and R. Smith-Bindman, "We Are Giving Ourselves Cancer," *New York Times*, January 31, 2014, http://www.nytimes.com/2014/01/31/opinion/we-are-giving-ourselves-cancer.html.

67. C. Libov, "Radiation from Needless Medical Tests Can Give You Cancer," *Newsmax Health*, April 24, 2012, http://www.newsmax-health.net/headline_health/radiation_medical_tests_/2012/04/24/446 984.html.

68. C. K. Cassel and J. A. Guest, "Choosing Wisely Helping Physicians and Patients Make Smart Decisions About Their Care," *Journal of the American Medical Association* 307, no. 17 (2012): 1801–1802.

69. "Choosing Wisely: Five Things Physicians and Patients Should Question," ABIM Foundation, accessed August 19, 2014, http://www.choosingwisely.org/doctor-patient-lists/.

70. V. M. Rao and D. C. Levin, "The Overuse of Diagnostic Imaging and the Choosing Wisely Initiative," *Annals of Internal Medicine* 157, no. 8 (2012): 574–577.

71. L. T. Krogsbøll et al., "General Health Checks in Adults for Reducing Morbidity and Mortality from Disease: Cochrane Systematic Review and Meta-Analysis," *British Medical Journal* 345 (2012): e7191.

72. S. R. Johnson, "Reducing Wasteful Care," *Modern Healthcare*, August 24, 2013, http://www .modernhealthcare.com/article/20130824/MAGAZINE/308249974.

73. L. M. Schwartz and S. Woloshin, "Endless Screenings Don't Bring Everlasting Health," *New York Times*, April 17, 2012, http://www.nytimes.com/2012/04/17/health/views/endless-screenings-dont-bring -everlasting-health.html.

74. B. L. Jacobs et al., "Use of Advanced Treatment Technologies Among Men at Low Risk of Dying from Prostate Cancer," *Journal of the American Medical Association* 309, no. 24 (2013): 2587–2595.

75. "Simple Treatments, Ignored," *New York Times*, September 9, 2012, http://www.nytimes.com /2012/09/09/opinion/sunday/simple-treatments-ignored.html.

76. J. H. Wasfy, "Sometimes 'Unnecessary' Medical Tests Save Lives," *Washington Post*, October 3, 2013, http://www.washingtonpost.com/opinions/sometimes-unnecessary-medical-tests-save-lives/2013 /10/03/74777dce-27b6-11e3-b75d-5b7f66349852_story.html.

77. E. Rosenthal, "Let's (Not) Get Physicals," *New York Times*, June 3, 2012, http://www.nytimes .com/2012/06/03/sunday-review/lets-not-get-physicals.html.

78. "Heart Rhythm Society's Choosing Wisely List Disappoints," *Medscape*, February 12, 2014, http://www.medscape.com/viewarticle/820477.

79. E. Picano et al., "The Appropriate and Justified Use of Medical Radiation in Cardiovascular Imaging: A Position Document of the ESC Associations of Cardiovascular Imaging, Percutaneous Cardiovascular Interventions and Electrophysiology," *European Heart Journal* 35, no. 10 (2014): 665–672.

80. P. Kassing and R. Duszak, "Repeat Medical Imaging: A Classification System for Meaningful Policy Analysis and Research," *Neiman Report*, February 2013, http://www.acr.org/-/media/ACR/ Documents/PDF/Research/Brief 02/PolicyBriefHPI012013.pdf.

81. A. J. Einstein et al., "Patient-Centered Imaging: Shared Decision Making for Cardiac Imaging Procedures with Exposure to Ionizing Radiation," *Journal of the American College of Cardiology* 63, no. 15 (2013): 1480–1489.

82. A. M. Seaman, "Doctors Don't Often Tell Patients of CT Scan Risks," *Reuters*, 2013, http://www .reuters.com/assets/print?aid=USBRE92316120130304.

83. G. Schwitzer, "When Doctors Don't Discuss Harms of Screening Tests with Patients," *Health News Review*, October 22, 2013, http://www.healthnewsreview.org/2013/10/when-doctors-dont-discuss -harms-of-screening-tests-with-patients/.

84. L. Landro, "New Tracking of a Patient's Radiation Exposure," *Wall Street Journal*, May 21, 2013, http://online.wsj.com/article/SB10001424127887324767004578489413973896412.html.

85. C. O'Donoghue et al., "Aggregate Cost of Mammography Screening in the United States: Comparison of Current Practice and Advocated Guidelines," *Annals of Internal Medicine* 160 (2014): 145–153.

86. H. G. Welch, "Breast Cancer Screenings: What We Still Don't Know," *New York Times*, December 30, 2013, http://www.nytimes.com/2013/12/30/opinion/breast-cancer-screenings-what-we-still-dont -know.html.

87. G. Kolata, "Vast Study Casts Doubts on Value of Mammograms," *New York Times*, February 12, 2014, http://www.nytimes.com/2014/02/12/health/study-adds-new-doubts-about-value-of -mammograms.html.

88. A. Bleyer and H. G. Welch, "Effect of Three Decades of Screening Mammography on Breast-Cancer Incidence," *New England Journal of Medicine* 367, no. 21 (2012): 1998–2005.

89. J. G. Elmore and C. P. Gross, "The Cost of Breast Cancer Screening in the United States: A Picture Is Worth . . . a Billion Dollars?," *Annals of Internal Medicine* 160 (2014): 203–204.

90. A. B. Miller et al., "Twenty-five Year Follow-Up for Breast Cancer Incidence and Mortality of the Canadian National Breast Screening Study: Randomised Screening Trial," *British Medical Journal* 348 (2014): g366.

91. J. A. Paulos, "Weighing the Positives," *Scientific American*, December 28, 2011, http://www .nature.com/scientificamerican/journal/v306/n1/full/scientificamerican0112-20.html.

92. N. Biller-Andorno and P. Jüni, "Abolishing Mammography Screening Programs? A View from the Swiss Medical Board," *New England Journal of Medicine* 340, no. 21 (2014): 1965–1967.

93. D. H. Newman, "Ignoring the Science on Mammograms," *New York Times*, November 28, 2012, http://well.blogs.nytimes.com/2012/11/28/ignoring-the-science-on-mammograms/.

94. J. C. Dooren and R. Winslow, "U.S. Panel Recommends Lung-Cancer Screening," *Wall Street Journal*, December 30, 2013, http://online.wsj.com/news/articles/SB1000142405270230459160457929 0843407880628.

95. D. V. Makarov et al., "Prostate Cancer Imaging Trends After a Nationwide Effort to Discourage Inappropriate Prostate Cancer Imaging," *Journal of the National Cancer Institute* 105, no. 17 (2013): 1306–1313.

96. J. Dorrier, "California Startup, Tribogenics, Develops Smart Phone Sized Portable X-Ray Machines," *Singularity Hub*, November 16, 2013, http://singularityhub.com/2013/11/16/southern-california -startup-tribogenics-develops-smart-phone-sized-portable-x-ray-machines/.

97. J. B. Haun et al., "Micro-NMR for Rapid Molecular Analysis of Human Tumor Samples," *Science Translational Medicine* 3, no. 71 (2011): 1–14.

98. N. Ungerleider, "An X-Ray Machine the Size of an iPhone That Looks Like a Star Trek Tricorder," *Fast Company*, December 8, 2011, http://www.fastcompany.com/1799596/x-ray-machine-size -iphone-looks-star-trek-tricorder.

99. P. Gwynne, "Seeing into the Future," *Nature* 502 (2013): S96–S97.

100. M. Kaku, *Physics of the Future* (Toronto, Canada: Doubleday, 2011), 60–62.

101. Ibid., 60.

102. Ibid., 62.

103. M. J. Leibo et al., "Is Pocket Mobile Echocardiography the Next-Generation Stethoscope? A Cross-sectional Comparison of Rapidly Acquired Images With Standard Transthoracic Echocardiography," *Annals of Internal Medicine* 155, no. 1 (2011): 33–38.

104. S. D. Solomon and F. Saldana, "Point-of-Care Ultrasound in Medical Education—Stop Listening and Look," *New England Journal of Medicine* 370 (2014): 1083–1085.

105. A. Flint, "Patients Should Be Able to Share Their Medical Imaging Studies," *neuroicudoc*, August 21, 2013, http://www.neuroicudoc.com/2013/08/patients-should-be-able-to-share-their.html.

106. J. Lee, "Share Ware," *Modern Healthcare*, November 24, 2012, http://www.modernhealthcare .com/article/20121124/MAGAZINE/311249953/?template=printpicart.

107. A. J. Johnson et al., "Access to Radiologic Reports via a Patient Portal: Clinical Simulations to Investigate Patient Preferences," *Journal of the American College of Radiology* 9, no. 4 (2012): 256–263.

108. A. Eisenberg, "Those Scan Results Are Just an App Away," *New York Times*, October 16, 2011, http://www.nytimes.com/2011/10/16/business/medical-apps-to-assist-with-diagnoses-cleared-by-fda .html.

109. D. McCormick et al., "Giving Office-Based Physicians Electronic Access to Patients' Prior Imaging and Lab Results Did Not Deter Ordering of Tests," *Health Affairs* 31, no. 3 (2012): 488–496.

110. T. McMahon, "The Smartphone Will See You Now: How Apps and Social Media Are Revolutionizing Medicine," *Macleans*, March 4, 2013, http://www2.macleans.ca/2013/03/04/the-smartphone -will-see-you-now.

111. "Turning Mobile Phones into 3D Scanners," Computer Vision and Geometry Group, accessed August 13, 2014, http://cvg.ethz.ch/mobile/.

112. J. Lademann, "Optical Methods of Imaging in the Skin," *Journal of Biomedical Optics* 18, no. 6 (2013): 061201-1.

113. W. Sohn et al., "Endockscope: Using Mobile Technology to Create Global Point of Service Endoscopy," *Journal of Endourology* 27, no. 9 (2013): 1154–1160.

114. K. Streams, "How to Turn a Smartphone Into a Digital Microscope Using Inexpensive Materials," *Laughing Squid,* 2013, http://laughingsquid.com/how-to-turn-a-smartphone-into-a-digital-microscope-using-inexpensive-materials/.

Chapter 7

1. R. Taylor et al., "Promoting Health Information Technology: Is There a Case for More-Aggressive Government Action?," *Health Affairs* 24, no. 5 (2005): 1234–1245.

2. J. Hoffman, "What the Therapist Thinks About You," *New York Times,* July 7, 2014, http://well.blogs.nytimes.com/2014/07/07/what-the-therapist-thinks-about-you/?_php=true&_type=blogs&ref=health&_r=0.

3. J. Kopman, "Electronic Health Records: Doctors Want to Keep Patients Out," *Everyday Health,* March 26, 2013, http://www.everydayhealth.com/healthy-living/electronic-health-records-doctors-want-to-keep-patients-out-7727.aspx.

4. L. Mearian, "U.S. Doctors Don't Believe Patients Need Full Access to Health Records," *Infoworld,* March 8, 2013, http://www.infoworld.com/print/214131.

5. B. N. Shenkin and D.C. Warner, "Giving the Patient His Medical Record: A Proposal to Improve the System," *New England Journal of Medicine* 289, no. 13 (1973): 688–692.

6. J. Katz, *The Silent World of Doctor and Patient* (Baltimore, MD: Johns Hopkins University Press, 1984), 4.

7. T. Delbanco et al., "Inviting Patients to Read Their Doctors' Notes: A Quasi-experimental Study and a Look Ahead," *Annals of Internal Medicine* 157, no. 7 (2012): 461–471.

8. J. Thew, "Opening Up About Medical Records: OpenNotes Gives Patients Access to Provider Notes," *HL7 Health,* January 28, 2014, http://www.hl7standards.com/blog/2014/01/28/open-notes/?utm_conte%C97b9&utm_medium=social&utm_source=twitter.com&utm_campaign=buffer.

9. M. Coren, "You Can Now Find Out What Your Doctor Is Writing Down in That File," *Fast Company,* July 23, 2013, http://www.fastcoexist.com/1682595/you-can-now-find-out-what-your-doctor-is-writing-down-in-that-file.

10. L. Landro, "Health-Care Providers Want Patients to Read Medical Records, Spot Errors," *Wall Street Journal,* June 9, 2014, http://online.wsj.com/articles/health-care-providers-want-patients-to-read-medical-records-spot-errors-1402354902.

11. J. Walker et al., "The Road Towards Fully Transparent Medical Records," *New England Journal of Medicine* 370 (2013): 6–8.

12. "More Than Forty Percent of U.S. Consumers Willing to Switch Physicians to Gain Online Access to Electronic Medical Records, According to Accenture Survey," *Accenture Newsroom,* September 16, 2013, http://newsroom.accenture.com/news/more-than-40-percent-of-us-consumers-willing-to-switch-physicians-to-gain-online-access-to-electronic-medical-records-according-to-accenture-survey.htm.

13. S. Reddy, "When Email Is Part of the Doctor's Treatment," *Wall Street Journal,* March 25, 2013, http://online.wsj.com/article/SB10001424127887324373204578376863506224702.html.

14. T. F. Bishop et al., "Electronic Communication Improves Access, but Barriers to Its Widespread Adoption Remain," *Health Affairs* 32, no. 8 (2013): 1361–1367.

15. F. N. Pelzman, "I'm Your Doctor, What Is Your Email?," *Med Page Today,* December 20, 2013, http://www.medpagetoday.com/PatientCenteredMedicalHome/PatientCenteredMedicalHome/43527?isalert=1.

16. "The Blue Button," in *Wikipedia,* accessed August 13, 2014, http://en.wikipedia.org/wiki/The_Blue_Button.

17. M. Beck, "Next in Tech: App Helps Patients Track Care," *Wall Street Journal*, December 16, 2013, http://online.wsj.com/news/articles/SB10001424052702303330204579248420368822400.

18. J. Savacool, "How Do You Measure Up? New Health Gadgets Can Tell You," *USA Today*, January 5, 2014, http://www.usatoday.com/story/news/nation/2014/01/05/fitness-health-monitors-ces/4301611/.

19. E. Stawicki, "Your Smartphone Might Hold Key to Your Medical Records," *Kaiser Health News*, June 17, 2013, http://www.kaiserhealthnews.org/Stories/2013/June/17/electronic-health-records-blue -button.aspx?p=1.

20. "With Major Pharmacies on Board, Is the Blue Button About to Scale Nation-wide?," *E Pluribus Unum*, February 7, 2014, http://e-pluribusunum.com/2014/02/07/major-pharmacies-blue-button-scale/.

21. D. Butler, "Human Genome at Ten: Science After the Sequence," *Nature* 465 (2010): 1000–1001.

22. R. Hillestad et al., "Can Electronic Medical Record Systems Transform Health Care? Potential Health Benefits, Savings, and Costs," *Health Affairs* 24, no. 5 (2005): 1103–1117.

23. R. Abelson and J. Creswell, "In Second Look, Few Savings from Digital Health Records," *New York Times*, January 11, 2013, http://www.nytimes.com/2013/01/11/business/electronic-records-systems -have-not-reduced-health-costs-report-says.html.

24. B. Wanamaker and D. Bean, "Why EHRs Are Not (Yet) Disruptive," *Christensen Institute Blog*, August 8, 2013, http://www.christenseninstitute.org/why-ehrs-are-not-yet-disruptive/.

25. R. Abelson, J. Creswell, and G. Palmer, "Medicare Bills Rise as Records Turn Electronic," *New York Times*, September 22, 2012, http://www.nytimes.com/2012/09/22/business/medicare-billing-rises -at-hospitals-with-electronic-records.html.

26. D. Ofri, "The Doctor Will See Your Electronic Medical Record Now," *Slate*, August 5, 2013, http://mobile.slate.com/blogs/future_tense/2013/08/05/study_reveals_doctors_are_spending_even_less _time_with_patients.html.

27. E. White, "Do Doctors Spend Too Much Time Looking at Computer Screen?," *Northwestern University News*, January 23, 2014, http://www.northwestern.edu/newscenter/stories/2014/01/do-doctors -spend-too-much-time-looking-at-computer-screen.html.

28. J. P. Weiner, S. Yeh, and D. Blumenthal, "The Impact of Health Information Technology and e-Health on the Future Demand for Physician Services," *Health Affairs* 32, no. 1 (2013): 1998–2004.

29. B. Monegain, "EHRs to Redefine the Role of Doctor," *Healthcare IT News*, January 27, 2014, http://www.healthcareitnews.com/news/ehrs-redefine-role-doctor.

30. K. Hafner, "A Busy Doctor's Right Hand, Ever Ready to Type," *New York Times*, January 14, 2014, http://www.nytimes.com/2014/01/14/health/a-busy-doctors-right-hand-ever-ready-to-type.html.

31. A. J. Bank, "In Praise of Medical Scribes," *Wall Street Journal*, April 6, 2014, http://online.wsj .com/news/articles/SB10001424052702304418404579469371577995400.

32. Anonymous, "The Disturbing Confessions of a Medical Scribe," *KevinMD.com*, March 9, 2014, http://www.kevinmd.com/blog/2014/03/confessions-medical-scribe.html.

33. R. Abelson, "Medicare Is Faulted on Shift to Electronic Records," *New York Times*, November 29, 2012, http://www.nytimes.com/2012/11/29/business/medicare-is-faulted-in-electronic-medical -records-conversion.html.

34. R. Abelson and J. Creswell, "Report Finds More Flaws in Digitizing Patient Files," *New York Times*, January 8, 2014, http://www.nytimes.com/2014/01/08/business/report-finds-more-flaws-in -digitizing-patient-files.html.

35. "Data Glitches Are Hazardous to Your Health," *Scientific American*, October 15, 2013, http:// www.nature.com/scientificamerican/journal/v309/n5/full/scientificamerican1113-10.html.

36. B. Ahier, "Nearly Half of Physicians Believe EHRs Are Making Patient Care Worse," *HIT Consultant*, February 13, 2014, http://hitconsultant.net/2014/02/13/nearly-half-of-physicians-believe-ehrs -are-making-patient-care-worse/.

37. A. Allen, "Electronic Health Records: A 'Clunky' Transition," *Politico*, June 15, 2014, http://www .politico.com/story/2014/06/health-care-electronic-records-107881.html.

38. S. Baum, "EHRs May Turn Small Errors Into Big Ones," *MedCity News*, December 16, 2012, http://www.medpagetoday.com/PracticeManagement/InformationTechnology/36474.

39. A. Jha, "The Wrong Question on Electronic Health Records," *Health Policy*, September 18, 2012, https://blogs.sph.harvard.edu/ashish-jha/the-wrong-question-on-electronic-health-records/.

40. D. F. Sittig and H. Singh, "Electronic Health Records and National Patient-Safety Goals," *New England Journal of Medicine* 367, no. 19 (2012): 1854–1860.

41. National Council on Patient Information and Education, "Accelerating Progress in Prescription Medicine Adherence: The Adherence Action Agenda," Be Medicine Smart, October 2013, http://www.bemedicinesmart.org/report.html.

42. K. Bole, "Reimagining Pharmacy Care," *UCSF News*, March 5, 2014, http://www.ucsf.edu/news/2014/02/112201/reimagining-pharmacy-care.

43. A. W. Mathews, "Beep! It's Your Medicine Nagging You," *Wall Street Journal*, February 28, 2010, http://online.wsj.com/news/articles/SB10001424052748703431604575095771390040944.

44. K. Langhauser, "A New Era in Medication Adherence," *Pharma Manufacturing*, December 13, 2013, http://www.pharmamanufacturing.com/articles/2013/dec-digital-insights/.

45. J. Comstock, "Medication Adherence: Whose Problem Is It?," *MobiHealthNews*, November 12, 2013, http://mobihealthnews.com/27258/medication-adherence-whose-problem-is-it/.

46. J. Brownlee, "How Ideo Helped Reinvent the Pillbox," *Fast Company*, February 6, 2014, http://www.fastcodesign.com/3026096/how-ideo-helped-reinvent-the-pillbox.

47. B. Dolan, "Study: GlowCaps Up Adherence to 98 Percent," *MobiHealthNews*, June 23, 2010, http://mobihealthnews.com/8069/study-glowcaps-up-adherence-to-98-percent/.

48. P. Pitts, "America's 'Other Drug Problem'—Medication Adherence," *Drugwonks*, January 21, 2014, http://drugwonks.com/blog/america-s-other-drug-problem-medication-adherence.

49. "ASCP Fact Sheet," American Society of Consultant Pharmacists, accessed August 13, 2014, http://www.ascp.com/articles/about-ascp/ascp-fact-sheet.

50. Z. Moukheiber, "A Digital Health Acquisition to Watch," *Forbes*, January 13, 2014, http://www.forbes.com/sites/zinamoukheiber/2014/01/13/a-digital-health-acquisition-to-watch/.

51. A. Schwartz, "A Cell Phone in a Pill Bottle, to Text You to Remember Your Meds," *Fast Company*, May 6, 2014, http://www.fastcoexist.com/1681935/a-cell-phone-in-a-pill-bottle-to-text-you-to-remember-your-meds.

52. T. Aungst, "Smartphones Are Revolutionizing Pill Identification," *iMedicalApps*, January 23, 2014, http://www.imedicalapps.com/2014/01/smartphones-revolutionizing-pill-identification/.

53. N. Versel, "Patient-Generated Data Is the Future of Care, VA Official Says," *MobiHealthNews*, July 18, 2013, http://mobihealthnews.com/23924/patient-generated-data-is-the-future-of-care-va-official-says/.

54. "Two Strategies for the Integration of Patient-Generated Data into the EMR. Which Road to Travel?," *cHealth Blog*, January 7, 2014, http://chealthblog.connectedhealth.org/2014/01/07/two-strategies-for-the-integration-of-patient-generated-data-into-the-emr-which-road-to-travel/.

55. J. Conn, "Staying Connected," *Modern Healthcare*, January 18, 2014, http://www.modernhealthcare.com/article/20140118/MAGAZINE/301189929/.

56. C. Zimmer, "Linking Genes to Diseases by Sifting Through Electronic Medical Records," *New York Times*, November 28, 2013, http://www.nytimes.com/2013/11/28/science/linking-genes-to-diseases-by-sifting-through-electronic-medical-records.html.

57. I. L. Katzan and R. A. Rudick, "Time to Integrate Clinical and Research Informatics," *Science Translational Medicine* 4, no. 162 (2012): 1–4.

58. J. S. Kahn, V. Aulakh, and A. Bosworth, "What It Takes: Characteristics of the Ideal Personal Health Record," *Health Affairs* 28, no. 2 (2009): 369–376.

59. R. Rowley, "What Is the Future of EHRs?," *RobertTrowleyMD.com*, January 22, 2014, http://robertrowleymd.com/2014/01/22/future-ehrs/.

60. B. Crounse, "Do We Need to Re-imagine the Electronic Medical Record?," *MSDN Blogs*, January 27, 2014, http://blogs.msdn.com/b/healthblog/archive/2014/01/27/do-we-need-to-re-imagine-the-electronic-medical-record.aspx.

61. I. Kohane, "Why You Should Demand More Surveillance—of Your Health Records," *Common Health*, June 21, 2013, http://commonhealth.wbur.org/2013/06/more-surveillance-health-records.

62. M. Smith et al., "Best Care at Lower Cost," Institute of Medicine of the National Academies, September 6, 2012, http://www.iom.edu/Reports/2012/Best-Care-at-Lower-Cost-The-Path-to-Continuously-Learning-Health-Care-in-America.aspx.

63. M. McCormack, "We'd All Be Better Off with Our Health Records on Facebook," *Quartz*, December 27, 2013, http://qz.com/161727/wed-all-be-better-off-with-our-health-records-on-facebook/.

64. N. Dawson, "Evernote Is My EMR," *e-patients.net*, January 23, 2014, http://e-patients.net/archives/2014/01/evernote-is-my-emr.html?utm_s%C9mpaign=Feed%3A+E-patients+%28e-patients%29&utm_content=Twitterrific.

65. S. A. Levingston, "Practice Fusion Wants to Be Free," *Bloomberg Businessweek*, February 6, 2014, http://www.businessweek.com/articles/2014-02-06/practice-fusions-medical-records-technology-is-free-for-doctors.

66. D. Hernandez, "How Medical Tech Promises to Save Lives," *USA Today*, June 14, 2014, http://www.usatoday.com/story/news/nation/2014/06/14/medical-technology-va-healthcare-emr/10369071/.

Chapter 8

1. U. E. Reinhardt, "The Disruptive Innovation of Price Transparency in Health Care," *Journal of the American Medical Association* 310, no. 18 (2013): 1927–1928.

2. T. Rosenberg, "The Cure for the $1,000 Toothbrush," *New York Times*, August 13, 2013, http://opinionator.blogs.nytimes.com/2013/08/13/the-cure-for-the-1000-toothbrush/.

3. S. Brill, "Bitter Pill: Why Medical Bills Are Killing Us," *TIME*, April 4, 2013, http://time.com/198/bitter-pill-why-medical-bills-are-killing-us/.

4. "Inside 'Bitter Pill': Steven Brill Discusses His TIME Cover Story," *TIME*, February 22, 2013, http://healthland.time.com/2013/02/20/bitter-pill-inside-times-cover-story-on-medical-bills/print/.

5. C. Miller, "Some Hospitals Set Charges at More Than 10 Times Their Costs," *Healthcare Intelligence Network*, January 13, 2014, http://hin.com/Healthcare_Business_Weekly_Update/2014/01/13/some-hospitals-set-charges-at-more-than-10-times-their-costs/.

6. C. White, J. D. Reschovsky, and A. M. Bond, "Understanding Differences Between High- and Low-Price Hospitals: Implications for Efforts to Rein In Costs," *Health Affairs* 33, no. 2 (2014): 324–331.

7. E. Rosenthal, "Let's (Not) Get Physicals," *New York Times*, June 3, 2012, http://www.nytimes.com/2012/06/03/sunday-review/lets-not-get-physicals.html.

8. E. Rosenthal, "A Push to Sell Testosterone Gels Troubles Doctors," *New York Times*, October 16, 2013, http://www.nytimes.com/2013/10/16/us/a-push-to-sell-testosterone-gels-troubles-doctors.html.

9. E. Rosenthal, "American Way of Birth, Costliest in the World," *New York Times*, July 1, 2013, http://www.nytimes.com/2013/07/01/health/american-way-of-birth-costliest-in-the-world.html.

10. E. Rosenthal, "As Hospital Prices Soar, a Stitch Tops $500," *New York Times*, December 3, 2013, http://www.nytimes.com/2013/12/03/health/as-hospital-costs-soar-single-stitch-tops-500.html.

11. E. Rosenthal, "The $2.7 Trillion Medical Bill: Colonoscopies Explain Why U.S. Leads the World in Health Expenditures," *New York Times*, June 2, 2013, http://www.nytimes.com/2013/06/02/health/colonoscopies-explain-why-us-leads-the-world-in-health-expenditures.html.

12. E. Rosenthal, "For Medical Tourists, Simple Math," *New York Times*, August 4, 2013, http://www.nytimes.com/2013/08/04/health/for-medical-tourists-simple-math.html.

13. E. Rosenthal, "Good Deals on Pills? It's Anyone's Guess," *New York Times*, November 10, 2013, http://www.nytimes.com/2013/11/10/sunday-review/good-deals-on-pills-its-anyones-guess.html.

14. E. Rosenthal, "The Growing Popularity of Having Surgery Overseas," *New York Times*, August 7, 2013, http://www.nytimes.com/2013/08/07/us/the-growing-popularity-of-having-surgery-overseas.html.

15. E. Rosenthal, "The Soaring Cost of a Simple Breath," *New York Times*, October 13, 2013, http://www.nytimes.com/2013/10/13/us/the-soaring-cost-of-a-simple-breath.html.

16. E. Rosenthal, "Think the E.R. Is Expensive? Look at How Much It Costs to Get There," *New York Times*, December 5, 2013, http://www.nytimes.com/2013/12/05/health/think-the-er-was-expensive-look-at-the-ambulance-bill.html.

17. E. Rosenthal, "Health Care's Road to Ruin," *New York Times*, December 22, 2013, http://www.nytimes.com/2013/12/22/sunday-review/health-cares-road-to-ruin.html.

18. E. Rosenthal, "When Health Costs Harm Your Credit," *New York Times*, March 9, 2014, http://www.nytimes.com/2014/03/09/sunday-review/when-health-costs-harm-your-credit.html.

19. E. Rosenthal, "Patients' Costs Skyrocket; Specialists' Incomes Soar," *New York Times*, January 1, 2014, http://www.nytimes.com/2014/01/19/health/patients-costs-skyrocket-specialists-incomes-soar.html.

20. E. Rosenthal, "Even Small Medical Advances Can Mean Big Jumps in Bills," *New York Times*, April 6, 2014, http://www.nytimes.com/2014/04/06/health/even-small-medical-advances-can-mean-big-jumps-in-bills.html.

21. M. B. Rothberg, "The $50,000 Physical," *Journal of the American Medical Association* 311, no. 21 (2014): 2175.

22. C. Bettigole, "The Thousand-Dollar Pap Smear," *New England Journal of Medicine* 369, no. 16 (2013): 1486–1487.

23. S. Lupkin, "Reddit User Posts $55,000 Hospital Bill for Appendectomy," *Good Morning America Yahoo News*, January 1, 2014, http://gma.yahoo.com/reddit-user-posts-55-000-hospital-bill-appendectomy-123853510.html.

24a. "The Anatomy of a Hospital Bill," *Wall Street Journal*, February 24, 2014, http://online.wsj.com/news/articles/SB10001424052702303496804579367244016430848.

24b. J. Nocera, "The $300,000 Drug," *New York Times*, July 18, 2014, http://www.nytimes.com/2014/07/19/opinion/joe-nocera-cystic-fibrosis-drug-price.html.

24c. R. Y. Hsia, Y. Akosa Antwi, and J. P. Nath, "Variation in Charges for 10 Common Blood Tests in California Hospitals: A Cross-Sectional Analysis," *British Medical Journal Open* 4 (2014): e005482.

25. R. Meyer, "American Healthcare Costs Are Completely Out of Line With the Rest of the Modern World," *World of DTC Marketing*, accessed January 29, 2014, http://worldofdtcmarketing.com/american-healthcare-costs-completely-line-rest-modern-world/cost-of-healthcare-in-the-u-s/.

26. R. S. Mathis, "Behind What Doesn't Make Sense," *Science* 342 (2013): 196.

27. T. Lieberman, "America's Healthcare Prices Are Absurd. So, Now What?," *Columbia Journalism Review*, February 25, 2014, http://www.cjr.org/the_second_opinion/elisabeth_rosenthal_on_covering_americas_rising_medical_costs.php?page=all.

28. R. Bayer et al., "Confronting the Sorry State of U.S. Health," *Science* 341 (2013): 962–963.

29. T. E. Board, "The Shame of American Health Care," *New York Times*, November 18, 2013, http://www.nytimes.com/2013/11/18/opinion/the-shame-of-american-health-care.html.

30. O. Khazan, "Expensive Healthcare Doesn't Help Americans Live Longer," *Atlantic*, December 2013, http://www.theatlantic.com/health/print/2013/12/expensive-healthcare-doesn-t-help-americans-live-longer/282343/.

31. "Best Care at Lower Cost The Path to Continuously Learning Health Care in America," Institute of Medicine of the National Academies, September 2012, http://www.iom.edu/~/media/Files/Report Files/2012/Best-Care/Best Care at Lower Cost_Recs.pdf.

32. R. J. Samuelson, "Health Care's Heap of Wasteful Spending," *Washington Post*, September 9, 2012, http://www.washingtonpost.com/opinions/health-cares-heap-of-waste/2012/09/13/ee62aa62-fdb6-11e1-b153-218509a954e1_print.html.

33. U. E. Reinhardt, "Waste vs. Value in American Health Care," *New York Times*, September 13, 2013, http://economix.blogs.nytimes.com/2013/09/13/waste-vs-value-in-american-health-care/.

34. T. Parker-Pope, "Overtreatment Is Taking a Harmful Toll," *New York Times*, August 27, 2012, http://well.blogs.nytimes.com/2012/08/27/overtreatment-is-taking-a-harmful-toll/.

35. N. E. Morden et al., "Choosing Wisely—The Politics and Economics of Labeling Low-Value Services," *New England Journal of Medicine* 370 (2014): 589–592.

36. A. L. Schwartz et al., "Measuring Low-Value Care in Medicare," *JAMA Internal Medicine* 174, no. 4 (2014): 1067–1076.

37. "Survey: Physicians are Aware That Many Medical Tests and Procedures Are Unnecessary, See Themselves as Solution," Robert Wood Johnson Foundation, April 2014, http://www.rwjf.org/en/about-rwjf/newsroom/newsroom-content/2014/04/survey--physicians-are-aware-that-many-medical-tests-and-procedu.html.

38. J. Appleby, "Hospitals Promote Screenings That Experts Say Many People Do Not Need," *Washington Post*, May 13, 2014, http://www.washingtonpost.com/national/health-science/hospitals-promote-screenings-that-experts-say-most-people-should-not-receive/2013/05/13/aaecb272-9ae2-11e2-9bda-edd1a7fb557d_story.html.

39. S. Garber et al., "Redirecting Innovation in US Health Care," The RAND Corporation, 2014, http://www.rand.org/pubs/research_reports/RR308.html.

40. R. Sihvonen et al., "Arthroscopic Partial Meniscectomy versus Sham Surgery for a Degenerative Meniscal Tear," *New England Journal of Medicine* 369, no. 26 (2013): 2515–2524.

41. S. Eappen et al., "Relationship Between Occurrence of Surgical Complications and Hospital Finances," *Journal of the American Medical Association* 309, no. 15 (2013): 1599–1606.

42. "Physician, Heal Thyself," *The Economist*, February 1, 2014, http://www.economist.com/node /21595431/print.

43. R. Vigen et al., "Association of Testosterone Therapy With Mortality, Myocardial Infarction, and Stroke in Men With Low Testosterone Levels," *Journal of the American Medical Association* 310, no. 17 (2013): 1829–1836.

44. A. Schwarz, "The Selling of Attention Deficit Disorder," *New York Times*, December 15, 2013, http://www.nytimes.com/2013/12/15/health/the-selling-of-attention-deficit-disorder.html.

45. J. E. Brody, "A Check on Physicals," *New York Times*, January 21, 2013, http://well.blogs.nytimes .com/2013/01/21/a-check-on-physicals/.

46. R. C. Rabin, "A Glut of Antidepressants," *New York Times*, August 12, 2013, http://well.blogs .nytimes.com/2013/08/12/a-glut-of-antidepressants/.

47. S. VanDriest et al., "Clinically Actionable Genotypes Among 10,000 Patients with Preemptive Pharmacogenomic Testing," *Clinical Pharmacology & Therapeutics* 95, no. 4 (2014): 423–431.

48. H. G. Welch, "Testing What We Think We Know," *New York Times*, August 20, 2012, http:// www.nytimes.com/2012/08/20/opinion/testing-standard-medical-practices.html.

49. M. Bassett, "Global Medical Imaging Market to Hit $32 Billion by 2014," *Fierce Medical Imaging*, July 11, 2013, http://www.fiercemedicalimaging.com/story/global-medical-imaging-market-hit-32 -billion-2014/2013-07-11.

50. B. Owens, "Enhanced Medical Vision," *Nature* 502 (2013): S82–S83.

51. R. F. Redberg and R. Smith-Bindman, "We Are Giving Ourselves Cancer," *New York Times*, January 31, 2014, http://www.nytimes.com/2014/01/31/opinion/we-are-giving-ourselves-cancer.html.

52. R. Pomerance, "The Less-Is-More Approach to Health Care," *US News and World Report*, March 5, 2013, http://health.usnews.com/health-news/health-wellness/articles/2013/03/05/the-less-is-more -approach-to-health-care.

53. M. Beck, "Study Raises Doubts Over Robotic Surgery," *Wall Street Journal*, February 19, 2013, http://online.wsj.com/article/SB10001424127887323764804578314182573530720.html.

54. J. N. Mirkin et al., "Direct-To-Consumer Internet Promotion of Robotic Prostatectomy Exhibits Varying Quality of Information," *Health Affairs* 31, no. 4 (2012): 760–769.

55. R. Langreth, "Robot Surgery Damaging Patients Rises with Marketing," *Bloomberg*, October 8, 2013, http://www.bloomberg.com/news/print/2013-10-08/robot-surgery-damaging-patients-rises-with -marketing.html.

56. "Proton Therapy," *Wikipedia*, accessed August 13, 2014, http://en.wikipedia.org/wiki/Proton _therapy#Treatment_centers.

57. A. Chandra, J. Holmes, and J. Skinner, "Is This Time Different? The Slowdown in Healthcare Spending," Brookings Panel on Economic Activity, Fall 2013, http://www.brookings.edu/~/media/ Projects/BPEA/Fall 2013/2013b_chandra_healthcare_spending.pdf.

58. S. Havele, "Why Patients Need to Be Treated like Consumers," *Rock Health*, January 28, 2014, http://rockhealth.com/2014/01/why-patients-need-to-be-treated-like-consumers-qa-noah-lang/.

59. B. Mannino, "Do You Really Need an Annual Physical?," *Fox Business*, August 24, 2012, http:// www.foxbusiness.com/personal-finance/2012/08/24/do-really-need-annual-physical/.

60. L. T. Krogsbøll et al., "General Health Checks in Adults for Reducing Morbidity and Mortality from Disease: Cochrane Systematic Review and Meta-analysis," *British Medical Journal* 345 (2012): e7191.

61. E. Klein, "The Two Most Important Numbers in American Health Care," *Washington Post*, September 19, 2013, http://www.washingtonpost.com/blogs/wonkblog/wp/2013/09/19/the-two-most -important-numbers-in-american-health-care/?print=1.

62. S. Lohr, "Salesforce Takes Its Cloud Model to Health Care," *New York Times*, June 26, 2014, http://bits.blogs.nytimes.com/2014/06/26/salesforce-takes-its-cloud-model-to-health-care/.

63. "End-Of-Life Care: A Challenge in Terms Of Costs and Quality," *Kaiser Health News*, June 4, 2013, http://www.kaiserhealthnews.org/Daily-Reports/2013/June/04/end-of-life-care.aspx.

64. G. W. Neuberg, "The Cost of End-of-Life Care: A New Efficiency Measure Falls Short of AHA/ACC Standards," *Circulation: Cardiovascular Quality and Outcomes* 2 (2009): 127–133.

65. "International Health Policy Survey in Eleven Countries," The Commonwealth Fund, November 2013, http://www.commonwealthfund.org/~/media/Files/Publications/In the Literature/2013/Nov/PDF_Schoen_2013_IHP_survey_chartpack_final.pdf.

66. D. Voran, "Will the Tech Bubble Break," *Information Week*, January 3, 2014, http://www.informationweek.com/healthcare/mobile-and-wireless/medicine-will-the-tech-bubble-break/d/d-id/1113295?print=yes.

67. "Sun, Shopping and Surgery," *The Economist*, December 9, 2010, http://www.economist.com/node/17680806/print.

68. "Plastic Surgery in South Korea: A Popular Look," *The Economist*, April 26, 2011, http://www.economist.com/blogs/banyan/2011/04/plastic_surgery_south_korea.

69. R. Pearl, "Offshoring American Health Care: Higher Quality At Lower Costs?," *Forbes*, March 27, 2014, http://www.forbes.com/sites/robertpearl/2014/03/27/offshoring-american-health-care-higher-quality-at-lower-costs/print/.

70. K. Okike et al., "Survey Finds Few Orthopedic Surgeons Know the Costs of the Devices They Implant," *Health Affairs* 33, no. 1 (2014): 103–109.

71. J. Gold, "How Much Does a New Hip Cost? Even The Surgeon Doesn't Know," *Kaiser Health News*, January 6, 2014, http://capsules.kaiserhealthnews.org/index.php/2014/01/how-much-does-a-new-hip-cost-even-the-surgeon-doesnt-know/.

72. B. Friedman, "Displaying the Cost of Lab Tests for Physicians in Their EHRs," *Lab Soft News*, January 7, 2014, http://labsoftnews.typepad.com/lab_soft_news/2014/01/displaying-the-cost-of-lab-tests-for-physicians-in-the-ehr.html.

73. T. Worstall, "Bending The Health Care Cost Curve: Fire the Doctors," *Forbes*, September 5, 2012, http://www.forbes.com/sites/timworstall/2012/09/05/bending-the-health-care-cost-curve-fire-the-doctors/print/.

74. "Medical Price Transparency Law Rolls Out: Physicians Must Be Able to Estimate Costs for Patients," Massachusetts Medical Society, January 2014, http://blog.massmed.org/index.php/2014/01/mass-medical-price-transparency-law-rolls-out-physicians-must-be-able-to-estimate-costs-for-patients/.

75. "Yale Office-Based Medicine Curriculum," Yale School of Medicine, accessed August 13, 2014, http://yobm.yale.edu/index.aspx.

76. T. Gower, "Should Doctors Consider Medical Costs?," *Boston Globe*, April 12, 2014, http://www.bostonglobe.com/ideas/2014/04/12/should-doctors-consider-medical-costs/GPJM1h30qtz6zpfzrxQGoL/story.html.

77. P. A. Ubel, "Doctor, First Tell Me What It Costs," *New York Times*, November 4, 2013, http://www.nytimes.com/2013/11/04/opinion/doctor-first-tell-me-what-it-costs.html.

78. P. A. Ubel, A. P. Abernethy, and S. Y. Zafar, "Full Disclosure—Out-of-Pocket Costs as Side Effects," *New England Journal of Medicine* 368, no. 16 (2013): 1484–1486.

79. C. Moriates, N. T. Shah, and V. M. Arora, "First, Do No (Financial) Harm," *Journal of the American Medical Association* 310, no. 6 (2013): 577–578.

80. A. Bond, "Can You Afford Your Medicine? Doctors Don't Ask," *New York Times*, May 1, 2014, http://well.blogs.nytimes.com/2014/05/01/doctors-not-asking-about-money/?ref=health.

81. D. Ofri, "Why Doctors Are Reluctant to Take Responsibility for Rising Medical Costs," *The Atlantic*, August 2013, http://www.theatlantic.com/health/print/2013/08/why-doctors-are-reluctant-to-take-responsibility-for-rising-medical-costs/278623/.

82. M. S. Patel et al., "Teaching Residents to Provide Cost-Conscious Care: A National Survey of Residency Program Directors," *JAMA Internal Medicine* 174, no. 3 (2013): 470–472.

83. R. Srivastava, "How Can We Save on Healthcare Costs If Doctors Are Kept in the Dark?," *The Guardian*, March 14, 2014, http://www.theguardian.com/commentisfree/2014/mar/14/how-can-we-save-on-healthcare-costs-if-doctors-are-kept-in-the-dark/print.

84. J. H. Cochrane, "What to Do When ObamaCare Unravels," *Wall Street Journal*, December 25, 2013, http://online.wsj.com/news/articles/SB10001424052702304866904579265932490593594.

85. M. J. DeLaMerced, "Oscar, a New Health Insurer, Raises $30 Million," *New York Times*, January 7, 2014, http://dealbook.nytimes.com/2014/01/07/oscar-a-new-health-insurer-raises-30-million/.

86. "The Geek Guide to Insurance," *The Economist*, April 5, 2014, http://www.economist.com/node /21600147/print.

87. C. Ornstein, "Can't Get Through to Your Health Insurer? Vent on Twitter," *ProPublica*, January 29, 2014, http://www.propublica.org/article/cant-get-through-to-your-health-insurer-vent-on-twitter.

88. T. Rosenberg, "Revealing a Health Care Secret: The Price," *New York Times*, July 31, 2013, http:// opinionator.blogs.nytimes.com/2013/07/31/a-new-health-care-approach-dont-hide-the-price/.

89. R. Kocher, "Last Week's Medicare Millionaires Story Was Only the Beginning," *Dallas News*, April 15, 2014, http://www.dallasnews.com/opinion/sunday-commentary/20140415-last-weeks -medicare-millionaires-story-was-only-the-beginning.ece.

90. N. Brennan, P. H. Conway, and M. Tavenner, "The Medicare Physician-Data Release—Context and Rationale," *New England Journal of Medicine*, July 10, 2014, http://www.nejm.org/doi/full/10.1056 /NEJMp1405026.

91. M. Beck, "How to Bring the Price of Health Care Into the Open," *Wall Street Journal*, February 23, 2014, http://online.wsj.com/news/articles/SB10001424052702303650204579375242842086688.

92. "Within Digital Health, Healthcare Cost Transparency Is an Increasingly Hot Area Among VCs," *CB Insights*, September 12, 2013, http://www.cbinsights.com/blog/trends/healthcare-cost -transparency.

93. "Price Transparency an Essential Building Block for a High-Value, Sustainable Health Care System," National Governors Association, accessed August 13, 2014, http://statepolicyoptions.nga.org/ policy_article/price-transparency-essential-building-block-high-value-sustainable-health-care-section.

94. B. Coluni, "Save $36 Billion in US Healthcare Spending Through Price Transparency," *Thompson Reuters*, February 2012, http://spu.edu/depts/hr/documents/health_plan_price_transparency.pdf.

95. D. Cutler and L. Dafny, "Designing Transparency Systems for Medical Care Prices," *New England Journal of Medicine* 362, no. 10 (2011): 894–895.

96. J. Millman, "Price Transparency Stinks in Health Care. Here's How the Industry Wants to Change That," *Washington Post*, April 16, 2014, http://www.washingtonpost.com/blogs/wonkblog/wp /2014/04/16/price-transparency-stinks-in-health-care-heres-how-the-industry-wants-to-change-that/.

97. M. Trilli, "Price Transparency in U.S. Healthcare: A New Market," Aite Group, June 5, 2013, http://www.aitegroup.com/report/price-transparency-us-healthcare-new-market.

98. T. Murphy, "Patients, Firms Shop for Better Health Care Deals," *ABC News*, October 26, 2013, http://e-healthynewsdaily.blogspot.com/2013/10/patients-firms-shop-for-better-health.html.

99. D. Munro, "Healthcare's Story of the Year for 2013—Pricing Transparency," *Forbes*, December 15, 2013, http://www.forbes.com/sites/danmunro/2013/12/15/healthcares-story-of-the-year-for-2013 -pricing-transparency/print/.

100. K. Phillips, "A Trend: Private Companies Provide Health Care Price Data," *Health Affairs Blog*, January 8, 2014, http://healthaffairs.org/blog/2014/01/08/a-trend-private-companies-provide-health -care-price-data/print/.

101. A. D. Sinaiko and M. B. Rosenthal, "Increased Price Transparency in Health Care—Challenges and Potential Effects," *New England Journal of Medicine* 364, no. 10 (2011): 891–894.

102a. M. K. McGee, "Mobile App Helps Consumers Shop for Healthcare," *Information Week*, April 2, 2012, http://www.informationweek.com/news/healthcare/patient/232800146?printer_friendly=this -page.

102b. S. G. Boodman, "Like Priceline for Patients: Doctors Compete for Business via Online Bids for Surgery," *Washington Post*, August 4, 2014, http://www.washingtonpost.com/national/health-science/ like-priceline-for-patients-doctors-compete-for-business-via-online-bids-for-surgery/2014/08/01 /030d3576-f7e4-11e3-a606-946fd632f9f1_story.html.

103. G. Perna, "Uwe Reinhardt: The Year of Hospital Pricing Transparency (Part 1)," *Healthcare Informatics*, December 13, 2013, http://www.healthcare-informatics.com/print/article/uwe-reinhardt-year -hospital-pricing-transparency-part-1.

104. M. Gamble, "Survey: 32% of Patients Ask About Cost Before Appointment or Hospital Visit," *Becker's Hospital Review*, January 9, 2014, http://www.beckershospitalreview.com/racs-/-icd-9-/-icd-10/ survey-32-of-patients-ask-about-cost-before-appointment-or-hospital-visit.html.

105. M. P. Mikluch, "On the Use of Knowledge in the U.S. Health Care System," *Charles Street Symposium*, 2013, http://www.podemska.com/on-the-use-of-knowledge-in.pdf.

106. N. Omigui et al., "Outmigration for Coronary Bypass Surgery in an Era of Public Dissemination of Clinical Outcomes," *Circulation* 93, no. 1 (1996): 27–33.

107a. R. Kolker, "Heartless," *New York Magazine*, 2014, http://nymag.com/nymetro/health/features /14788/.

107b. S.-j Wu et al., "Price Transparency for MRIs Increased Use of Less Costly Providers and Triggered Provider Competition," *Health Affairs* 33, no. 8 (2014): 1391–1398.

107c. S. Kliff, "When Health Care Prices Stop Being Hidden, and Start Getting Real," *Vox*, August 18, 2014, http://www.vox.com/2014/8/5/5970685/when-health-care-prices-stop-being-hidden-and-start -getting-real.

107d. E. Rosenthal, "Why We Should Know the Price of Medical Tests," *New York Times*, August 5, 2014, http://well.blogs.nytimes.com/2014/08/05/why-we-should-know-the-price-of-medical-tests/.

108. J. H. Hibbard et al., "An Experiment Shows That a Well-Designed Report on Costs and Quality Can Help Consumers Choose High-Value Health Care," *Health Affairs* 31, no. 3 (2012): 560–568.

109. J. A. Guest and L. Quincy, "Consumers Gaining Ground in Health Care," *Journal of the American Medical Association* 310, no. 18 (2013): 1939–1940.

110. "DocAdvisor," *The Economist*, July 26, 2014, http://www.economist.com/node/21608767/print.

Chapter 9

1. R. Cook, *Cell* (New York, NY: Penguin, 2014), 216.

2. M. Miliard, "Q&A: Eric Dishman on Patient Engagement," *Healthcare IT News*, April 10, 2012, http://www.healthcareitnews.com/eric-dishman-interview.

3. J. Hempel, "IBM's Massive Bet on Watson," *Fortune*, September 19, 2013, http://fortune.com /2013/09/19/ibms-massive-bet-on-watson/.

4. D. Rotman, "How Technology Is Destroying Jobs," *MIT Technology Review*, June 12, 2013, http://www.technologyreview.com/featuredstory/515926/how-technology-is-destroying-jobs/.

5. W. B. Arthur, *The Nature of Technology* (New York, NY: Penguin, 2009).

6. E. Brynjolfsson and A. McAfee, *Race Against the Machine* (Lexington, MA: Digital Frontier Press, 2011).

7. Cook, *Cell*, 30.

8. Ibid., 216–217.

9. R. Cook and E. Topol, "Cook and Topol: How Digital Medicine Will Soon Save Your Life," *Wall Street Journal*, February 21, 2014, http://online.wsj.com/news/articles/SB10001424052702303973704579351080028045594.

10. "A Survey of America's Physicians: Practice Patterns and Perspectives," The Physicians Foundation, September 21, 2012, http://www.physiciansfoundation.org/healthcare-research/a-survey-of -americas-physicians-practice-patterns-and-perspectives.

11. P. Carrera, "Do-It-Yourself Health Care," *Health Affairs* 32, no. 6 (2013): 1173.

12. K. Uhlig et al., "Self-Measured Blood Pressure Monitoring in the Management of Hypertension: A Systematic Review and Meta-Analysis," *Annals of Internal Medicine* 159, no. 3 (2013): 185–194.

13. K. L. Margolis et al., "Effect of Home Blood Pressure Telemonitoring and Pharmacist Management on Blood Pressure Control: A Cluster Randomized Clinical Trial," *Journal of the American Medical Association* 310, no. 1 (2013): 46–56.

14. S. Nundy et al., "Mobile Phone Diabetes Project Led to Improved Glycemic Control and Net Savings for Chicago Plan Participants," *Health Affairs* 33, no. 2 (2014): 265–272.

15. L. Kish, "The Blockbuster Drug of the Century: An Engaged Patient," *HL7 Standards*, August 28, 2012, http://www.hl7standards.com/blog/2012/08/28/drug-of-the-century/.

16. S. Dentzer, "Rx for the 'Blockbuster Drug' of Patient Engagement," *Health Affairs* 32, no. 2 (2013): 202.

17. L. Ricciardi et al., "A National Action Plan to Support Consumer Engagement via E-Health," *Health Affairs* 32, no. 2 (2013): 376–384.

18. J. H. Hibbard and J. Greene, "What the Evidence Shows About Patient Activation: Better Health Outcomes and Care Experiences; Fewer Data on Costs," *Health Affairs* 32, no. 2 (2013): 207–214.

19. S. Bouchard, "Harnessing the Power of Retail Clinics," *Healthcare Finance News,* April 25, 2014, http://www.healthcarefinancenews.com/news/harnessing-power-retail-clinics.

20. M. Hamilton, "Why Walk-in Health Care Is a Fast-Growing Profit Center for Retail Chains," *Washington Post,* April 4, 2014, http://www.washingtonpost.com/business/why-walk-in-health-care-is-a-fast-growing-profit-center-for-retail-chains/2014/04/04/a05f7cf4-b9c2-11e3-96ae-f2c36d2b1245_story.html.

21. S. Reddy, "Drugstores Play Doctor: Physicals, Flu Diagnosis, and More," *Wall Street Journal,* April 7, 2014, http://online.wsj.com/news/articles/SB1000142405270230481900457948741238535 9986.

22. K. Koplovitz, "Healthcare IT—An Investment Choice for the Future," *Forbes,* February 2, 2014, http://www.forbes.com/sites/kaykoplovitz/2014/02/04/healthcare-it-an-investment-choice-for-the-future/.

23. M. Beck and T. W. Martin, "Pediatrics Group Balks at Rise of Retail Health Clinics," *Wall Street Journal,* February 24, 2014, http://online.wsj.com/news/article_email/SB100014240527023048347045 79400962328393876-lMyQjAxMTA0MDIwNDEyNDQyWj - printMode.

24. B. Japsen, "As Walgreen Plays Doctor, Family Physicians Bristle," *Forbes,* April 6, 2013, http://www.forbes.com/sites/brucejapsen/2013/04/06/as-walgreen-plays-doctor-family-physicians-bristle/print/.

25. M. Healy, "Docs Oppose Retail-Based Clinics for Kids' Care," *USA Today,* February 24, 2014, http://www.usatoday.com/story/news/nation/2014/02/24/pediatrician-retail-health-clinics/5688603/.

26. M. Beck, "At VHA, Doctors, Nurses Clash on Oversight," *Wall Street Journal,* January 26, 2014, http://online.wsj.com/news/articles/SB10001424052702304856504579340603947983912.

27. "The Future of Nursing: Leading Change, Advancing Health Report Recommendations," Institute of Medicine, November 17, 2010, http://www.iom.edu/Reports/2010/The-Future-of-Nursing-Leading-Change-Advancing-Health/Recommendations.aspx.

28. C. Gounder, "The Case for Changing How Doctors Work," *New Yorker,* October 1, 2013, http://www.newyorker.com/online/blogs/currency/2013/10/changing-how-doctors-work.html?printable=true&currentPage=all.

29. S. Jauhar, "Nurses Are Not Doctors," *New York Times,* April 30, 2014, http://www.nytimes.com/2014/04/30/opinion/nurses-are-not-doctors.html.

30. O. Khazan, "The Case for Seeing a Nurse Instead of a Doctor," *The Atlantic,* April 2014, http://www.theatlantic.com/health/print/2014/04/the-case-for-seeing-a-nurse-instead-of-a-doctor/361111/.

31. L. Uscher-Pines and A. Mehrotra, "Analysis of Teladoc Use Seems to Indicate Expanded Access to Care for Patients Without Prior Connection to a Provider," *Health Affairs* 33, no. 2 (2014): 258–264.

32. "How Long Will You Wait to See a Doctor?," *CNN Money,* accessed August 19, 2014, http://money.cnn.com/interactive/economy/average-doctor-wait-times/.

33. E. Rosenthal, "The Health Care Waiting Game," *New York Times,* July 6, 2014, http://www.nytimes.com/2014/07/06/sunday-review/long-waits-for-doctors-appointments-have-become-the-norm.html.

34. T. Morrow, "How Virtual Health Assistants Can Reshape Healthcare," *Forbes,* March 13, 2013, http://www.forbes.com/sites/ciocentral/2013/03/13/how-virtual-health-assistants-can-reshape-healthcare/print/.

35. T. Morrow, "Virtual Health Assistants: A Prescription for Retail Pharmacies," *Drug Store News,* July 18, 2013, http://www.drugstorenews.com/article/virtual-health-assistants-prescription-retail-pharmacies.

36. T. McMahon, "The Smartphone Will See You Now," *MacLean's Magazine,* March 4, 2013, 46–49.

37. A. Carrns, "Visiting the Doctor, Virtually," *New York Times,* February 13, 2013, http://bucks.blogs.nytimes.com/2013/02/13/visiting-the-doctor-virtually/.

38. T. Wasserman, "The Doctor Will See You Now—On Your Cellphone," *Mashable,* December 10, 2013, http://mashable.com/2013/12/10/doctor-on-demand-app/.

39. R. Xu, "The Doctor Will See You Onscreen," *New Yorker*, March 10, 2014, http://www.newyorker.com/online/blogs/currency/2014/03/the-doctor-will-see-you-onscreen.html?printable=true&currentPage=all.

40. A. Sifferlin, "The Doctor Will Skype You Now," *TIME*, January 13, 2014, http://content.time.com/time/subscriber/printout/0,8816,2161682,00.html.

41. K. Bourzac, "The Computer Will See You Now," *Nature* 502 (2013): 592–594.

42. "The Robots Are Coming. How Many of Us Will Prosper from the Second Machine Age?," *Raw Story*, January 4, 2014, http://www.rawstory.com/rs/2014/01/04/the-robots-are-coming-how-many-of-us-will-prosper-from-the-second-machine-age/.

43. J. Marte, "The Doctor Visit of the Future May Be a Phone Call," *Market Watch*, March 3, 2014, http://www.marketwatch.com/story/the-doctor-will-facetime-you-now-2014-03-03/print?guid=D2E3D006-A2D6-11E3-BC16-00212803FAD6.

44. L. Landro, "A Better Online Diagnosis Before the Doctor Visit," *Wall Street Journal*, July 22, 2013, http://online.wsj.com/article/SB10001424127887324328904578621743278445114.html.

45. S. Koven, "Doctors, Patients, and Computer Screens," *Boston Globe*, February 24, 2014, http://www.bostonglobe.com/lifestyle/health-wellness/2014/02/24/practice-doctors-patients-and-computer-screens/JMMYaCDtf3mnuQZGfkMVyL/story.html.

46. L. Landro, "The Doctor's Team Will See You Now," *Wall Street Journal*, February 17, 2014, http://online.wsj.com/news/articles/SB10001424052702304899704579389203539061082.

47. T. W. Martin, "When Your M.D. Is an Algorithm," *Wall Street Journal*, April 11, 2013, http://online.wsj.com/article/SB10001424127887324010704578414992125798464.html.

48. A. Vaterlaus-Staby, "Is Data the Doctor of the Future?," *PSFK*, March 11, 2014: http://www.psfk.com/2014/03/data-doctor-future-future-health.html#!bGg2V0.

49. S. Bader, "The Doctor's Office of the Future: Coffeeshop, Apple Store, and Fitness Center," *Fast Company*, December 11, 2013, http://www.fastcoexist.com/3023255/futurist-forum/the-doctors-office-of-the-future-coffeeshop-apple-store-and-fitness-center.

50. A. Hamilton, "Could ePatient Networks Become the Superdoctors of the Future?," *Fast Company*, September 28, 2014, http://www.fastcoexist.com/1680617/could-epatient-networks-become-the-superdoctors-of-the-future.

51. S. D. Hall, "The Idea of Virtual Doctor Visits Is Growing on Us," *Fierce Health IT*, March 7, 2013, http://www.fiercehealthit.com/node/19095/print.

52. S. Mace, "Developing Telemedicine Options," *Health Leaders Media*, April 11, 2014, http://www.healthleadersmedia.com/print/MAG-303102/Developing-Telemedicine-Options.

53. K. Lee, "'Telehealth' Evolving Doctor-Patient Services with Online Interactions," *NECN*, January 21, 2014, http://www.necn.com/01/21/14/Telehealth-evolving-doctor-patient-servi/landing.html?blockID=861974.

54. C. Lowe, "The Future of Doctors," TeleCare Aware, January 23, 2014, http://telecareaware.com/the-future-of-doctors/.

55. R. Pearl, "Kaiser Permanente Northern California: Current Experiences with Internet, Mobile, and Video Technologies," *Health Affairs* 33, no. 2 (2014): 251–257.

56. D. Raths, "Kaiser N. Calif. Topped 10 Million Virtual Visits in 2013," *Healthcare Informatics*, February 11, 2013, http://www.healthcare-informatics.com/print/blogs/david-raths/kaiser-n-calif-topped-10-million-virtual-visits-2013.

57. "Why Telemedicine Is the Future of the Health Care Industry," *The Week*, April 23, 2014, http://theweek.com/article/index/260330/why-telemedicine-is-the-future-of-the-health-care-industry.

58. D. Liu, "Vinod Khosla: Technology Will Replace 80 Percent of Docs," *Health Care Blog*, August 31, 2014, http://thehealthcareblog.com/blog/2012/08/31/vinod-khosla-technology-will-replace-80-percent-of-docs/.

59. L. Gannes, "Doctor on Demand App Gives $40 Medical Consultations from the Comfort of Your Smartphone," *All Things D*, December 10, 2013, http://allthingsd.com/?p=377886&ak_action=printable.

60. "MedLion Direct Primary Care Partners with Helpouts by Google to Give Patients Live Video Appointments," *PRWeb*, April 2, 2014, http://www.prweb.com/releases/2014MedLionGoogleHelpouts/04/prweb11730367.htm.

61. E. A. Moore, "For $49, a Doctor Will See You Now—Online," *CNET,* October 9, 2013, http://news.cnet.com/8301-17938_105-57606794-1/for-$49-a-doctor-will-see-you-now-online/.

62. A. Nixon, "Virtual Doctor's Office Visits via Telemedicine to be Norm," *TribLive,* October 31, 2013, http://triblive.com/business/headlines/4976316-74/doctor-patients-telemedicine?printerfriendly=true.

63. J. Bellamy, "Telemedicine: Click and the Doctor Will See You Now," *Science Based Medicine,* May 1, 2014, http://www.sciencebasedmedicine.org/telemedicine-click-and-the-doctor-will-see-you-now/.

64. W. H. Frist, "Connected Health and the Rise of the Patient-Consumer," *Health Affairs* 33, no. 2 (2014): 191–193.

65. L. Freeman, "Patients Skipping Waiting Room in Favor of Visiting Doctor Online," *23 ABC,* August 9, 2013, http://www.turnto23.com/web/kero/lifestyle/health/patients-skipping-waiting-room-in-favor-of-visiting-doctor-online-1.

66. R. Flinn, "Video Dial-a-Doctor Seen Easing Shortage in Rural U.S.," *Bloomberg Businessweek,* September 5, 2012, http://www.businessweek.com/printer/articles/319338?type=bloomberg.

67. C. Farr, "Former Apple CEO Backs Virtual Doctor's Office to Create the 'Consumer Era' of Medicine," *Venture Beat,* January 22, 2014, http://venturebeat.com/2014/01/22/former-apple-ceo-backs-virtual-doctors-office-to-create-the-consumer-era-of-medicine/.

68. R. Empson, "With $1.2M from Greylock, Yuri Milner and 500 Startups, First Opinion Lets You Text a Doctor Anytime," *TechCrunch,* January 14, 2014, http://techcrunch.com/2014/01/14/with-1-2m-from-greylock-yuri-milner-and-500-startups-first-opinion-lets-you-text-a-doctor-anytime/.

69. O. Kharif, "Telemedicine: Doctor Visits via Video Calls," *Bloomberg Businessweek,* February 27, 2014, http://www.businessweek.com/articles/2014-02-27/health-insurers-add-telemedicine-services-to-cut-costs.

70. W. Khawar, "For $69 and Your Smart Phone in Hand, a Board Certified Dermatologist Will Look at Your Rash," *iMedical Apps,* August 19, 2013, http://www.imedicalapps.com/2013/08/smartphone-dermatologist-rash/.

71. L. Dignan, "Expanding Amazon's Mayday Button: Five New Uses to Ponder," *ZDNet,* January 3, 2014, http://www.zdnet.com/expanding-amazons-mayday-button-five-new-uses-to-ponder-7000024741/.

72. D. Pogoreic, "MDs, AT&T Alum Look to Test the Market for Virtual Concierge Care in California via Crowdfunding," *MedCity News,* March 4, 2014, http://medcitynews.com/2014/03/crowdfunding-lean-mhealth-startup-att-mhealth-alum-test-market-virtual-concierge-care/.

73. "How Digital Checkups Provide Better Patient Care [Future of Health]," *PSFK,* March 6, 2014, http://www.psfk.com/2014/03/remote-health.html.

74. L. H. Schwamm, "Telehealth: Seven Strategies to Successfully Implement Disruptive Technology and Transform Health Care," *Health Affairs* 33, no. 2 (2014): 200–206.

75. C. Brown, "Bringing Home the Value of Telehealth," *Business Innovation,* February 18, 2014, http://www.business2community.com/business-innovation/bringing-home-value-telehealth-0783860#!bGhsGA.

76. C. Farr, "Google Jumps into the Healthcare Field with Video Service Helpouts," *MedCity News,* November 20, 2013, http://medcitynews.com/2013/11/google-jumps-healthcare-field-video-service-helpouts/.

77. J. Roettgers, "Google's Helpouts Could Be the Company's Secret Weapon to Take on Healthcare," *Tech News and Analysis,* November 4, 2013, http://gigaom.com/2013/11/04/googles-helpouts-could-be-the-companys-secret-weapon-to-take-on-healthcare/.

78. D. Tahir, "Verizon Introduces Virtual Visits, New Telehealth Offering," *Modern Healthcare,* June 25, 2014, http://www.modernhealthcare.com/article/20140625/NEWS/306259948.

79. "For $50 a Month, These Health Advisors Will Answer All Your Paranoid Medical Questions," *Fast Company,* April 17, 2014, http://www.fastcoexist.com/3029237/for-50-a-month-these-health-advisors-will-answer-all-your-paranoid-medical-questions.

80. G. Clapp, "Meet Better—Your Personal Health Assistant," Better, April 15, 2014, http://www.getbetter.com/blog/2014/4/15/meet-better-your-personal-health-assistant.

81. N. Ungerleider, "The Mayo Clinic's New Doctor-in-an-iPhone," *Fast Company,* April 18, 2014, http://www.fastcompany.com/3029304/the-mayo-clinics-new-doctor-in-an-iphone.

82. L. Rao, "Better Raises $5M from Chamath Palihapitiya and Mayo Clinic to Be Your Personal Health Advocate," *TechCrunch*, April 16, 2014, http://techcrunch.com/2014/04/16/better-raises-5m -from-chamath-palihapitiya-and-mayo-clinic-to-be-your-personal-health-advocate/.

83. B. Dolan, "Mayo Clinic–Backed Better Launches Personal Health Assistant Service," *Mobi-HealthNews*, April 16, 2014, http://mobihealthnews.com/32130/mayo-clinic-backed-better-launches -personal-health-assistant-service/.

84a. G. Pittman, "Virtual Visits to Doctor May Be Cheaper Than and as Effective as In-Person Visits," *Washington Post*, January 18, 2013, http://www.washingtonpost.com/national/health-science/virtual -visits%C9n-visits/2013/01/18/8237c028-601e-11e2-a389-ee565c81c565_print.html.

84b. C. Schmidt, "Uber-Inspired Apps Bring a Doctor Right to Your Door," *CNN*, July 31, 2014, http://www.cnn.com/2014/07/31/health/doctor-house-call-app/.

85. L. H. Schwamm, "Telehealth: Seven Strategies to Successfully Implement Disruptive Technology and Transform Healthcare," *Health Affairs* 33, no. 2 (2014): 200–206.

86a. H. Gregg, "WellPoint's Telemedicine Service Saves Patients $71 per Visit," *Beckers Hospital Review*, March 6, 2014, http://www.beckershospitalreview.com/healthcare-information-technology/ wellpoint-s-telemedicine-service-saves-patients-71-per-visit/print.html.

86b. "Technology, Media & Telecommunications Predictions," Deloitte Global Report, 2014, http:// www2.deloitte.com/global/en/pages/technology-media-and-telecommunications/articles/tmt -predictions-2014.html.

86c. L. Mearian, "Almost One in Six Doctor Visits Will Be Virtual This Year," *Computer World*, August 9, 2014, http://www.computerworld.com.au/article/552031/almost_one_six_doctor_visits_will _virtual_year/.

87. D. F. Maron, "Virtual Doctor Visits Gaining Steam in 'Geneticist Deserts,'" *Scientific American*, April 21, 2014, http://www.scientificamerican.com/article/virtual-doctor-visits-gaining-steam/?print=true.

88. "Genetic Counseling via Telephone as Effective as In-person Counseling," Lombardi News Release Archive, January 22, 2014, http://explore.georgetown.edu/documents/74419/?PageTemplateID =141.

89. J. Adler-Milstein, J. Kvedar, and D. W. Bates, "Telehealth Among US Hospitals: Several Factors, Including State Reimbursement and Licensure Policies, Influence Adoption," *Health Affairs* 33, no. 2 (2014): 207–215.

90. R. Kocher, "Doctors Without State Borders: Practicing Across State Lines," *Health Affairs*, February 18, 2014, http://healthaffairs.org/blog/2014/02/18/doctors-without-state-borders-practicing-across -state-lines/.

91. M. Ravindranath, "Daschle, Former Senators Form Alliance to Lobby for New Telehealth Rules," *Washington Post*, March 1, 2014, http://www.washingtonpost.com/business/on-it/daschle-former-senato %C9h-rules/2014/03/01/194bc356-98ef-11e3-80ac-63a8ba7f7942_story.html.

92a. R. Pear, "Medical Boards Draft Plan to Ease Path to Out-of-State and Online Treatment," *New York Times*, June 30, 2014, http://www.nytimes.com/2014/06/30/us/medical-boards-draft-plan-to-ease -path-to-out-of-state-and-online-treatment.html.

92b. R. Steinbrook, "Interstate Medical Licensure: Major Reform of Licensing to Encourage Medical Practice in Multiple States," *Journal of the American Medical Association* 312, no. 7 (2014): 695–696.

93. Z. Landman, "Mobile Health Lets Doctors Practice Like It's 1950," *Huffington Post*, November 12, 2013, http://www.huffingtonpost.com/zachary-landman/mobile-health-lets-doctor_b_4262299 .html.

94. I. Gal, "Israeli Invention May Spare Visit to Doctor," *Y Net News*, November 4, 2013, http://www .ynetnews.com/articles/0,7340,L-4443648,00.html.

95a. "New Medical Tech Company, MedWand Solutions, LLC, Set to Revolutionize Telemedicine," PRWeb press release, April 28, 2014, http://www.prweb.com/releases/2014/04/prweb11799903.htm.

95b. R. Matheson, "Mental-Health Monitoring Goes Mobile," *MIT News*, July 16, 2014, http:// newsoffice.mit.edu/2014/mental-health-monitoring-goes-mobile-0716.

96. M. Wardrop, "Doctors Told to Prescribe Smartphone Apps to Patients," *Telegraph*, February 22, 2012, http://www.telegraph.co.uk/health/healthnews/9097647/Doctors-told-to-prescribe-smartphone -apps-to-patients.html.

97. S. Curtis, "Digital Doctors: How Mobile Apps Are Changing Healthcare," *Telegraph,* December 4, 2013, http://www.telegraph.co.uk/technology/news/10488778/Digital-doctors-how-mobile-apps-are -changing-healthcare.html.

98. "How Speech-Recognition Software Got So Good," *The Economist,* April 22, 2014, http://www .economist.com/node/21601175/print.

99. J. Conn, "IT Experts Push Translator Systems to Convert Doc-Speak into ICD-10 Codes," *Modern Healthcare,* May 3, 2014, http://www.modernhealthcare.com/article/20140503/MAGAZINE/305 039969/1246/.

100. R. Rosenberger, "Siri, Take This Down: Will Voice Control Shape Our Writing?," *The Atlantic,* August 2012, http://www.theatlantic.com/technology/print/2012/08/siri-take-this-down-will-voice -control-shape-our-writing/259624/.

101. E. Brynjolfsson and A. McAfee, *The Second Machine Age* (New York: W.W. Norton & Co., 2014).

102. K. Kelly, "Better Than Human: Why Robots Will—and Must—Take Our Jobs," *Wired,* December 24, 2012, http://www.wired.com/gadgetlab/2012/12/ff-robots-will-take-our-jobs/all/.

103. D. Bethel, "Doctor Dinosaur: Physicians May Not Be Exempt from Extinction," *KevinMD.com,* November 9, 2013, http://www.kevinmd.com/blog/2013/11/physicians-exempt-extinction.html.

104. E. Wicklund, "Korean Doctors Fight Back Against mHealth," *mHealth News,* November 27, 2013, http://www.mhealthnews.com/blog/korean-doctors-fight-back-against-mhealth.

105. J. D. Rockoff, "Robots vs. Anesthesiologists," *Wall Street Journal,* October 9, 2013, http://online .wsj.com/article/SB10001424052702303983904579093252573814132.html.

106a. R. Bradley, "Rethinking Health Care with PatientsLikeMe," *Fortune,* April 15, 2013, http:// fortune.com/2013/04/15/rethinking-health-care-with-patientslikeme/.

106b. "The Computer Will See You Now," *The Economist,* August 16, 2014, http://www.economist.com /news/science-and-technology/21612114-virtual-shrink-may-sometimes-be-better-real-thing-computer -will-see.

106c. G. M. Lucas, J. Gratch, A. King, and L.-P. Morency, "It's Only a Computer: Virtual Humans Increase Willingness to Disclose," *Computers in Human Behavior* 37 (2014): 94–100.

106d. "Physician Shortages to Worsen Increase in Residency Training," American Association of Medical Colleges, 2014, https://www.aamc.org/download/153160/data/physician_shortages_to_worsen_ without_increases_in_residency_tr.pdf.

106e. J. Eden, D. Berwick, and G. Wilensky, "Graduate Medical Education That Meets the Nation's Health Needs," in *Institute of Medicine* (Washington D.C.: The National Academies Press, 2014), http:// www.nap.edu/openbook.php?record_id=18754.

107. S. Gottlieb and E. J. Emanuel, "No, There Won't Be a Doctor Shortage," *New York Times,* December 5, 2013, http://www.nytimes.com/2013/12/05/opinion/no-there-wont-be-a-doctor-shortage .html.

108. J. Parkinson, "I Was Invited to a Private Breakfast with...," *New Yorker,* November 8, 2013, http:// blog.jayparkinsonmd.com/post/66394909190/i-was-invited-to-attend-a-private-breakfast-with.

109. "The Doctor Will Email You Now, and Patients Like It," *Science Blog,* August 6, 2013, http:// scienceblog.com/65398/the-doctor-will-email-you-now-and-patients-like-it/.

110. "The Doctor Will E-mail You Now," *Consumer Reports,* December 2013, http://www .consumerreports.org/cro/magazine/2014/01/the-doctor-will-email-you-now/index.htm.

111. J. Bresnick, "42% of Docs Fear mHealth Will Lessen Their Power Over Patients," *EHR Intelligence,* October 23, 2013, http://ehrintelligence.com/2013/10/23/42-of-docs-fear-mhealth-will-lessen -their-power-over-patients/.

112. "The Dream of the Medical Tricorder," *The Economist,* November 29, 2012, http://www .economist.com/news/technology-quarterly/21567208-medical-technology-hand-held-diagnostic -devices-seen-star-trek-are-inspiring.

113. E. J. Topol and M. R. Splinter, "Stuck in the Past: Why Are Doctors Still Using the Stethoscope and Manila Folder?," *Medscape,* December 10, 2013, http://www.medscape.com/viewarticle/817495 _print.

114. D. M. Knowlan, "Looking Back and Looking Forward: The White Coat Lecture," *Baylor University Medical Center Proceedings* 27, no. 1 (2014): 63–65.

115. "ICU Sonography Tutorial 9—Lung Ultrasound," Critical Echo, accessed August 13, 2014, http://www.criticalecho.com/content/tutorial-9-lung-ultrasound.

116. cyberPhil, "Why Not Teach Ultrasound in Medical School?," *Dr. Philip Gardiner's Blog,* January 9, 2013, http://www.philipgardiner.me.uk/2013/01/why-not-teach-medical-ultrasound-in-medical -school/.

117. J. A. Krisch, "R.I.P., Stethoscope?," *Popular Mechanics,* January 23, 2014, http://www .popularmechanics.com/science/health/med-tech/rip-stethoscope-16414909?utm_medium =referral&utm_source=pulsenews.

118. B. P. Nelson and J. Narula, "How Relevant Is Point-of-Care Ultrasound in LMIC?," *Global Heart* 8, no. 4 (2013): 287–288.

119. B. P. Nelson and A. Sanghvi, "Point-of-Care Cardiac Ultrasound: Feasibility of Performance by Noncardiologists," *Global Heart* 8, no. 4 (2013): 293–297.

120. A. Relman, "A Coming Medical Revolution," *New York Review of Books,* October 25, 2014, http:// www.nybooks.com/articles/archives/2012/oct/25/coming-medical-revolution/?pagination =false&printpage=true.

121. E. Rosenthal, "Apprehensive, Many Doctors Shift to Jobs with Salaries," *New York Times,* February 14, 2014, http://www.nytimes.com/2014/02/14/us/salaried-doctors-may-not-lead-to-cheaper -health-care.html.

122. D. Drake, "The Health-Care System Is So Broken, It's Time for Doctors to Strike," *The Daily Beast,* April 29, 2014, http://www.thedailybeast.com/articles/2014/04/29/the-health-care-system-is-so -broken-it-s-time-for-doctors-to-strike.html.

123. D. Shannon, "Why I Left Medicine: A Burnt-Out Doctor's Decision To Quit," *Common Health,* October 18, 2013, http://commonhealth.wbur.org/2013/10/why-i-left-medicine-a-burnt-out-doctors -decision-to-quit.

124. D. F. Craviotto, "A Doctor's Declaration of Independence," *Wall Street Journal,* April 28, 2014, http://online.wsj.com/news/articles/SB10001424052702304279904579518273176775310.

125. D. Ofri, "The Epidemic of Disillusioned Doctors," *TIME,* July 2, 2013, http://ideas.time.com /2013/07/02/the-epidemic-of-disillusioned-doctors/print/.

126. A. W. Mathews, "Hospitals Prescribe Big Data to Track Doctors at Work," *Wall Street Journal,* July 11, 2013, http://online.wsj.com/article/SB10001424127887323551004578441154292068308.html.

127. V. McEvoy, "Why 'Metrics' Overload Is Bad Medicine," *Wall Street Journal,* February 12, 2014, http://online.wsj.com/news/articles/SB10001424052702303293604579253971350304330?mod=WSJ _Opinion_LEFTTopOpinion.

128. R. Abelson and S. Cohen, "Sliver of Medicare Doctors Get Big Share of Payouts," *New York Times,* April 9, 2014, http://www.nytimes.com/2014/04/09/business/sliver-of-medicare-doctors-get-big -share-of-payouts.html.

129. R. Gunderman, "For the Young Doctor About to Burn Out," *The Atlantic,* February 21, 2014, http://www.theatlantic.com/health/archive/2014/02/for-the-young-doctor-about-to-burn-out/284005/.

130. D. Drake, "How Being a Doctor Became the Most Miserable Profession," *The Daily Beast,* April 14, 2014, http://www.thedailybeast.com/articles/2014/04/14/how-being-a-doctor-became-the-most -miserable-profession.html.

131. L. Radnofsky, "Medicare to Publish Trove of Data on Doctors," *Wall Street Journal,* April 2, 2014, http://online.wsj.com/news/articles/SB10001424052702303847804579477923585256790.

132. S. Dhand, "The Human Side of Medicine That No Computer Can Ever Touch," *KevinMD.com,* November 27, 2013, http://www.kevinmd.com/blog/2013/11/human-side-medicine-computer-touch .html.

133. D. Diamond, "Hospitals Lost Jobs—Again," *Advisory Board Daily Briefing,* August 2, 2013, http://www.advisory.com/Daily-Briefing/Blog/2013/08/Hospitals-lost-jobs-again.

134. J. Weiner, "What Big Data Can't Tell Us, but Kolstad's Paper Suggests," *Penn LDI,* April 24, 2014, http://ldi.upenn.edu/voices/2014/04/24/what-big-data-can-t-tell-us-but-kolstad-s-paper-suggests.

135. L. Rosenbaum, "What Big Data Can't Tell Us About Health Care," *New Yorker,* April 23, 2014, http://www.newyorker.com/online/blogs/currency/2014/04/the-medicare-data-dump-and-the-cost-of -care.html?printable=true&currentPage=all.

136. J. T. Kolstad, "Information and Quality When Motivation Is Intrinsic: Evidence from Surgeon Report Cards," National Bureau of Economic Research, February 2013, http://www.nber.org/papers/w18804.

137. C. Ornstein, "Beyond Ratings: More Tools Coming to Pick Your Doctor," *ProPublica*, April 8, 2014, http://www.propublica.org/article/beyond-ratings-more-tools-coming-to-pick-your-doctor.

138. Z. Moukheiber, "Grand Rounds Wants to Find the Right Doctor for You," *Forbes*, April 8, 2014, http://www.forbes.com/sites/zinamoukheiber/2014/04/08/grand-rounds-wants-to-find-the-right-doctor-for-you/.

139. L. Abrams, "Study: Hospitals with More Facebook 'Likes' Have Lower Mortality Rates," *The Atlantic*, March 2013, http://www.theatlantic.com/health/print/2013/03/study-hospitals-with-more-facebook-likes-have-lower-mortality-rates/273697/.

140. L. Abrams, "Why We're Still Waiting on the 'Yelpification' of Health Care," *The Atlantic*, October 2012, http://www.theatlantic.com/health/print/2012/10/why-were-still-waiting-on-the-yelpification-of-health-care/263815/.

141. D. Streitfeld, "Physician, Review Thyself," *New York Times*, March 4, 2014, http://bits.blogs.nytimes.com/2014/03/04/physician-review-thyself/?smid=tw-share.

142. "Consumer Reports Teams with Massachusetts Group to Rate Nearly 500 Primary Care Doctors' Practices," *Consumer Reports*, May 31, 2012, http://c354183.r83.cf1.rackcdn.com/MHQP%20Consumer%20Reports%20Insert%202012.pdf.

143. R. Gunderman, "Why Doctor Ratings Are Misleading," *The Atlantic*, April 2014, http://www.theatlantic.com/health/print/2014/04/why-doctor-ratings-are-misleading/360476/.

144. C. Doyle, L. Lennox, and D. Bell, "A Systematic Review of Evidence on the Links Between Patient Experience and Clinical Safety and Effectiveness," *British Medical Journal* 3 (2013): e001570.

145. J. Rossen, "Insult and Injury: How Doctors Are Losing the War Against Trolls," *BuzzFeed*, April 3, 2014, http://www.buzzfeed.com/jakerossen/insult-and-injury-inside-the-webs-one-sided-war-on-doctors.

146. J. J. Fenton et al., "The Cost of Satisfaction," *Archives of Internal Medicine* 172, no. 5 (2012): 405–411.

147. O. Khazan, "Why Aren't Doctors More Tech-Savvy?," *The Atlantic*, January 21, 2014, http://www.theatlantic.com/health/archive/2014/01/why-arent-doctors-more-tech-savvy/283178/.

148. J. Bendix, "Can the Doctor-Patient Relationship Survive?," *Medical Economics*, December 10, 2013, http://medicaleconomics.modernmedicine.com/medical-economics/news/can-doctor-patient-relationship-survive?page=full.

149. R. Harrell, "Why a Patient's Story Matters More Than a Computer Checklist," *NPR*, November 17, 2013, http://www.npr.org/blogs/health/2013/11/17/242366259/why-a-patient-s-story-matters-more-than-a-computer-checklist.

150. I. Bau, "Health 2.0 v.2013: Integration and Patient Outcomes Are Still Driving Health Technology—but So Should Empathy, Caring, and Communication," *Health Policy Consultation Services—Resources for Patient-Centered & Equitable Care*, October 4, 2013, http://ignatiusbau.com/?s=integration+patient+outcomes+health.

151. S. Guglani, "Compassionate Care: A Force for Change," *The Lancet* 382 (2013): 676.

152. E. Topol, "Machinations of the Machine Age," commencement address at Temple University, 2014, http://www.temple.edu/medicine/tusm_grad_speech_topol.htm.

153. "The Future of Jobs: The Onrushing Wave," *The Economist*, January 16, 2014, http://www.economist.com/news/briefing/21594264-previous-technological-innovation-has-always-delivered-more-long-run-employment-not-less.

Chapter 10

1. "The Future of Healthcare: Virtual Physician Visits & Bedless Hospitals," *Lab Soft News*, April 1, 2013, http://labsoftnews.typepad.com/lab_soft_news/2013/04/the-future-of-healthcare-less-emphasis-on-hospital-visits.html.

2. D. DiSanzo, "Op/Ed: Hospital of the Future Will Be a Health Delivery Network," *US News & World Report*, January 14, 2014, http://health.usnews.com/health-news/hospital-of-tomorrow/articles/2014/01/14/oped-hospital-of-the-future-will-be-a-health-delivery-network.

3. J. Comstock, "Revisiting How Christensen's 'Disruption Innovation' in Healthcare Means De-centralization," *MobiHealthNews*, March 26, 2014, http://mobihealthnews.com/31470/revisiting-how-christensens-disruption-innovation-in-healthcare-means-decentralization/.

4. E. Topol et al., "A Randomized Controlled Trial of Hospital Discharge Three Days After Myo-cardial Infarction in the Era of Reperfusion," *New England Journal of Medicine* 318 (1988): 1083–1088.

5. "American Hospital Association Annual Survey of Hospitals," in *Hospital Statistics, 1976, 1981, 1999–2011 editions* (Chicago, IL: American Hospital Association).

6. J. T. James, "A New, Evidence-Based Estimate of Patient Harms Associated with Hospital Care," *Journal of Patient Safety* 9, no. 3 (2013): 122–128.

7. L. L. Leape et al., "Perspective: A Culture of Respect, Part 2: Creating a Culture of Respect," *Academic Medicine* 87, no. 7 (2012): 853–858.

8. M. Makary, "How to Stop Hospitals from Killing Us," *Wall Street Journal*, September 21, 2012, http://online.wsj.com/news/articles/SB10000872396390444620104578008263334441352.

9. M. Makary, *Unaccountable: What Hospitals Won't Tell You and How Transparency Can Revolutionize Health Care* (New York, NY: Bloomsbury, 2012).

10. L. Landro, "Hospital Horrors," *Wall Street Journal*, October 3, 2012, http://online.wsj.com/news/articles/SB10000872396390444709004577652201640230514.

11. L. Hand, "Healthcare-Associated Infections Still Major Issue, CDC Says," *Medscape*, March 26, 2014, http://www.medscape.com/viewarticle/822612.

12. S. Sternberg, "Medical Errors Harm Huge Number of Patients," *US News & World Report*, August 28, 2012, http://health.usnews.com/health-news/articles/2012/08/28/medical-errors-harm-huge-number-of-patients?page=4.

13. S. S. Magill et al., "Multistate Point-Prevalence Survey of Health Care–Associated Infections," *New England Journal of Medicine* 370 (2014): 1198–1208.

14. W. Hudson, "1 in 25 Patients Gets Infection in Hospital," *CNN*, March 26, 2014, http://www.cnn.com/2014/03/26/health/hospital-infections/.

15. C. Russell, "The Alarming Rate of Errors in the ICU," *The Atlantic*, August 28, 2012, http://www.theatlantic.com/health/archive/2012/08/the-alarming-rate-of-errors-in-the-icu/261650/.

16. T. Weber, C. Ornstein, and M. Allen, "Why Can't Medicine Seem to Fix Simple Mistakes?," *ProPublica*, July 20, 2012, http://www.propublica.org/article/why-cant-medicine-seem-to-fix-simple-mistakes.

17. "Survive Your Hospital Stay," *Consumer Reports*, May 2014, http://www.consumerreports.org/content/cro/en/consumer-reports-magazine/z2014/May/surviveYourStayAtTheHospital.print.html.

18. "Hospitals Are Still Awful: Movement Toward Patient Centered Care and Eric Topol's Idea," *ACP Hospitalist*, February 26, 2013, http://blog.acphospitalist.org/2013/02/hospitas-are-still-awful-movement.html.

19. E. Rosenthal, "Is This a Hospital or a Hotel?," *New York Times*, September 22, 2013, http://www.nytimes.com/2013/09/22/sunday-review/is-this-a-hospital-or-a-hotel.html.

20. Intel, "Intel Research: Global Innovation Barometer," *Il Sole 24*, November 2010, http://www.ilsole24ore.com/pdf2010/Editrice/ILSOLE24ORE/ILSOLE24ORE/Online/_Oggetti_Correlati/Documenti/Tecnologie/2013/11/Intel-Innovation-Barometer-Overview-FINAL.pdf.

21. B. Sadick, "The Hospital Room of the Future," *Wall Street Journal*, November 17, 2013, http://online.wsj.com/news/articles/SB10001424052702303442004579119922380316310.

22. "Patient Room 2020 Prototype," *NXT News*, accessed August 13, 2013, http://nxthealth.org/portfolio/patient-room-2020-prototype/.

23. J. Flaherty, "What Would the Ideal Hospital Look Like in 2020?," *Wired*, July 19, 2013, http://www.wired.com/design/2013/07/hospital-of-the-future/.

24. B. Nycum, "Why Don't New Hospital Designs Include the Patient?," *Huffington Post*, December 20, 2013, http://www.huffingtonpost.ca/benjie-nycum/hospital-design_b_4482067.html.

25. I. Bau, "Health 2.0 v.2013: Integration and Patient Outcomes Are Still Driving Health Technology—but So Should Empathy, Caring, and Communication," *Health Policy Consultation Services—Resources for Patient-Centered & Equitable Care*, October 4, 2013, http://ignatiusbau.com/?s=integration+patient+outcomes+health.

26. J.-Y. Park et al., "Lessons Learned from the Development of Health Applications in a Tertiary Hospital," *Telemedicine and e-Health* 20, no. 3 (2014): 215–222.

27. N. Fisher, "Global Study Finds Majority Believe Traditional Hospitals Will Be Obsolete in the Near Future," *Forbes,* December 9, 2013, http://www.forbes.com/sites/theapothecary/2013/12/09/global -study-finds-majority-believe-traditional-hospitals-will-be-obsolete-in-the-near-future/.

28. P. S. McLeod, "New Outpatient Treatment Paradigm Spurs Construction of 'Bedless Hospitals'; Trend May Reshape Clinical Pathology Laboratory Testing," *Dark Daily,* April 1, 2013, http://www .darkdaily.com/new-outpatient-treatment-paradigm-spurs-construction-of-bedless-hospitals-trend-may -reshape-clinical-pathology-laboratory-testing-40113#axzz3Arr352HN.

29. F. Palumbo et al., "Sensor Network Infrastructure for a Home Care Monitoring System," *Sensors* 14 (2014): 3833–3860.

30. G. Orwell, "How the Poor Die," 1946, accessed August 13, 2013, http://orwell.ru/library/articles /Poor_Die/english/e_pdie.

31. "Hospital Operators and Obamacare: Prescription for Change," *The Economist,* June 29, 2013, http://www.economist.com/node/21580181/print.

32. D. Chase, "What's the Role of a Hospital in 10 Years?," *Forbes,* July 24, 2013, http://www.forbes .com/sites/davechase/2013/07/24/whats-the-role-of-a-hospital-in-10-years/print/.

33. T. C. Tsai and A. K. Jha, "Hospital Consolidation, Competition, and Quality: Is Bigger Necessarily Better?," *Journal of the American Medical Association* 312, no. 1 (2014): 29–30.

Chapter 11

1. N. Limaye and C. I. Barash, "The Modern Social Contract Between the Patient, the Healthcare Provider, and Digital Medicine," *Journal of Socialomics* 3, no. 1 (2014): 1000105.

2. G. Satell, "In 2014, Every Business Will Be Disrupted by Open Technology," *Forbes,* December 14, 2014, http://www.forbes.com/sites/gregsatell/2013/12/14/in-2014-every-business-will-be-disrupted -by-open-technology/print/.

3. M. Harden, "Big Data for Healthcare: End of the Zombie Film Genre," *Wired,* March 20, 2014, http://www.wired.com/insights/2014/03/big-data-healthcare-end-zombie-film-genre/.

4a. J. Akst, "Networking Medicine," *The Scientist,* March 2, 2014, http://www.the-scientist.com /?articles.view/articleNo/34585/title/Networking-Medicine/.

4b. J. Stein, "Arrogance is Good: In Defense of Silicon Valley," *Bloomberg Business Week,* August 7, 2014, http://www.businessweek.com/articles/2014-08-07/silicon-valley-tech-entrepreneurs-behind-the -stereotype.

5. "3scale Infrastructure for the Programmable Web," 3scale, June 2011, http://www.3scale.net/wp -content/uploads/2012/06/What-is-an-API-1.0.pdf.

6. D. G. McNeil, "A New Test for Malaria, No Blood Required," *New York Times,* January 7, 2014, http://www.nytimes.com/2014/01/07/science/a-new-test-for-malaria-no-blood-required.html.

7. M. M. Waldrop, "Campus 2.0," *Nature* 495 (2013): 160–163.

8. N. Heller, "Has the Future of College Moved Online?," *New Yorker,* May 20, 2013, http://www .newyorker.com/reporting/2013/05/20/130520fa_fact_heller?printable=true&currentPage=all.

9. "When Waiting Is Not an Option," *The Economist,* May 13, 2012, http://www.economist.com/ node/21554157/print.

10. J. Weiner, "What Big Data Can't Tell Us, but Kolstad's Paper Suggests," *Penn LDI,* April 24, 2014, http://ldi.upenn.edu/voices/2014/04/24/what-big-data-can-t-tell-us-but-kolstad-s-paper -suggests.

11. "How Speech-Recognition Software Got So Good," *The Economist,* April 22, 2014, http://www .economist.com/node/21601175/print.

12. T. Lewin, "Master's Degree Is New Frontier of Study Online," *New York Times,* August 18, 2013, http://www.nytimes.com/2013/08/18/education/masters-degree-is-new-frontier-of-study-online.html.

13. M. M. Waldrop, "Massive Open Online Courses, aka MOOCs, Transform Higher Education and Science," *Scientific American,* March 13, 2013, http://www.scientificamerican.com/article/massive -open-online-courses-transform-higher-education-and-science/.

14. A. Schwartz, "Larry Page Wants to Open Up Anonymous Medical Records for All Researchers to Use," *Fast Company*, March 19, 2014, http://www.fastcoexist.com/3027942/larry-page-wants-to-open -up-anonymous-medical-records-for-all-researchers-to-use.

15. G. Ferenstein, "Larry Page's Wish to Make All Health Data Public Has Big Benefits—and Big Risks," *TechCrunch*, March 19, 2014, http://techcrunch.com/2014/03/19/larry-pages-wish-to-make-all -health-data-public-has-big-benefits-and-big-risks/.

16. "Larry Page: 'Making Our Medical Records Open for Sharing Will Save 100,000 Lives a Year,'" *mHealth Insight: The blog of a 3G Doctor*, March 20, 2014, http://mhealthinsight.com/2014/03/20/larry -page-making-our-medical-records-open-for-sharing-will-save-100000-lives-a-year/.

17. E. Callaway, "UK Push to Open Up Patients' Data," *Nature* 502 (2013): 283.

18. "Intel Research: Global Innovation Barometer," *Il Sole 24*, November 2010, http://www .ilsole24ore.com/pdf2010/Editrice/ILSOLE24ORE/ILSOLE24ORE/Online/_Oggetti_Correlati/ Documenti/Tecnologie/2013/11/Intel-Innovation-Barometer-Overview-FINAL.pdf.

19. S. Baum, "Survey: 90% of People Will Share Health Data, 26% Don't Care About Privacy," *MedCity News*, April 25, 2014, http://medcitynews.com/2014/04/comes-sharing-personal-healthcare -data-survey-shows-comfort-level-rising/.

20. "Personal Data for the Public Good: New Opportunities to Enrich Understanding of Individual and Population Health," Health Data Exploration Project, March 2014, http://www.rwjf.org/content/ dam/farm/reports/reports/2014/rwjf411080.

21. J. Bresnick, "Most Patients Are Willing to Share Health Data, Engage Online," *EHR Intelligence*, April 29, 2014, http://ehrintelligence.com/2014/04/29/most-patients-are-willing-to-share-health-data -engage-online/.

22. J. Comstock, "PatientsLikeMe Signs Five-Year Data Access Deal with Genentech," *MobiHealth-News*, April 2014, http://mobihealthnews.com/31960/patientslikeme-signs-five-year-data-access-deal -with-genentech/.

23. M. P. Ball et al., "Harvard Personal Genome Project: Lessons from Participatory Public Research," *Genome Medicine* 6 (2014): 10.

24. A. Sun, "From Volunteers, a DNA Database," *New York Times*, April 29, 2014, http://www .nytimes.com/2014/04/29/science/from-volunteers-a-dna-database.html.

25. M. J. Ackerman, "Confidential Patient Consult Forms for Kim Goodsell," 2012, unpublished: Mayo Clinic Cardiology.

26. R. Abelson and S. Cohen, "Sliver of Medicare Doctors Get Big Share of Payouts," *New York Times*, April 9, 2014, http://www.nytimes.com/2014/04/09/business/sliver-of-medicare-doctors-get-big -share-of-payouts.html.

27. H. Vogt, "Using Free Wi-Fi to Connect Africa's Unconnected," *Wall Street Journal*, April 13, 2014, http://online.wsj.com/news/articles/SB10001424052702303287804579447323711745040.

28. M. Kaganovich, "The Cloud Will Cure Cancer," *TechCrunch*, March 29, 2012, http://techcrunch .com/2012/03/29/cloud-will-cure-cancer/.

29. R. Winslow, "Patients Share DNA for Cures," *Wall Street Journal*, September 16, 2013, http:// online.wsj.com/article/SB10001424127887323342404579079453190552312.html.

30. J. Kotz, "Bringing Patient Data into the Open," *Science-Business eXchange*, June 21, 2012, http:// www.nature.com/scibx/journal/v5/n25/full/scibx.2012.644.html.

31. R. Winslow, "'Big Data' for Cancer Care," *Wall Street Journal*, March 26, 2013, http://online.wsj .com/news/articles/SB10001424127887323466204578384732911187000.

32a. J. C. Lechleiter, "How to Win the Super Bowl Against Cancer," *Wall Street Journal*, February 3, 2014, http://online.wsj.com/news/articles/SB10001424052702303519404579351053655838512.

32b. M. Helft, "Can Big Data Cure Cancer?," *Fortune*, July 24, 2014, http://fortune.com/2014/07/24 /can-big-data-cure-cancer/.

33. T. Hay, "Ad-Tech Entrepreneurs Build Cancer Database," *Wall Street Journal*, June 18, 2014, http://online.wsj.com/articles/ad-tech-entrepreneurs-build-cancer-database-1403134613.

34. P. C. Boutros et al., "Global Optimization of Somatic Variant Identification in Cancer Genomes with a Global Community Challenge," *Nature Genetics* 46, no. 4 (2014): 318–319.

35. D. Marbach et al., "Wisdom of Crowds for Robust Gene Network Inference," *Nature Methods* 9 (2012): 796–804.

36. A. Hartocollis, "Cancer Centers Racing to Map Patients' Genes," *New York Times*, April 22, 2013, http://www.nytimes.com/2013/04/22/health/patients-genes-seen-as-future-of-cancer-care.html.

37a. H. Fineman, "Meet Patrick Soon-Shiong, The LA Billionaire Reinventing Your Health Care," *Huffington Post,* December 1, 2013, http://www.huffingtonpost.com/2013/12/01/patrick-soon-shiong _n_4351344.html?view=print&comm_ref=false.

37b. M. Herper, "World's Richest Doctor Buys World's Most Powerful DNA Sequencer," *Forbes,* July 31, 2014, http://www.forbes.com/sites/matthewherper/2014/07/31/worlds-richest-doctor-buys-worlds -most-powerful-dna-sequencer/.

38. R. M. Plenge et al., "Crowdsourcing Genetic Prediction of Clinical Utility in the Rheumatoid Arthritis Responder Challenge," *Nature Genetics* 45, no. 5 (2013): 468–469.

39. A. Moody, "The Big Picture," *Nature* 502 (2013): S95.

40. T. Ray, "In Tackling the VUS Challenge, Are Public Databases the Solution or a Liability for Labs?," *Genome Web*, February 12, 2014, http://www.genomeweb.com/print/1348716.

41. K. Lambertson and S. F. Terry, "Free the Data," *Genetic Testing and Molecular Biomarkers* 18, no. 1 (2014): 1–2.

42. "Share Alike," *Nature* 490 (2012): 143–144.

43. H. Rehm et al., "How Genetic Data Sharing Will Revolutionize Healthcare," *Footnote1,* January 31, 2014, http://footnote1.com/how-genetic-data-sharing-will-revolutionize-healthcare/.

44. M. Andrews, "Decline on Autopsies May Obscure Understanding of Disease," *Los Angeles Times*, May 17, 2011, http://articles.latimes.com/print/2011/may/17/health/la-he-healthcare-autopsies-201105 17.

45. C. VanDerWerf, "Explainer: Can You Just Die Suddenly?," *The Conversation*, April 9, 2014, https://theconversation.com/explainer-can-you-just-die-suddenly-25423.

46. J. Erdmann, "Telltale Hearts," *Nature Medicine* 19 (2013): 1361–1364.

47. A. D. Marcus, "'Hackathons' Aim to Solve Health Care's Ills," *Wall Street Journal*, April 4, 2014, http://online.wsj.com/news/articles/SB10001424052702304179704579461284247758424.

48. B. Palmer, "Are Hackathons the Future of Medical Innovation?," *Slate*, April 10, 2014, http://www .slate.com/articles/business/crosspollination/2014/04/medical_hackathons_is_this_the_future_of_health _care_innovation.html.

49. Z. Moukheiber, "Grand Rounds Wants to Find the Right Doctor for You," *Forbes*, April 8, 2014, http://www.forbes.com/sites/zinamoukheiber/2014/04/08/grand-rounds-wants-to-find-the-right-doctor -for-you/.

50. N. LaPorte, "Medical Care Aided by the Crowd," *New York Times*, April 14, 2013, http://www .nytimes.com/2013/04/14/business/watsi-a-crowdfunding-site-offers-help-with-medical-care.html.

51. S. Lupkin, "Boy Author Raises $750K for Sick Friend," *ABC News*, February 27, 2014, http:// abcnews.go.com/blogs/health/2014/02/27/boy-author-raises-750k-for-sick-friend/.

52. J. Robinson, "Healbe Hustle: The Full Story of How a Failed Russian Cake Shop Owner Humiliated Indiegogo and Took 'the Crowd' for Over $1M," *Pando*, April 12, 2014, http://pando.com/2014 /04/12/healbe-hustle-the-full-story-of-how-a-failed-russian-cake-shop-owner-humiliated-indiegogo-and -took-the-crowd-for-over-1m/.

53. J. Cafariello, "They Told Us This Would Happen," *Wealth Daily*, April 8, 2014, http://www .wealthdaily.com/articles/they-told-us-this-would-happen/5112.

54. O. Khazan, "Have You Contributed to a Health Scam?," *The Atlantic*, June 16, 2014, http://www .theatlantic.com/health/archive/2014/06/can-you-spot-the-fake-health-gadget/372788/.

55. D. F. Craviotto, "A Doctor's Declaration of Independence," *Wall Street Journal*, April 28, 2014, http://online.wsj.com/news/articles/SB10001424052702304279904579518273176775310.

56. C. Weaver, M. Beck, and R. Winslow, "Doctor-Pay Trove Shows Limits of Medicare Billing Data," *Wall Street Journal*, April 9, 2014, http://online.wsj.com/news/articles/SB100014240527023038 73604579492012568434456.

57. N. Brennan, P. H. Conway, and M. Tavenner, "The Medicare Physician-Data Release—Context and Rationale," *New England Journal of Medicine* 371 (2014): 99–101, http://www.nejm.org/doi/full/10 .1056/NEJMp1405026.

58. P. T. O'Gara, "Caution Advised: Medicare's Physician-Payment Data Release," *New England Journal of Medicine* 371 (2014): 101–103, http://www.nejm.org/doi/full/10.1056/NEJMp1405322.

59. L. Radnofsky, "Medicare to Publish Trove of Data on Doctors," *Wall Street Journal*, April 2, 2014, http://online.wsj.com/news/articles/SB10001424052702303847804579477923585256790.

60. C. Weaver, T. McGinty, and L. Radnofsky, "Small Slice of Doctors Account for Big Chunk of Medicare Costs," *Wall Street Journal*, April 9, 2014, http://online.wsj.com/news/articles/SB1000142405 2702303456104579490043350808268.

61. L. Rosenbaum, "What Big Data Can't Tell Us About Health Care," *New Yorker*, April 23, 2014, http://www.newyorker.com/online/blogs/currency/2014/04/the-medicare-data-dump-and-the-cost-of -care.html?printable=true&currentPage=all.

62. D. Tahir, "Nobody Blames Doctors for High Medical Costs. That's About to Change," *New Republic*, April 10, 2014, http://www.newrepublic.com/article/117327/what-medicare-pays-doctors-hhs -releases-data-reimbursements.

63. S. Herron, "Ten Things to Know About Drug Adverse Events," openFDA, accessed August 13, 2014, https://open.fda.gov/update/ten-things-to-know-about-adverse-events/.

64. F. S. Collins et al., "PCORnet: Turning a Dream into Reality," *Journal of the American Medical Informatics Association*, May 12, 2014, http://jamia.bmj.com/content/early/2014/05/12/amiajnl-2014 -002864.full.

65. J. Bellamy, "Telemedicine: Click and the Doctor Will See You Now," *Science Based Medicine*, May 1, 2014, http://www.sciencebasedmedicine.org/telemedicine-click-and-the-doctor-will-see-you-now/.

66. E. C. Hayden, "Geneticists Push for Global Data-Sharing," *Nature* 498 (2013): 16–17.

67. E. Callaway, "Global Genomic Data-Sharing Effort Kicks Off," *Nature News & Comment*, March 6, 2014, http://www.nature.com/news/global-genomic-data-sharing-effort-kicks-off-1.14826.

68. B. M. Kuehn, "Alliance Aims for Standardized, Shareable Genomic Data," *Journal of the American Medical Association* 310, no. 3 (2013): 248–249.

69. G. Kolata, "Accord Aims to Create Trove of Genetic Data," *New York Times*, June 6, 2013, http:// www.nytimes.com/2013/06/06/health/global-partners-agree-on-sharing-trove-of-genetic-data.html.

70. P. Waldron, "UC Santa Cruz Researcher Leads Cancer's Digital Revolution," *San Jose Mercury News*, January 2, 2014, http://www.mercurynews.com/breaking-news/ci_24836309/uc-santa-cruz -researcher-leads-cancers-digital-revolution.

71. "Global Genomics Harmony," *Genome Web*, March 7, 2014, http://www.genomeweb.com/print /1359101.

72. V. Swarup and D. H. Geschwind, "Alzheimer's Disease: From Big Data to Mechanism," *Nature* 500 (2013): 34–35.

73. H. Rhinn et al., "Integrative Genomics Identifies APOE ε4 Effectors in Alzheimer's Disease," *Nature* 500, no. 7460 (2013): 45–50.

74. V. Marx, "Genomics in the Clouds," *Nature Methods* 10, no. 10 (2013): 941–945.

75. "Brought to Book: Academic Journals Face a Radical Shake-Up," *The Economist*, July 21, 2012, http://www.economist.com/node/21559317/print.

76. F. Berman and V. Cerf, "Who Will Pay for Public Access to Research Data?," *Science* 341 (2013): 616–617.

77. J. Esposito, "Open Access and Professional Societies," *Scholarly Kitchen*, August 1, 2013, http:// scholarlykitchen.sspnet.org/2013/08/01/open-access-and-professional-societies/.

78. M. W. Carroll, "Creative Commons and the Openness of Open Access," *New England Journal of Medicine* 368, no. 9 (2013): 789–791.

79. M. Frank, "Open but Not Free—Publishing in the 21st Century," *New England Journal of Medicine* 368, no. 9 (2013): 787–789.

80. C. Haug, "The Downside of Open-Access Publishing," *New England Journal of Medicine* 368, no. 9 (2013): 791–793.

81. J. Priem, "Beyond the Paper," *Nature* 495 (2013): 437–440.

82. J. Wilbanks, "A Fool's Errand," *Nature* 485 (2013): 440–441.

83. "We Paid for the Research, So Let's See It," *New York Times*, February 26, 2013, http://www .nytimes.com/2013/02/26/opinion/we-paid-for-the-scientific-research-so-lets-see-it.html.

84. I. Sample, "Nobel Winner Declares Boycott of Top Science Journals," *The Guardian*, December 9, 2013, http://www.theguardian.com/science/2013/dec/09/nobel-winner-boycott-science-journals/ print.

85. R. Schekman, "How Journals like *Nature, Cell* and *Science* Are Damaging Science," *The Guardian,* December 9, 2013, http://www.theguardian.com/commentisfree/2013/dec/09/how-journals-nature-science-cell-damage-science/print.

86. M. Eisen, "The Impact of Randy Schekman Abandoning *Science* and *Nature* and *Cell*," *Michael Eisen.org,* December 10, 2013, http://www.michaeleisen.org/blog/?p=1495.

87. J. Conn, "IT Experts Push Translator Systems to Convert Doc-Speak into ICD-10 Codes," *Modern Healthcare,* May 3, 2014, http://www.modernhealthcare.com/article/20140503/MAGAZINE/305039969/1246/.

88. S. Curry, "Push Button for Open Access," *The Guardian,* November 18, 2013, http://www.theguardian.com/science/2013/nov/18/open-access-button-push/print.

89. A. Swan, "How to Hasten Open Access," *Nature* 495 (2013): 442.

90. J. Novet, "Academia.edu Slammed with Takedown Notices from Journal Publisher Elsevier," *Venture Beat,* December 6, 2013, http://venturebeat.com/2013/12/06/academia-edu-slammed-with-takedown-notices-from-journal-publisher-elsevier/.

91. A. J. Wolpert, "For the Sake of Inquiry and Knowledge—The Inevitability of Open Access," *New England Journal of Medicine* 368, no. 9 (2013): 785–787.

92. D. Shotton, "Open Citations," *Nature* 502 (2013): 295–297.

93. "The Patent Bargain: An Open-Source Patent Database Highlights the Need for More Transparency Worldwide," *Nature* 504 (2013): 187–188.

94. E. Musk, "All Our Patent Are Belong to You," *Tesla Motors Blog,* June 12, 2014, http://www.teslamotors.com/blog/all-our-patent-are-belong-you.

95. W. Oremus, "Tesla Is Opening Its Patents to All. That's Not as Crazy as It Sounds," *Slate,* June 12, 2014, http://www.slate.com/blogs/future_tense/2014/06/12/tesla_opens_patents_to_public_what_is_elon_musk_thinking.html.

96. C. L. Treasure, J. Avorn, and A. S. Kesselheim, "What Is the Public's Right to Access Medical Discoveries Based on Federally Funded Research?," *Journal of the American Medical Association* 311, no. 9 (2014): 907–908.

97. D. G. McNeil, "Car Mechanic Dreams Up a Tool to Ease Births," *New York Times,* November 14, 2013, http://www.nytimes.com/2013/11/14/health/new-tool-to-ease-difficult-births-a-plastic-bag.html.

98. A. Tucker, "Jack Andraka, the Teen Prodigy of Pancreatic Cancer," *Smithsonian Magazine,* December 2012, http://www.smithsonianmag.com/science-nature/jack-andraka-the-teen-prodigy-of-pancreatic-cancer-135925809/?no-ist.

99. G. Cuda-Kroen, "Patients Find Each Other Online to Jump-Start Medical Research," *NPR,* May 28, 2012, http://www.npr.org/blogs/health/2012/05/28/153706146/patients-find-each-other-online-to-jump-start-medical-research?ps=sh_stcatimg.

100. G. Marcus, "Open-Sourcing a Treatment for Cancer," *New Yorker,* February 27, 2014, http://www.newyorker.com/online/blogs/elements/2014/02/open-sourcing-cancer.html?printable=true&currentPage=all.

101. J. N. Honeyman et al., "Detection of a Recurrent DNAJB1-PRKACA Chimeric Transcript in Fibrolamellar Hepatocellular Carcinoma," *Science* 343, no. 6174 (2014): 1010–1014.

102. A. D. Marcus, "Frustrated ALS Patients Concoct Their Own Drug," *Wall Street Journal,* April 15, 2012, http://online.wsj.com/news/articles/SB10001424052702304818404577345953943484054?mg=reno64-wsj.

103. D. L. Scher, "Crowdsourced Clinical Studies: A New Paradigm in Health Care?," *Digital Health Corner,* March 30, 2012, http://davidleescher.com/2012/03/30/crowdsourced-clinical-studies-a-new-paradigm-in-health-care/.

104. A. Hamilton, "Could ePatient Networks Become the Superdoctors of the Future?," *Fast Coexist,* September 28, 2012, http://www.fastcoexist.com/1680617/could-epatient-networks-become-the-superdoctors-of-the-future.

105. L. Scanlon, "Genentech and PatientsLikeMe Enter Patient-Centric Research Collaboration," *PatientsLikeMe,* April 7, 2014, http://news.patientslikeme.com/print/node/470.

106. N. Zeliadt, "Straight Talk with . . . Jamie Heywood," *Nature Medicine* 20, no. 5 (2014): 457.

107. A. Opar, "New Tools Automatically Match Patients with Clinical Trials," *Nature Medicine* 19, no. 7 (2013): 793.

108. T. Stynes, "Cholesterol Drug Trial Uses New Approach to Recruit Patients," *Wall Street Journal*, December 19, 2013, http://online.wsj.com/news/articles/SB1000142405270230486690457926827012 3589210.

109. A. J. Parchman et al., "Trial Prospector: An Automated Clinical Trials Eligibility Matching Program," *Journal of Clinical Oncology* 31 (2013): abstr 6538.

110. J. Walker, "Data Mining to Recruit Sick People," *Wall Street Journal*, 2013, http://online.wsj.com /news/articles/SB10001424052702303722104579240140554518458 - printMode.

111. B. Goldacre, "RandomiseMe: Our Fun New Website That Lets Anyone Design and Run a Randomised Controlled Trial," *Bad Science*, December 16, 2013, http://www.badscience.net/2013/12/ randomiseme-our-fun-new-website-that-lets-anyone-design-and-run-a-randomised-controlled-trial/.

112. H. M. Krumholz et al., "A Historic Moment for Open Science: The Yale University Open Data Access Project and Medtronic," *Annals of Internal Medicine* 158 (2013): 910–911.

113. M. Herper, "No More Secrets: Medtronic Shows How Open Science Might Work in the Real World," *Forbes*, June 19, 2013, http://www.forbes.com/sites/matthewherper/2013/06/19/no-more-secrets -medtronic-shows-how-open-science-might-work-in-the-real-world/.

114. J. S. Ross and H. M. Krumholz, "Ushering in a New Era of Open Science Through Data Sharing," *Journal of the American Medical Association* 309, no. 13 (2013): 1355–1356.

115. H. M. Krumholz, "Give the Data to the People," *New York Times*, February 3, 2014, http://www .nytimes.com/2014/02/03/opinion/give-the-data-to-the-people.html.

116. R. E. Kuntz, "The Changing Structure of Industry-Sponsored Clinical Research: Pioneering Data Sharing and Transparency," *Annals of Internal Medicine* 158, no. 12 (2013): 914–915.

117. R. Winslow and J. D. Rockoff, "J&J to Share Drug Research Data in Pact with Yale," *Wall Street Journal*, January 30, 2014, http://online.wsj.com/news/articles/SB1000142405270230374360457935122 61144315256.

118. "Discussion Framework for Clinical Trial Data Sharing Guiding Principles, Elements, and Activities," Institute of Medicine, January 22, 2014, http://www.iom.edu/Reports/2014/Discussion -Framework-for-Clinical-Trial-Data-Sharing.aspx.

119. L. Marsa, "Health Care's Big Data Mandate," *The Atlantic*, December 16, 2013, http://www .theatlantic.com/sponsored/cvs-innovation-care/2013/12/health-cares-big-data-mandate/78/?sr_source =linkedin.

120. M. Langley and J. D. Rockoff, "Drug Companies Join NIH in Study of Alzheimer's, Diabetes, Rheumatoid Arthritis, Lupus," *Wall Street Journal*, February 3, 2014, http://online.wsj.com/news/articles /SB10001424052702303519404579353442155924498 - printMode.

121. J. Comstock, "UCLA Pilots Mobile Vision Testing App for Patients with Diabetes," *MobiHealthNews*, April 23, 2014, http://mobihealthnews.com/32369/ucla-pilots-mobile-vision-testing-app-for -patients-with-diabetes/.

122. V. Marx, "My Data Are Your Data," *Nature Biotechnology* 30, no. 6 (2012): 509–511.

123. P. Cameron et al., "Crowdfunding Genomics and Bioinformatics," *Genome Biology* 14 (2013): 134.

124. K. Murphy, "Crowdfunding Tips for Turning Inspiration into Reality," *New York Times*, January 23, 2014, http://www.nytimes.com/2014/01/23/technology/personaltech/crowdfunding-tips-for-turning -inspiration-into-reality.html.

125. B. L. Ranard et al., "Crowdsourcing—Harnessing the Masses to Advance Health and Medicine, a Systematic Review," *Journal of General Internal Medicine* 29, no. 1 (2013): 187–203.

126. S. Novella, "CureCrowd—Crowdsourcing Science," *Science Based Medicine*, May 7, 2014, http:// www.sciencebasedmedicine.org/curecrowd-crowdsourcing-science/.

127. "Open-Source Medical Devices: When Code Can Kill or Cure," *The Economist*, May 31, 2012, http://www.economist.com/node/21556098.

Chapter 12

1. L. Fox, "Snowden and His Accomplices," *Wall Street Journal*, April 14, 2014, http://online.wsj .com/news/articles/SB10001424052702303603904579495391321958008.

2. N. Bilton, "Entering the Era of Private and Semi-Anonymous Apps," *New York Times,* February 7, 2014, http://bits.blogs.nytimes.com/2014/02/07/entering-the-era-of-private-and-semi-anonymous -apps/?ref=technology.

3. S. Halpern, "Partial Disclosure," *New York Review of Books,* July 10, 2014, http://www.nybooks .com/articles/archives/2014/jul/10/glenn-greenwald-partial-disclosure/?pagination=false&printpage=true.

4. D. Frum, "We Need More Secrecy," *The Atlantic,* May 2014, http://www.theatlantic.com/ magazine/print/2014/05/we-need-more-secrecy/359820/.

5. "A Robust Health Data Infrastructure," Agency for Health Care Research and Quality, April 2014, http://healthit.gov/sites/default/files/ptp13-700hhs_white.pdf.

6. H. Kahn, "Who Really Owns Your Personal Data?," *Details,* May 1, 2013, http://www.details .com/culture-trends/critical-eye/201305/sharing-biodata-on-apps-and-devices?printable=true.

7. L. Mearian, "How Big Data Will Save Your Life," *Computer World,* April 25, 2013, http://www .computerworld.com/s/article/print/9238593/How_big_data_will_save_your_life?taxonomyName =Big+Data&taxonomyId=221.

8. E. B. Larson, "Building Trust in the Power of 'Big Data' Research to Serve the Public Good," *Journal of the American Medical Association* 309, no. 23 (2013): 2443–2444.

9. J. Ball and S. Ackerman, "NSA Loophole Allows Warrantless Search for US Citizens' Emails and Phone Calls," *The Guardian,* August 9, 2013, http://www.theguardian.com/world/2013/aug/09/nsa -loophole-warrantless-searches-email-calls/print.

10. J. Glanz, J. Larson, and A. W. Lehren, "Spy Agencies Tap Data Streaming from Phone Apps," *New York Times,* January 28, 2014, http://www.nytimes.com/2014/01/28/world/spy-agencies-scour -phone-apps-for-personal-data.html.

11. J. Angwin, *Dragnet Nation: A Quest for Privacy, Security, and Freedom In a World of Relentless Surveillance* (New York, NY: Henry Holt and Co., 2014).

12. J. Angwin, "Has Privacy Become a Luxury Good?," *New York Times,* March 4, 2014, http://www .nytimes.com/2014/03/04/opinion/has-privacy-become-a-luxury-good.html.

13. M. Wood, "Sweeping Away a Search History," *New York Times,* April 3, 2014, http://www .nytimes.com/2014/04/03/technology/personaltech/sweeping-away-a-search-history.html.

14. T. Gara, "What Google Knows About You," *Wall Street Journal,* April 27, 2014, http://blogs.wsj .com/indiarealtime/2014/04/27/googles-all-seeing-eye-does-it-see-into-me-clearly-or-darkly/tab/print/.

15. M. Sopfner, "Why We Fear Google," *Frankfurter Allgemeine Feuilleton,* April 17, 2014, http:// www.faz.net/-gsf-7oid8.

16. D. Talbot, "Ultraprivate Smartphones: New Models Built with Security and Privacy in Mind Reflect the Zeitgeist of the Snowden Era," *MIT Technology Review,* April 23, 2014, http://www .technologyreview.com/featuredstory/526496/ultraprivate-smartphones/.

17. G. Schmidt, "Cellphone Cases to Prepare You for Anything, Even a Flat Tire," *New York Times,* April 24, 2014, http://www.nytimes.com/2014/04/24/technology/personaltech/cellphone-cases-to -prepare-you-for-anything-even-a-flat-tire.html.

18. K. Wagstaff, "Anonymous, Inc.: The Corporate Set Embraces Digital Ephemerality," *Wall Street Journal,* May 29, 2014, http://online.wsj.com/articles/anonymous-inc-the-corporate-set-embraces-digital -ephemerality-1401378250.

19. E. Mills, "Obama Unveils Consumer Privacy Bill of Rights," *CNET,* February 22, 2012, http:// www.cnet.com/news/obama-unveils-consumer-privacy-bill-of-rights/.

20. S. Lohr, "White House Tech Advisers: Online Privacy Is a 'Market Failure,'" *New York Times,* May 5, 2014, http://bits.blogs.nytimes.com/2014/05/05/white-house-tech-advisers-online-privacy-is -a-market-failure/.

21. S. Lyon, "Obama's Orwellian Image Control," *New York Times,* December 12, 2013, http://www .nytimes.com/2013/12/12/opinion/obamas-orwellian-image-control.html.

22. T. Simonite, "Five Things Obama's Big Data Experts Warned Him About," *MIT Technology Review,* May 1, 2014, http://www.technologyreview.com/view/527071/five-things-obamas-big-data -experts-warned-him-about/.

23. "Report to the President: Big Data and Privacy: A Technological Perspective," President's Council of Advisors on Science and Technology, May 2014, http://www.whitehouse.gov/sites/default/files/ microsites/ostp/PCAST/pcast_big_data_and_privacy_-_may_2014.pdf.

24. "Big Data: Seizing Opportunities, Preserving Values," Executive Office of the President, May 1, 2014, http://www.whitehouse.gov/sites/default/files/docs/big_data_privacy_report_may_1_2014 .pdf.

25. A. C. Madrigal, "I'm Being Followed: How Google—and 104 Other Companies—Are Tracking Me on the Web," *The Atlantic,* February 2014, http://www.theatlantic.com/technology/print/2012/02/ im-being-foll%C951-and-104-other-companies-151-are-tracking-me-on-the-web/253758/.

26. S. Wolfram, "Data Science of the Facebook World," *Stephen Wolfram Blog,* April 24, 2014, http:// blog.stephenwolfram.com/2013/04/data-science-of-the-facebook-world/.

27. D. Mann, "1984 in 2014," *EP Studios Software,* April 21, 2014, http://www.epstudiossoftware .com/?p=1411.

28. H. Kelly, "After Boston: The Pros and Cons of Surveillance Cameras," *CNN,* April 26, 2013, http://www.cnn.com/2013/04/26/tech/innovation/security-cameras-boston-bombings/.

29. S. Clifford and Q. Hardy, "Attention, Shoppers: Store Is Tracking Your Cell," *New York Times,* July 15, 2013, http://www.nytimes.com/2013/07/15/business/attention-shopper-stores-are-tracking-your -cell.html.

30. C. Duhigg, "How Companies Learn Your Secrets," *New York Times,* February 19, 2012, http:// www.nytimes.com/2012/02/19/magazine/shopping-habits.html.

31. K. Hill, "How Target Figured Out a Teen Girl Was Pregnant Before Her Father Did," *Forbes,* February 16, 2014, http://www.forbes.com/sites/kashmirhill/2012/02/16/how-target-figured-out-a-teen -girl-was-pregnant-before-her-father-did/print/.

32. C. C. Miller and S. Sengupta, "Selling Secrets of Phone Users to Advertisers," *New York Times,* October 6, 2013, http://www.nytimes.com/2013/10/06/technology/selling-secrets-of-phone-users-to -advertisers.html.

33a. D. Talbot, "Now Your Phone's Tilt Sensor Can Identify You," *MIT Technology Review,* May 1, 2014, http://www.technologyreview.com/news/527031/now-your-phones-tilt-sensor-can-identify-you/.

33b. Q. Hardy, "How Urban Anonymity Disappears When All Data Is Tracked," *New York Times Bits,* April 19, 2014, http://bits.blogs.nytimes.com/2014/04/19/how-urban-anonymity-disappears-when-all -data-is-tracked/?_php=true&_type=blogs&_r=0.

34. B. Morais, "Through a Face Scanner Darkly," *New Yorker,* January 31, 2014, http://www .newyorker.com/online/blogs/elements/2014/02/through-a-face-scanner-darkly.html?printable =true&currentPage=all.

35. N. Singer, "When No One Is Just a Face in the Crowd," *New York Times,* February 2, 2014, http://www.nytimes.com/2014/02/02/technology/when-no-one-is-just-a-face-in-the-crowd.html.

36. "The Face Recognition Algorithm That Finally Outperforms Humans," *Medium,* April 22, 2014, https://medium.com/the-physics-arxiv-blog/2c567adbf7fc.

37. D. Cardwell, "At Newark Airport, the Lights Are On, and They're Watching You," *New York Times,* February 18, 2014, http://www.nytimes.com/2014/02/18/business/at-newark-airport-the-lights -are-on-and-theyre-watching-you.html.

38. "Clever Cities: The Multiplexed Metropolis," *The Economist,* September 15, 2014, http://www .economist.com/node/21585002/print.

39. "Biometric Technology Identifies One of the Boston Marathon Bombers," *Homeland Security News Wire,* May 28, 2013, http://www.homelandsecuritynewswire.com/dr20130527-biometric -technology-identifies-one-of-the-boston-marathon-bombers.

40. D. Eggers, *The Circle* (San Francisco, CA: McSweeney's Books, 2013).

41. M. Atwood, "When Privacy Is Theft," *New York Review of Books,* November 21, 2013, http:// www.nybooks.com/articles/archives/2013/nov/21/eggers-circle-when-privacy-is-theft/?pagination =false&printpage=true.

42. J. Nocera, "A World Without Privacy," *New York Times,* October 15, 2013, http://www.nytimes .com/2013/10/15/opinion/nocera-a-world-without-privacy.html.

43. A. Townsend, *Smart Cities: Big Data, Civic Hackers, and the Quest for a New Utopia* (New York, NY: W. W. Norton & Co., 2013).

44. S. Kroft, "The Data Brokers: Selling Your Personal Information," *CBS News,* March 9, 2014, http://www.cbsnews.com/news/the-data-brokers-selling-your-personal-information/.

45. A. E. Marwick, "How Your Data Are Being Deeply Mined," *New York Review of Books*, January 9, 2014, http://www.nybooks.com/articles/archives/2014/jan/09/how-your-data-are-being-deeply-mined /?pagination=false&printpage=true.

46. N. Singer, "A Student-Data Collector Drops Out," *New York Times,* April 27, 2014, http://www .nytimes.com/2014/04/27/technology/a-student-data-collector-drops-out.html.

47. J. Lanier, "How Should We Think About Privacy?," *Scientific American* 309, no. 5 (2013): 64–71.

48. D. M. Jackson, "When Meta Met Data," *New York Times*, October 4, 2013, http://www.nytimes .com/2013/10/06/magazine/when-meta-met-data.html?pagewanted=all.

49. R. J. Rosen, "Stanford Researchers: It Is Trivially Easy to Match Metadata to Real People," *The Atlantic*, December 2013, http://www.theatlantic.com/technology/print/2013/12/stanford-researchers-it -is-trivially-easy-to-match-metadata-to-real-people/282642/.

50. T. Lahey, "A Watchful Eye in Hospitals," *New York Times*, February 17, 2014, http://www .nytimes.com/2014/02/17/opinion/a-watchful-eye-in-hospitals.html.

51. S. D. Hall, "Medical Identity Theft Up 20% Since 2012," *Fierce Health IT,* September 12, 2013, http://www.fiercehealthit.com/story/how-to-prevent-medical-identity-theft/2013-09-12.

52. M. Ollove, "The Rise of Medical Identity Theft in Healthcare," *Kaiser Health News*, February 7, 2014, http://www.kaiserhealthnews.org/Stories/2014/February/07/Rise-of-indentity-theft.aspx.

53. M. Madden, "More Online Americans Say They've Experienced a Personal Data Breach," *Pew Research*, April 14, 2014, http://www.pewresearch.org/fact-tank/2014/04/14/more-online-americans-say -theyve-experienced-a-personal-data-breach/.

54. "Better Information Means Better Care," NHS, January 14, 2014, http://www.england.nhs.uk/ wp-content/uploads/2014/01/cd-leaflet-01-14.pdf.

55. "Careless.data," *Nature* 507 (2014): 7.

56. B. Goldacre, "Care.data Is in Chaos. It Breaks My Heart," *The Guardian*, February 28, 2014, http://www.theguardian.com/commentisfree/2014/feb/28/care-data-is-in-chaos/print.

57. E. Callaway, "UK Push to Open Up Patients' Data," *Nature* 502 (2013): 283.

58. L. Donnelly, "Patient Records Should Not Have Been Sold, NHS Admits," *Telegraph,* February 24, 2014, http://www.telegraph.co.uk/health/nhs/10659147/Patient-records-should-not-have-been-sold -NHS-admits.html.

59. R. Ramesh, "NHS Patient Data to Be Made Available for Sale to Drug and Insurance Firms," *The Guardian*, January 19, 2014, http://www.theguardian.com/society/2014/jan/19/nhs-patient-data -available-companies-buy/print.

60. J. Best, "Big Doubts on Big Data: Why I Won't Be Sharing My Medical Data with Anyone—yet," *ZDNet,* February 19, 2014, http://www.zdnet.com/uk/big-doubts-on-big-data-why-i-wont-be-sharing -my-medical-data-with-anyone-yet-7000026497/.

61. S. Knapton, "Health Records of Every NHS Patient to Be Shared in Vast Database," *Telegraph,* January 10, 2014, http://www.telegraph.co.uk/news/10565160/Health-records-of-every-NHS-patient-to -be-shared-in-vast-database.html.

62. C. Manson, "Could Controversial Data Sharing Be Good for Patient Health?," *The Guardian*, April 22, 2014, http://www.theguardian.com/healthcare-network/2014/apr/22/controversial-data -sharing-good-patient-health/print.

63. J. Comstock, "Health App Makers Face Privacy and Security Regulation from Many Quarters," *MobiHealthNews*, January 28, 2014, http://mobihealthnews.com/29336/health-app-makers-face-privacy -and-security-regulation-from-many-quarters/.

64. H. Smith, "mHealth and HIPAA Breaches—Where Are They?," *What's Harold In*, February 16, 2014, http://whats.harold.in/2014/02/mhealth-and-hipaa-breaches-where-are.html.

65. J. L. Hall, and D. McGraw, "For Telehealth to Succeed, Privacy and Security Risks Must Be Identified and Addressed," *Health Affairs* 33, no. 2 (2014): 216–221.

66. "Privacy Rights Clearinghouse Releases Study: Mobile Health and Fitness Apps: What Are the Privacy Risks?," Privacy Rights Clearinghouse, July 15, 2013, http://www.privacyrights.org/mobile -medical-apps-privacy-alert.

67. A. Carrns, "Free Apps for Nearly Every Health Problem, but What About Privacy?," *New York Times*, September 12, 2013, http://www.nytimes.com/2013/09/12/your-money/free-apps-for-nearly-every-health-problem-but-what-about-privacy.html.

68. A. Campbell, "Dispatch Software for Trucking: How GPS Tracking Systems Affect Performance," *Trucking Office*, August 21, 2013, http://www.truckingoffice.com/2013/dispatch-software-for-trucking-how-gps-tracking-systems-affect-performance.

69. N. Greenfieldboyce, "Indie Truckers: Keep Big Brother Out of My Cab," *NPR*, April 20, 2011, http://www.npr.org/2011/04/20/135507979/indie-truckers-keep-big-brother-out-of-my-cab.

70. B. Greene, "How Your Boss Can Keep You on a Leash," *CNN*, February 2, 2014, http://www.cnn.com/2014/02/02/opinion/greene-corporate-surveillance/index.html?iref=allsearch.

71. H. J. Wilson, "Wearable Gadgets Transform How Companies Do Business," *Wall Street Journal*, October 20, 2013, http://online.wsj.com/news/articles/SB10001424052702303796404579099203059125112.

72. T. Simonite, "Using a Smartphone's Eyes and Ears to Log Your Every Move," *MIT Technology Review*, July 4, 2013, http://www.technologyreview.com/news/516566/using-a-smartphones-eyes-and-ears-to-log-your-every-move/.

73. L. Eadicicco, "What Fitbit and Nest Are Doing with Your Data," *Slate*, April 19, 2014, http://www.slate.com/blogs/business_insider/2014/04/19/fitbit_nest_data_how_the_companies_are_making_money_off_you.html.

74. A. Pai, "Nielsen: 46 Million People Used Fitness Apps in January," in *MobiHealthNews*, April 17, 2014, http://mobihealthnews.com/32183/nielsen-46-million-people-used-fitness-apps-in-january/.

75. T. Klosowski, "Lots of Health Apps Are Selling Your Data. Here's Why," *Lifehacker*, May 9, 2014, http://lifehacker.com/lots-of-health-apps-are-selling-your-data-heres-why-1574001899.

76. C. Rubin, "Your Trainer Saw That," *New York Times*, April 17, 2014, http://www.nytimes.com/2014/04/17/fashion/devices-like-fitbit-and-up24-being-used-by-gyms-to-track-clients-fitness-activity.html.

77. T. Lee, "Hackers Break into Networks of 3 Big Medical Device Makers," *SF Gate*, February 8, 2014, http://m.sfgate.com/news/article/Hackers-break-into-networks-of-3-big-medical-5217780.php.

78. R. Pierson, "FDA Urges Protection of Medical Devices from Cyber Threats," *Medscape*, 2013, http://www.medscape.com/viewarticle/806269_print.

79. A. Sarvestani, "Boston Children's Hospital Faces Cyber Threats—Are the Medical Devices Safe?," *Mass Device*, April 24, 2014, http://www.massdevice.com/news/boston-childrens-hospital-faces-cyber-threats-are-medical-devices-safe?page=show.

80. D. Talbot, "Encrypted Heartbeats Keep Hackers from Medical Implants," *MIT Technology Review*, September 16, 2013, http://www.technologyreview.com/news/519266/encrypted-heartbeats-keep-hackers-from-medical-implants/.

81. K. Zetter, "It's Insanely Easy to Hack Hospital Equipment," *Wired*, April 25, 2014, http://www.wired.com/2014/04/hospital-equipment-vulnerable/.

82. L. Hood, "Your Body Is the Next Frontier in Cybercrime," *The Conversation*, October 1, 2013, https://theconversation.com/your-body-is-the-next-frontier-in-cybercrime-18771.

83. J. A. Finkle, "A Security Firm Has Hired the Diabetic Who Hacked into His Own Insulin Pump to Show How It Could Be Used to Kill People," *Business Insider*, May 30, 2014, http://www.businessinsider.com/r-rapid7-hires-jay-radcliffe-diabetic-who-hacked-his-insulin-pump-2014-29.

84. N. Perlroth, "Heartbleed Highlights a Contradiction in the Web," *New York Times*, April 19, 2014, http://www.nytimes.com/2014/04/19/technology/heartbleed-highlights-a-contradiction-in-the-web.html.

85. N. Perlroth and Q. Hardy, "Heartbleed Flaw Could Reach Beyond Websites to Digital Devices, Experts Say," *New York Times*, April 11, 2014, http://www.nytimes.com/2014/04/11/business/security-flaw-could-reach-beyond-websites-to-digital-devices-experts-say.html.

86. R. Merkel, "How the Heartbleed Bug Reveals a Flaw in Online Security," *The Conversation*, April 11, 2014, https://theconversation.com/how-the-heartbleed-bug-reveals-a-flaw-in-online-security-25536.

87. "CyberRx Health Industry Cyber Threat Exercise, Spring 2014," HITRUST Alliance Inc., April 21, 2014, http://hitrustalliance.net/content/uploads/2014/05/CyberRX_Preliminary_Report.pdf.

88a. J. Conn, "Cybersecurity Test Finds Healthcare Communications Weak Links," *Modern Health-care*, April 21, 2014, http://www.modernhealthcare.com/article/20140421/NEWS/304219940/.

88b. E. D. Perakslis, "Cybersecurity in Health Care," *New England Journal of Medicine* 371, no. 5 (2014): 395–397.

88c. D. J. Nigrin, "When 'Hacktivists' Target Your Hospital," *New England Journal of Medicine* 371, no. 5 (2014): 393–395.

88d. N. Perlroth, "Hack of Community Health Systems Affects 4.5 Million Patients," *New York Times*, August 18, 2014, http://bits.blogs.nytimes.com/2014/08/18/hack-of-community-health-systems-affects -4-5-million-patients/?ref=health.

89. C. Wiltz, "Report: Healthcare Cybersecurity Appalling, Legislation Not Enough," MDDI, April 7, 2014, http://www.mddionline.com/article/report-healthcare-cybersecurity-legislation-not -enough.

90. L. Miller, "The Google of Spit," *New York Magazine,* April 22, 2014, http://nymag.com/news/ features/23andme-2014-4/.

91. Y. Erlich and A. Narayanan, "Routes for Breaching and Protecting Genetic Privacy," *Nature Reviews Genetics* 15 (2014): 409–421.

92. K. Peikoff, "Fearing Punishment for Bad Genes," *New York Times*, April 8, 2014, http://www .nytimes.com/2014/04/08/science/fearing-punishment-for-bad-genes.html.

93. B. M. Knoppers, "It's Yet to Be Shown That Discrimination Exists," *New York Times*, April 14, 2014, http://www.nytimes.com/roomfordebate/2014/04/14/dna-and-insurance-fate-and-risk/its-yet-to -be-shown-that-genetic-discrimination-exists.

94. Y. Joly, I. N. Feze, and J. Simard, "Genetic Discrimination and Life Insurance: A Systematic Review of the Evidence," *BMC Medicine* 11 (2013): 25.

95. A. S. Macdonald, "Risks Are Too Small for Insurers to Worry," *New York Times*, April 14, 2014, http://www.nytimes.com/roomfordebate/2014/04/14/dna-and-insurance-fate-and-risk/risks-are-too -small-for-insurers-to-worry.

96. G. Gruber, "Guarantee Privacy to Ensure Proper Treatment," *New York Times,* April 14, 2014, http://www.nytimes.com/roomfordebate/2014/04/14/dna-and-insurance-fate-and-risk/guarantee -privacy-to-ensure-proper-genetic-treatment.

97. M. Gymrek et al., "Identifying Personal Genomes by Surname Inference," *Science* 339 (2013): 321–324.

98. P. Aldhous, "Genetic Mugshot Recreates Faces from Nothing but DNA," *New Scientist*, March 20, 2014, http://www.newscientist.com/article/mg22129613.600-genetic-mugshot-recreates-faces-from -nothing-but-dna.html.

99. O. Solon, "Algorithm Identifies Rare Genetic Disorders from Family Pics," *Wired,* June 24, 2014, http://www.wired.co.uk/news/archive/2014-06/24/facial-identification-genetic-disorders.

100. M. Angrist, "Open Window: When Easily Identifiable Genomes and Traits Are in the Public Domain," *PLoS One* 9, no. 3 (2014): e92060.

101. S. E. Brenner, "Be Prepared for the Big Genome Leak," *Nature* 498 (2013): 139.

102. D. Hernandez, "Selling Your Most Personal Item: You," *Wired,* March 27, 2013, http://www .wired.com/business/2013/03/miinome-genetic-marketplace/.

103. J. E. Lunshof, G. M. Church, and B. Prainsack, "Raw Personal Data: Providing Access," *Science* 343 (2014): 373–374.

104. B. Dolan, "In-Depth: Consumer Health and Data Privacy Issues Beyond HIPAA," *MobiHealth-News,* May 23, 2014, http://mobihealthnews.com/33393/in-depth-consumer-health-and-data-privacy -issues-beyond-hipaa/.

105. S. Fairclough, "Physiological Data Must Remain Confidential," *Nature* 505 (2014): 263.

Chapter 13

1. E. Brynjolfsson and A. McAfee, *The Second Machine Age* (New York, NY: W.W. Norton & Co., 2013).

2. D. Hardawar, "Predictive Tech Is Getting Smarter and More Pervasive—but More Controversial, Too," *Venture Beat,* March 15, 2014, http://venturebeat.com/2014/03/15/predictive-tech-is-getting -smarter-and-more-pervasive-but-more-controversial-too/.

3. V. Khosla, "Do We Need Doctors Or Algorithms?," *TechCrunch*, January 10, 2012, http:// techcrunch.com/2012/01/10/doctors-or-algorithms/.

4. M. Kinsley, "Have You Lost Your Mind?," *New Yorker,* April 28, 2014, http://www.newyorker .com/reporting/2014/04/28/140428fa_fact_kinsley.

5. "A Survey of the Future of Medicine," *The Economist,* March 19, 1994, http://www.highbeam .com/doc/1G1-15236568.html.

6. E. Topol, "Individualized Medicine from Prewomb to Tomb," *Cell* 157 (2014): 241–253.

7a. M. Petronzio, "How One Woman Hid Her Pregnancy from Big Data," *Mashable*, April 26, 2014, http://mashable.com/2014/04/26/big-data-pregnancy/.

7b. D. Harris, "How Machine Learning is Saving Lives While Saving Hospitals Money," *Gigaom,* July 14, 2014, http://gigaom.com/2014/07/14/how-machine-learning-is-saving-lives-while-saving -hospitals-money/.

7c. M. Evans, "Data Collection Could Stump Next Phase of Predictive Analytics," *Modern Healthcare,* July 12, 2014, http://www.modernhealthcare.com/article/20140712/MAGAZINE/307129969 /?template=printpicart.

8. A. Pandey, K. Abdullah, and M. H. Drazner, "Impact of Vice President Cheney on Public Interest in Left Ventricular Assist Devices and Heart Transplantation," *American Journal of Cardiology* 113 (2014): 1529–1531.

9. C. Anderson, "The End of Theory: The Data Deluge Makes the Scientific Method Obsolete," *Wired*, June 23, 2008, http://archive.wired.com/science/discoveries/magazine/16-07/pb_theory.

10. D. Butler, "Web Data Predict Flu," *Nature* 456 (2008): 287–288.

11. S. Cook et al., "Assessing Google Flu Trends Performance in the United States During the 2009 Influenza Virus A (H1N1) Pandemic," *PLoS One* 6, no. 8 (2011): e23610.

12. J. Ginsberg et al., "Detecting Influenza Epidemics Using Search Engine Query Data," *Nature* 457 (2009): 1012–1015.

13. D. Lazer et al., "The Parable of Google Flu: Traps in Big Data Analysis," *Science* 343 (2014): 1203–1205.

14. A. C. Madrigal, "In Defense of Google Flu Trends," *The Atlantic,* March 2014, http://www .theatlantic.com/technology/print/2014/03/in-defense-of-google-flu-trends/359600/.

15. S. Lohr, "Google Flu Trends: The Limits of Big Data," *New York Times*, March 28, 2014, http:// bits.blogs.nytimes.com/2014/03/28/google-flu-trends-the-limits-of-big-data/.

16. B. Schiller, "Predicting Contagious Outbreaks Using Your Most Popular Friends," *Fast Company*, April 25, 2014, http://www.fastcoexist.com/3029058/predicting-contagious-outbreaks-using-your-most -popular-friends.

17. D. Butler, "When Google Got Flu Wrong," *Nature* 494 (2013): 155–156.

18. T. Harford, "Big Data: Are We Making a Big Mistake?," *Financial Times,* March 28, 2014, http:// www.ft.com/intl/cms/s/2/21a6e7d8-b479-11e3-a09a-00144feabdc0.html-axzz2yJNfSGDx.

19. M. Krenchel and C. Madsbjerg, "Your Big Data Is Worthless If You Don't Bring It Into the Real World," *Wired,* April 11, 2014, http://www.wired.com/2014/04/your-big-data-is-worthless-if-you-dont -bring-it-into-the-real-world/.

20. G. Marcus and E. Davis, "Eight (No, Nine!) Problems With Big Data," *New York Times*, April 7, 2014, http://www.nytimes.com/2014/04/07/opinion/eight-no-nine-problems-with-big-data.html.

21a. M. Garcia-Herranz et al., "Using Friends as Sensors to Detect Global-Scale Contagious Outbreaks," *PLoS One* 9, no. 4 (2014): e92413.

21b. "How A Computer Algorithm Predicted West Africa's Ebola Outbreak Before It Was Announced," Public Health Watch, August 10, 2014, http://publichealthwatch.wordpress.com/2014/08/10 /how-a-computer-algorithm-predicted-west-africas-ebola-outbreak-before-it-was-announced/.

21c. D. Spiegelhalter, "The Future Lies in Uncertainty," *Science* 345, no. 6194 (2014): 264–265.

22. N. Singer, "Listen to Pandora, and It Listens Back," *New York Times,* January 5, 2014, http://www .nytimes.com/2014/01/05/technology/pandora-mines-users-data-to-better-target-ads.html.

23. N. Singer, "When a Health Plan Knows How You Shop," *New York Times,* June 29, 2014, http://www.nytimes.com/2014/06/29/technology/when-a-health-plan-knows-how-you-shop.html.

24. S. Pettypiece and J. Robertson, "Hospitals Are Mining Patients' Credit Card Data to Predict Who Will Get Sick," *Businessweek,* July 3, 2014, http://www.businessweek.com/printer/articles/211245-hospitals-are-mining-patients-credit-card-data-to-predict-who-will-get-sick.

25. B. Molen, "Her Name Is Cortana. Her Attitude Is Almost Human," *Engadget,* June 4, 2014, http://www.engadget.com/2014/06/04/cortana-microsoft-windows-phone/.

26. M. Scott, "A Smartphone Keyboard App That Anticipates What You Want to Type," *New York Times,* June 16, 2014, http://www.nytimes.com/2014/06/16/technology/a-smartphone-keyboard-app-that-anticipates-what-you-want-to-type.html.

27. O. Malik, "The Coming Era of Magical Computing," *Fast Company,* November 18, 2013, http://www.fastcompany.com/3021153/technovore/om-malik-the-coming-era-of-magical-computing.

28. D. Nosowitz, "Can Gadgets Really Tell The Future?," *Fast Co. Design,* February 27, 2014, http://www.fastcodesign.com/3026853/can-gadgets-really-tell-the-future.

29. "Move Over, Siri," *The Economist,* November 30, 2013, http://www.economist.com/news/technology-quarterly/21590760-predictive-intelligence-new-breed-personal-assistant-software-tries/print.

30. "A Cure for the Big Blues," *The Economist,* January 11, 2014, http://www.economist.com/node/21593489/print.

31. S. E. Ante, "IBM Struggles to Turn Watson Computer into Big Business," *Wall Street Journal,* January 7, 2014, http://online.wsj.com/news/articles/SB10001424052702304887104579306881917668654.

32. J. Hempel, "IBM's Massive Bet on Watson," *CNN Money,* September 19, 2013, http://money.cnn.com/2013/09/19/technology/ibm-watson.pr.fortune/index.html?pw_log=in.

33. A. Bari, M. Chaouchi, and T. Jong, *Predictive Analytics for Dummies* (Hoboken, NJ: John Wiley & Sons, 2014), 129.

34. M. van Rijmenam, "How Machine Learning Could Result in Great Applications for Your Business," *Big Data-Startups Blog,* January 10, 2014, http://www.bigdata-startups.com/machine-learning-result-great-applications-business/.

35. N. Jones, "The Learning Machines," *Nature* 505 (2014): 146–148.

36. J. Markoff, "Scientists See Promise in Deep-Learning Programs," *New York Times,* November 24, 2012, http://www.nytimes.com/2012/11/24/science/scientists-see-advances-in-deep-learning-a-part-of-artificial-intelligence.html.

37. "Don't Be Evil, Genius," *The Economist,* February 1, 2014, http://www.economist.com/node/21595462/print.

38. J. Pearson, "Superintelligent AI Could Wipe Out Humanity, If We're Not Ready for It," *Motherboard,* April 23, 2014, http://motherboard.vice.com/read/super-intelligent-ai-could-wipe-out-humanity-if-were-not-ready-for-it.

39. E. Brynjolfsson and A. McAfee, "The Dawn of the Age of Artificial Intelligence," *The Atlantic,* February 2014, http://www.theatlantic.com/business/print/2014/02/the-dawn-of-the-age-of-artificial-intelligence/283730/.

40. S. Schneider, "The Philosophy of 'Her,'" *New York Times,* March 2, 2014, http://opinionator.blogs.nytimes.com/2014/03/02/the-philosophy-of-her/?ref=opinion.

41. A. Vance, "The Race to Buy the Human Brains Behind Deep Learning Machines," *Bloomberg Businessweek,* January 27, 2014, http://www.businessweek.com/printer/articles/180155-the-race-to-buy-the-human-brains-behind-deep-learning-machines.

42. G. Satell, "Why the Future of Technology Is All Too Human," *Forbes,* February 23, 2014, http://www.forbes.com/sites/gregsatell/2014/02/23/why-the-future-of-technology-is-all-too-human/.

43. D. Auerbach, "A.I. Has Grown Up and Left Home," *Nautilus,* December 19, 2013, http://nautil.us/issue/8/home/ai-has-grown-up-and-left-home.

44. D. Rowinski, "Google's Game of Moneyball in the Age of Artificial Intelligence," *Read Write,* January 29, 2014, http://readwrite.com/2014/01/29/google-artificial-intelligence-robots-cognitive-computing-moneyball - awesm=~our3BQPIj4IPFE.

45. T. Simonite, "An AI Chip to Help Computers Understand Images," *MIT Technology Review,* January 2, 2014, http://m.technologyreview.com/news/523181/an-ai-chip-to-help-computers-understand -images/.

46. D. Brooks, "What Machines Can't Do," *New York Times,* February 4, 2014, http://www.nytimes .com/2014/02/04/opinion/brooks-what-machines-cant-do.html.

47. S. Fletcher, "Machine Learning," *Scientific American* 309 (2013): 62–68.

48. G. Marcus, "Why Can't My Computer Understand Me?," *New Yorker,* August 14, 2013, http:// www.newyorker.com/online/blogs/elements/2013/08/why-cant-my-computer-understand-me.html ?printable=true&currentPage=all.

49a. D. Tweney, "Scientists Exploring Computers That Can Learn and Adapt," *Venture Beat,* December 29, 2013, http://venturebeat.com/2013/12/29/scientists-exploring-computers-that-can-learn-and -adapt/.

49b. J. Markhoff, "Computer Eyesight Gets A Lot More Accurate," *New York Times,* August 18, 2014, http://bits.blogs.nytimes.com/2014/08/18/computer-eyesight-gets-a-lot-more-accurate/?ref=technology.

50. M. M. Waldrop, "Smart Connections," *Nature* 503 (2013): 22–24.

51. "Supercomputers, The Human Brain and the Advent of Computational Biology," *Antisense Science,* March 29, 2014, http://antisensescienceblog.wordpress.com/2014/03/29/supercomputers-the -human-brain-and-the-advent-of-computational-biology/.

52. M. Starr, "Brain-Inspired Circuit Board 9000 Times Faster Than an Average PC," *CNET,* May 1, 2014, http://m.cnet.com.au/brain-inspired-circuit-board-9000-times-faster-than-an-average-pc-339 347168.htm?redir=1.

53. J. Markoff, "Brainlike Computers, Learning from Experience," *New York Times,* December 29, 2013, http://www.nytimes.com/2013/12/29/science/brainlike-computers-learning-from-experience .html.

54. E. M. Rusli, "Attempting to Code the Human Brain," *Wall Street Journal,* February 3, 2014, http://online.wsj.com/news/articles/SB10001424052702304851104579361191171330498.

55. N. B. Turk-Browne, "Functional Interactions as Big Data in the Human Brain," *Science* 342, no. 6158 (2013): 580–584.

56. D. M. Wenger and A. F. Ward, "The Internet Has Become the External Hard Drive for Our Memories," *Scientific American,* November 19, 2013, http://www.scientificamerican.com/article/the -internet-has-become-the-external-hard-drive-for-our-memories/.

57. "Neuromorphic Computing; The Machine of a New Soul," *The Economist,* August 1, 2013, http://www.economist.com/news/science-and-technology/21582495-computers-will-help-people -understand-brains-better-and-understanding-brains.

58. G. Marcus, "Hyping Artificial Intelligence, Yet Again," *New Yorker,* December 31, 2014, http:// www.newyorker.com/online/blogs/elements/2014/01/the-new-york-times-artificial-intelligence-hype -machine.html.

59. D. Basulto, "Artificial Intelligence Is the Next Big Tech Trend. Here's Why," *Washington Post,* March 25, 2014, http://www.washingtonpost.com/blogs/innovations/wp/2014/03/25/artificial -intelligence-is-the-next-big-tech-trend-heres-why//?print=1.

60. L. Dormehl, "Facial Recognition: Is the Technology Taking Away Your Identity?," *The Guardian,* May 4, 2014, http://www.theguardian.com/technology/2014/may/04/facial-recognition-technology -identity-tesco-ethical-issues/print.

61. M. S. Bartlett et al., "Automatic Decoding of Facial Movements Reveals Deceptive Pain Expressions," *Current Biology* 24 (2014): 738–743.

62. J. Hoffman, "Reading Pain in a Human Face," *New York Times,* April 28, 2014, http://well.blogs .nytimes.com/2014/04/28/reading-pain-in-a-human-face/.

63. S. Du, Y. Tao, and A. M. Martinez, "Compound Facial Expressions of Emotion," *PNAS Early Edition,* March 31, 2014, http://www.pnas.org/cgi/doi/10.1073/pnas.1322355111.

64. H. Ledford, "The Computer Will See You Now," *Nature News,* November 9, 2011, http://www .nature.com/news/the-computer-will-see-you-now-1.9324.

65. F. Manjoo, "Conjuring Images of a Bionic Future," *New York Times,* April 24, 2014, http://www .nytimes.com/2014/04/24/technology/personaltech/app-controlled-hearing-aid-improves-even-normal -hearing.html.

66. "What Is Bothering You Today?" Symptom Checker, the Award-winning Symcat App, accessed August 13, 2014, http://www.symcat.com/.

67a. P. Marks, "Watson in Your Pocket: Supercomputer Gets Own Apps," *New Scientist*, April 28, 2014, http://www.newscientist.com/article/dn25476-watson-in-your-pocket-supercomputer-gets-own-apps.html?full=true&print=true-.U1-0o17KR4E.

67b. H. Singh, "The Battle Against Misdiagnosis," *Wall Street Journal*, August 7, 2014, http://online.wsj.com/articles/hardeep-singh-the-battle-against-misdiagnosis-1407453373#printMode.

67c. J. Frieden, "Misdiagnosis. Can It Be Remedied?" *MedPage Today*, August 17, 2014, http://www.medpagetoday.com/PublicHealthPolicy/GeneralProfessionalIssues/47232.

68. J. O. Drife, "House," *British Medical Journal* 330 (2005): 1090.

69. "BMJ Backs HOUSE MD," *Z3*, January 17, 2007, http://z3.invisionfree.com/House_Fans/ar/t1817.htm.

70. C. J. Gill, L. Sabin, and C. H. Schmid, "Why Clinicians Are Natural Bayesians," *British Medical Journal* 330 (2005): 1080–1083.

71. R. N. Chitty, "Why Clinicians Are Natural Bayesians: Is There a Bayesian Doctor in the House?," *British Medical Journal* 330 (2005): 1390.

72. D. Hernandez, "Artificial Intelligence Is Now Telling Doctors How to Treat You," *Wired*, June 2, 2014, http://www.wired.com/2014/06/ai-healthcare/.

73. R. M. French, "Dusting Off the Turing Test," *Science* 336 (2012): 164–165.

74. G. Poste, "Bring on the Biomarkers," *Nature* 469 (2011): 156–157.

75. A. B. Jensen et al., "Temporal Disease Trajectories Condensed from Population-Wide Registry Data Covering 6.2 Million Patients," *Nature Communications*, June 24, 2014, http://www.readbyqxmd.com/read/24959948/temporal-disease-trajectories-condensed-from-population-wide-registry-data-covering-6-2-million-patients.

76. C. Mims, "Forget 'The Cloud'; 'The Fog' Is Tech's Future," *Wall Street Journal*, May 18, 2014, http://online.wsj.com/news/articles/SB10001424052702304908304579566662320279406.

77. M. Cottrell et al., "Fault Prediction in Aircraft Engines Using Self-Organizing Maps," 2009, accessed from arXiv, August 13, 2014, http://arxiv.org/pdf/0907.1368v1.pdf.

78. R. Pipke et al., "Feasibility of Personalized Nonparametric Analytics for Predictive Monitoring of Heart Failure Patients Using Continuous Mobile Telemetry," Proceedings of the 4th Conference on Wireless Health, 2013, Article No. 7, accessed from the ACM Digital Library, August 13, 2014, http://dl.acm.org/citation.cfm?id=2534107.

79. C. Smith, "The Digital Doctor Will See You Now: How Big Data Is Saving Lives," *Tech Radar*, June 18, 2014, http://www.techradar.com/news/computing/the-digital-doctor-will-see-you-now-how-big-data-is-saving-lives-1253870.

80. J. Hamblin, "Who Will Watch You Fall? A Radar Detection Program for the Elderly," *The Atlantic*, April 2014, http://www.theatlantic.com/health/print/2014/04/old-americans-on-radar/360833/.

81a. P. Clark, "Innovation: Floor Tiles That Can Monitor the Health of the Elderly," *Businessweek*, March 20, 2014, http://www.businessweek.com/articles/2014-03-20/intellimat-flooring-measures-health-based-on-footstep-patterns.

81b. D. Spector, "Microchips Will Be Implanted Into Healthy People Sooner Than You Think," *Business Insider*, August 8, 2014, http://www.businessinsider.com/microchip-implants-in-healthy-people-2014-7.

82. W. Koh et al., "Noninvasive In Vivo Monitoring of Tissue-Specific Global Gene Expression in Humans," in *PNAS Early Edition*, May 5, 2014, http://www.pnas.org/cgi/doi/10.1073/pnas.1405528111.

Chapter 14

1. S. Berkley, "How Cell Phones Are Transforming Health Care in Africa," *MIT Technology Review*, September 12, 2013, http://www.technologyreview.com/view/519041/how-cell-phones-are-transforming-health-care-in-africa/.

2. A. Caramenico, "Mobile Tech to End Health Disparities," *Fierce Health Payer*, February 13, 2014, http://www.fiercehealthpayer.com/node/23277/print.

3. C. J. L. Murray and A. D. López, "Measuring the Global Burden of Disease," *New England Journal of Medicine* 369 (2013): 448–457.

4. C. Murray et al., "The Global Burden of Disease: Generating Evidence, Guiding Policy," Institute for Health Metrics and Evaluation, July 23, 2013, http://www.healthdata.org/sites/default/files/files/policy_report/2013/GBD_GeneratingEvidence/IHME_GBD_GeneratingEvidence_FullReport.pdf.

5. L. O. Gostin, "Healthy Living Needs Global Governance," *Nature* 511 (2014): 147–149.

6. B. McKay, "Tuberculosis Affects Children More Than Previously Thought," *Wall Street Journal*, March 23, 2014, http://online.wsj.com/news/articles/SB10001424052702304179704579457780012223184.

7. M. Kessel, "Neglected Diseases, Delinquent Diagnostics," *Science Translational Medicine* 6, no. 226 (2014): 1–3.

8. J. G. Kahn, J. S. Yang, and J. S. Kahn, "'Mobile' Health Needs and Opportunities in Developing Countries," *Health Affairs* 29, no. 2 (2010): 252–258.

9. R. Richards-Kortum and M. Oden, "Devices for Low-Resource Health Care," *Science* 342 (2013): 1055–1057.

10. A. Wesolowski et al., "Quantifying the Impact of Human Mobility on Malaria," *Science* 267 (2012): 267–270.

11a. D. N. Breslauer et al., "Mobile Phone Based Clinical Microscopy for Global Health Applications," *PLoS One* 4, no. 7 (2009): e6320.

11b. S. A. Lee and C. Yang, "A Smartphone-Based Chip-Scale Microscope Using Ambient Illumination," *Lab Chip* 14 (2014): 3056–3063.

12. E. K. Sackmann, A. L. Fulton, and D. J. Beebe, "The Present and Future Role of Microfluidics in Biomedical Research," *Nature* 507 (2014): 181–189.

13. "Detecting Disease with a Smartphone Accessory," *Science Daily*, June 4, 2013, http://www.sciencedaily.com/releases/2013/06/130604113959.htm.

14. A. D. Warren et al., "Point-Of-Care Diagnostics for Noncommunicable Diseases Using Synthetic Urinary Biomarkers and Paper Microfluidics," *PNAS Early Edition*, February 19, 2014, http://www.pnas.org/content/early/2014/02/19/1314651111.

15. G. Miller, "How to Make a Microscope Out of Paper in 10 Minutes," *Wired*, March 7, 2014, http://www.wired.com/wiredscience/2014/03/paper-microscope/.

16. "The $1 Origami Microscope," *MIT Technology Review*, March 11, 2014, http://www.technologyreview.com/view/525471/the-1-origami-microscope/.

17. B. Ouyang, "50 Cent Origami Microscope for Third-World Diagnostics," *MedGadget*, March 11, 2014, http://www.medgadget.com/2014/03/50-cent-origami-microscope-for-third-world-diagnostics.html/print/.

18. K. Newby, "Stanford Bioengineer Develops a 50-Cent Paper Microscope," *Scope Blog*, March 10, 2014, http://scopeblog.stanford.edu/2014/03/10/stanford-bioengineer-develops-a-50-cent-paper-microscope/.

19. J. Cybulski, J. Clements, and M. Prakash, "Foldscope: Origami-Based Paper Microscope," arXiv, 2014, http://arxiv.org/pdf/1403.1211.pdf.

20. K. Newby, "Free DIY Microscope Kits to Citizen Scientists with Inspiring Project Ideas," *Scope Blog*, March 13, 2014, http://scopeblog.stanford.edu/2014/03/13/free-diy-microscope-kits-to-citizen-scientists-with-inspiring-project-ideas/.

21. F. Alam, "Birth of the DIY Malaria Detector," *Popular Science*, January 16, 2014, http://www.popsci.com/blog-network/biohackers/birth-diy-malaria-detector.

22. C. Scott, "New Inexpensive Skin Test in Development to Diagnose Malaria in an Instant," *Singularity Hub*, January 29, 2014, http://singularityhub.com/2014/01/29/new-inexpensive-skin-test-to-diagnose-malaria-in-an-instant/.

23. D. G. McNeil, "A New Test for Malaria, No Blood Required," *New York Times*, January 7, 2014, http://www.nytimes.com/2014/01/07/science/a-new-test-for-malaria-no-blood-required.html.

24. E. Y. Lukianova-Hleb et al., "Hemozoin-Generated Vapor Nanobubbles for Transdermal Reagent- and Needle-Free Detection of Malaria," *PNAS Early Edition*, December 30, 2013, http://www.pnas.org/content/early/2013/12/26/1316253111.abstract?sid=0d140ff1-05a8-4161-84db-ac74a789ba19.

25. B. Dolan, "MIT Startup Winner Envisions Wristworn, Malaria Diagnostic Device," *MobiHealth-News,* May 15, 2014, http://mobihealthnews.com/33193/mit-startup-winner-envisions-wristworn -malaria-diagnostic-device/.

26. C. Winter, "Nanobiosym's Gene-Radar Diagnoses Diseases Faster," *Bloomberg Businessweek,* December 12, 2013, http://www.businessweek.com/articles/2013-12-12/innovation-nanobiosyms-gene -radar-diagnoses-diseases-faster.

27. A. Proffitt, "QuantuMDx Launches MolDx Indiegogo Campaign," *Bio-IT World,* February 12, 2014, http://www.bio-itworld.com/2014/2/12/quantumdx-launches-moldx-indiegogo-campaign.html.

28. M. Perelman, "Biomeme Transforming Smartphones into Convenient, Low-Cost Labs for Quick DNA Diagnostics and On-Site Disease Tracking," presented at the Scripps Translational Science Institute on September 12, 2013.

29. T. Fong, "QuantuMDx Eyeing 2015 Launch of Handheld POC MDx Device," *Genome Web,* January 27, 2014, http://www.genomeweb.com/pcrsample-prep/quantumdx-eyeing-2015-launch -handheld-poc-mdx-device.

30. S. Baum, "Biomeme's Smartphone Lab to Identify Pathogens Sets Sights on Central America," *MedCity News,* April 3, 2014, http://medcitynews.com/2014/04/biomemes-smartphone-lab-identify -pathogens-sets-sights-central-america/.

31. "Pocket Diagnosis," University of Cambridge, accessed August 13, 2014, http://www.cam.ac.uk /research/news/pocket-diagnosis.

32. A. K. Yetisena et al., "A Smartphone Algorithm with Inter-Phone Repeatability for the Analysis of Colorimetric Tests," *Sensors and Actuators B: Chemical* 196 (2014): 156–160.

33. A. H. J. Kolk et al., "Breath Analysis as a Potential Diagnostic Tool for Tuberculosis," *International Journal of Tuberculosis and Lung Disease* 16, no. 6 (2012): 777–782.

34. G. Theron et al., "Feasibility, Accuracy, and Clinical Effect of Point-of-Care Xpert MTB/RIF Testing for Tuberculosis In Primary-Care Settings in Africa: A Multicentre, Randomised, Controlled Trial," *The Lancet* 383 (2014): 424–435.

35. J. I. Gordon et al., "The Human Gut Microbiota and Undernutrition," *Science Translational Medicine* 12, no. 4 (2012): 137ps12.

36. D. A. Relman, "Undernutrition—Looking Within for Answers," *Science* 339 (2013): 530–532.

37. M. I. Smith et al., "Gut Microbiomes of Malawian Twin Pairs Discordant for Kwashiorkor," *Science* 339 (2013): 548–554.

38. E. Yong, "Gut Microbes Contribute to Mysterious Malnutrition," *National Geographic,* January 30, 2013, http://phenomena.nationalgeographic.com/2013/01/30/gut-microbes-kwashiorkor -malnutrition/.

39. A. Anthony, "I Had the Bacteria in My Gut Analysed. And This May Be the Future of Medicine," *The Guardian,* February 11, 2014, http://www.theguardian.com/science/2014/feb/11/gut-biology-health -bacteria-future-medicine/print.

40. I. Trehan et al., "Antibiotics as Part of the Management of Severe Acute Malnutrition," *New England Journal of Medicine* 368, no. 5 (2013): 425–435.

41. D. Grady, "Malnourished Gain Lifesaver in Antibiotics," *New York Times,* January 31, 2013, http://www.nytimes.com/2013/01/31/health/antibiotics-can-save-lives-of-severely-malnourished -children-studies-find.html.

42. X. Didelot et al., "Transforming Clinical Microbiology with Bacterial Genome Sequencing," *Nature Reviews Genetics* 13, no. 9 (2012): 601–612.

43. E. Yong, "Searching for a 'Healthy' Microbiome," *PBS,* January 29, 2014, http://www.pbs.org/ wgbh/nova/next/body/microbiome-diversity/.

44. P. R. Dormitzer et al., "Synthetic Generation of Influenza Vaccine Viruses for Rapid Response to Pandemics," *Science Translational Medicine* 5, no. 185 (2013): 1–13.

45. "Cancer in the Developing World: Worse Than AIDS," *The Economist,* March 1, 2014, http:// www.economist.com/node/21597962/print.

46. B. O. Anderson, "Breast Cancer—Thinking Globally," *Science* 343 (2014): 1403.

47. A. Rutkin, "Cancer Diagnosis as Simple as a Pregnancy Test," *New Scientist,* February 24, 2014, http://www.newscientist.com/article/dn25110-cancer-diagnosis-as-simple-as-a-pregnancy-test.html.

48. B. Fung, "The Cancer Screening That Runs on Your Smartphone," *The Atlantic*, April 2014, http://www.theatlantic.com/health/print/2012/04/the-cancer-screening-that-runs-on-your-smartphone/256119/.

49. H. Hodson, "Solar DNA Tests Detect Cancer Without Electricity," *New Scientist*, February 21, 2014, http://www.newscientist.com/article/dn25103-solar-dna-tests-detect-cancer-without-electricity.html#.U_TF1EuWvlc.

50. A. Trafton, "A Paper Diagnostic for Cancer," *MIT News*, February 24, 2014, http://web.mit.edu/newsoffice/2014/a-paper-diagnostic-for-cancer-0224.html.

51. S. Young, "Cheaper Cancer Gene Tests, by the Drop," *MIT Technology Review*, February 25, 2014, http://www.technologyreview.com/news/524896/cheaper-cancer-gene-tests-by-the-drop/.

52. "The Sensor Project: At the Intersection of Innovation and Global Health," ECEM, accessed August 13, 2014, https://secure.e2rm.com/registrant/LoginRegister.aspx?eventid=141287&langpref=en-CA&Referrer=http%3a%2f%2fthesensorproject.org%2f.

53. "Imaging the World Is Helping to Make Progress Toward the United Nations' Millennium Development Goal 5," Imaging the World, November 4, 2013, http://imagingtheworld.org/imaging-the-world-itw-is-helping-to-make-progress-toward-the-united-nations-millennium-development-goal-5/.

54. S. Agarwal and A. Labrique, "Newborn Health on the Line: The Potential mHealth Applications," *Journal of the American Medical Association*, July 16, 2014, http://jama.jamanetwork.com/article.aspx?articleID=1883978.

55. R. Barclay, "Smartphone Device Can Detect Preeclampsia, Saving Lives Worldwide," *Healthline News*, March 9, 2014, http://www.healthline.com/health-news/tech-mobile-pulse-oximeter-for-preeclampsia-030914.

56. J. Comstock, "Small Trial Shows $50 Smartphone Endoscope Performs Well," *MobiHealthNews*, March 10, 2014, http://mobihealthnews.com/30756/small-trial-shows-50-smartphone-endoscope-performs-well/.

57. B. Lovejoy, "Stanford University Develops $90 iPhone Accessory to Replace Ophthalmology Kit Costing Tens of Thousands," *9 to 5 Mac*, March 17, 2014, http://9to5mac.com/2014/03/17/stanford-university-develops-90-iphone-accessory-to-replace-ophthalmology-kit-costing-tens-of-thousands/.

58. D. Myung et al., "Simple, Low-Cost Smartphone Adapter for Rapid, High Quality Ocular Anterior Segment Imaging: A Photo Diary," *Journal MTM* 3, no. 1 (2014): 2–8.

59a. M. Aderholt, "Researchers 3D Print Smartphone Compatible Microscope Lenses for 1 Penny," *3D Print*, April 27, 2014, http://3dprint.com/2721/3d-print-smartphone-microscope-lenses/.

59b. A. Nemiroskia et al., "Universal Mobile Electrochemical Detector Designed for Use in Resource-Limited Applications," *PNAS Early Edition*, August 4, 2014, www.pnas.org/cgi/doi/10.1073/pnas.1405679111.

59c. A. Simmonds, "Handheld Device Could Enable Low-Cost Chemical Tests," *Nature*, August 4, 2014, http://www.nature.com/news/handheld-device-could-enable-low-cost-chemical-tests-1.15662.

60. N. Crisp and L. Chen, "Global Supply of Health Professionals," *New England Journal of Medicine* 370 (2014): 950–957.

61. G. Graham, "Leveraging Mobile Technology for Improved Public Health: Empowering Communities with Increased Access and Connectivity," *Huffington Post*, February 11, 2014, http://www.huffingtonpost.com/dr-garth-graham/leveraging-mobile-technol_b_4725698.html?view=print&comm_ref=false.

62. A. Fallon, "Virtual Doctor Project: Telemedicine Project in Zambia," *Africa Health IT News*, January 9, 2014, http://africahealthitnews.com/blogs/telemedicine/virtual-doctor-project-telemedicine-project-zambia/.

63. "Digital Life in 2025," Pew Research Center, March 11, 2014, http://www.pewinternet.org/2014/03/11/digital-life-in-2025/.

64. E. Wyatt, "Most of U.S. Is Wired, but Millions Aren't Plugged In," *New York Times*, August 19, 2013, http://www.nytimes.com/2013/08/19/technology/a-push-to-connect-millions-who-live-offline-to-the-internet.html.

65. Y. Xiaohui et al., "mHealth in China and the United States," Center for Technology Innovation at Brookings, March 12, 2014, http://www.brookings.edu/research/reports/2014/03/12-mhealth-china-united-states-mobile-technology-health-care.

66. G. Slabodkin, "Homeless Patients May Benefit from mHealth," *FierceMobileHealthcare*, September 6, 2013, http://www.fiercemobilehealthcare.com/node/10399/print.

67. S. Jackson, "Cell Phones Help Poor Diabetics with Glucose Control," *FierceMobileHealthcare*, May 20, 2014, http://www.fiercemobilehealthcare.com/story/cell-phones-help-poor-diabetics-glucose -control/2011-05-20.

68. G. Slabodkin, "mHealth Improves Care for Urban Poor Populations," *FierceMobileHealthcare*, May 10, 2013, http://www.fiercemobilehealthcare.com/node/10250/print.

69. "The Rise of the Cheap Smartphone," *The Economist*, April 3, 2014, http://www.economist.com /node/21600134/print.

70. M. Honan, "Don't Diss Cheap Smartphones. They're About to Change Everything," *Wired*, May 16, 2014, http://www.wired.com/2014/05/cheap-smartphones/.

71. H. Vogt, "Using Free Wi-Fi to Connect Africa's Unconnected," *Wall Street Journal*, April 13, 2014, http://online.wsj.com/news/articles/SB10001424052702303287804579447323711745040.

72. M. Zuckerberg, "Mark Zuckerberg on a Future Where the Internet Is Available to All," *Wall Street Journal*, July 7, 2014, http://online.wsj.com/articles/mark-zuckerberg-on-a-future-where-the -internet-is-available-to-all-1404762276.

73. D. Fletcher, "Daniel Fletcher: Why Your iPhone Upgrade Is Good for the Poor," *Wall Street Journal*, September 20, 2013, http://online.wsj.com/news/articles/SB10001424127887324492604579083762147495666.

74. A. Minter, "Your iPhone's Afterlife," *Fast Company*, November 18, 2013, http://www.fastcompany .com/3021305/junkyard-planet-your-iphones-after-life.

75. A. Toor, "Cellphones Ignite a 'Reading Revolution' in Poor Countries," *The Verge*, April 23, 2014, http://www.theverge.com/2014/4/23/5643058/mobile-phone-reading-illiteracy-developing-countries -unesco.

Chapter 15

1. E. S. Andersen, *Joseph A. Schumpeter: A Theory of Social and Economic Evolution* (New York, NY: Palgrave McMillan, 2011).

2. R. Smith, "Teaching Medical Students Online Consultation with Patients," *BMJ Blogs*, February 14, 2014, http://blogs.bmj.com/bmj/2014/02/14/richard-smith-teaching-medical-students-online -consultation-with-patients/.

3. "Alan Turing," *Wikiquote*, accessed August 13, 2014, http://en.wikiquote.org/wiki/Alan _Turing.

4. "Ignaz Semmelweis," *Wikipedia*, accessed August 13, 2014, http://en.wikipedia.org/wiki/Ignaz _Semmelweis.

5. B. Ewigman et al., "Ethics and Routine Ultrasonography in Pregnancy," *American Journal of Obstetrics & Gynecology* 163, no. 1 (1990): 256–257.

6. S. J. Reiser, *Technological Medicine: The Changing World of Doctors and Patients* (New York, NY: Cambridge University Press, 2009), 12.

7. H. J. West, D. deBronkart, and G. D. Demetri, "A New Model: Physician-Patient Collaboration in Online Communities and the Clinical Practice of Oncology," Department of Thoracic Oncology, Swedish Cancer Institute, 2012, http://meetinglibrary.asco.org/sites/meetinglibrary.asco.org/files/ Educational Book/PDF Files/2012/zds00112000443.pdf.

8. P. Wicks, T. Vaughan, and J. Heywood, "Subjects No More: What Happens When Trial Participants Realize They Hold the Power?," *British Medical Journal* 348 (2014): g368.

9. "The New Patient Revolution Is Among Us . . .," *Smart Patients*, February 1, 2014, http://www .smartpatients.com/blog/the-new-patient-revolution/.

10. J. Aw, "Patients Who Question Their Doctors Are Changing the Face of Medicine—and Physicians Are Embracing the Shift," *National Post*, March 11, 2014, http://life.nationalpost.com/2014/03/11 /patients-who-question-their-doctors-are-changing-the-face-of-medicine-and-physicians-are-embracing -the-shift/.

11. F. Godlee, "Towards the Patient Revolution," *British Medical Journal* 348 (2014): g1209.

12. J. H. Hibbard and J. Greene, "What the Evidence Shows About Patient Activation: Better Health Outcomes and Care Experiences; Fewer Data on Costs," *Health Affairs* 32, no. 2 (2013): 207–214.

13. E. Hill, "Smart Patients," *The Lancet* 15 (2014): 140–141.

14. M. R. Katz, "Katz: 'Participatory Medicine' Encourages Partnership Between Patient and Provider," *Times Dispatch,* August 20, 2014, http://www.timesdispatch.com/opinion/their-opinion/columnists-blogs/guest-columnists/katz-participatory-medicine-encourages-partnership-between-patient-and-provider/article_7cb25dfd-cbfb-505d-b164-11b5c0b45fa9.html.

15. M. Miliard, "Q&A: Eric Dishman on Patient Engagement," *Healthcare IT News,* April 10, 2012, http://www.healthcareitnews.com/print/45046.

16. "Partnering with Patients to Drive Shared Decisions, Better Value, and Care Improvement," Institute of Medicine, August 2013, http://www.iom.edu/~/media/Files/Report Files/2013/Partnering-with-Patients/PwP_meetingsummary.pdf.

17. M. Gur-Arie, "How mHealth Will Change the Doctor-Patient Culture," *Kevin MD*, March 4, 2014, http://www.kevinmd.com/blog/2014/03/mhealth-change-doctorpatient-culture.html.

18. D. Shanahan, "A Brave New World—'Research with' Not 'Research on' Patients," *BioMed Central,* May 20, 2014, http://blogs.biomedcentral.com/bmcblog/2014/05/20/international-clinical-trials-day-2014/.

19. J. Comstock, "In-Depth: Providers' Inevitable Acceptance of Patient Generated Health Data," *MobiHealthNews,* March 21, 2014, http://mobihealthnews.com/31268/in-depth-providers-inevitable-acceptance-of-patient-generated-health-data/3/.

20. L. Rao, "One Medical Group Raises $40M to Help Reinvent the Doctor's Office," *TechCrunch,* April 17, 2014, http://techcrunch.com/2014/04/17/one-medical-group-raises-40m-to-help-reinvent-the-doctors-office/.

21. A. K. Rudansky, "How Patient Generated Data Changes Healthcare," *Information Week,* September 10, 2013, http://www.informationweek.com/healthcare/patient/how-patient-generated-data-changes-healt/240161051?printer_friendly=this-page.

22. B. Dolan and A. Pai, "In-Depth: Providers' Inevitable Acceptance of Patient Generated Health Data," *MobiHealthNews,* March 21, 2014, http://mobihealthnews.com/31268/in-depth-providers-inevitable-acceptance-of-patient-generated-health-data/2/.

23. J. Sarasohn-Kahn, "Why Having Access to Your Health Information Matters," *Healthcare DIY,* March 1, 2014, http://healthcarediy.com/technology/your-medical-records-are-your-medical-records/.

24. B. Dolan and A. Pai, "In-Depth: Providers' Inevitable Acceptance of Patient Generated Health Data," *MobiHealthNews,* March 21, 2014, http://mobihealthnews.com/31268/in-depth-providers-inevitable-acceptance-of-patient-generated-health-data/.

25. J. Markoff, "A Trip in a Self-Driving Car Now Seems Routine," *New York Times,* May 13, 2014, http://bits.blogs.nytimes.com/2014/05/13/a-trip-in-a-self-driving-car-now-seems-routine/?smid=tw-nytimesbits.

26. A. Salkever, "What Google's Driverless Car Future Might Really Look Like," *Read Write,* May 28, 2014, http://readwrite.com/2014/05/28/googles-driverless-car-future?awesm=readwr.it_p20r-awesm=~oFWmYrlzbbCpi0.

27. C. C. Miller, "When Driverless Cars Break the Law," *New York Times,* May 14, 2014, http://www.nytimes.com/2014/05/14/upshot/when-driverless-cars-break-the-law.html.

28. G. Sullivan, "Google's New Driverless Car Has No Brakes or Steering Wheel," *Washington Post,* May 28, 2014, http://www.washingtonpost.com/news/morning-mix/wp/2014/05/28/googles-new-driverless-car-has-no-brakes-or-steering-wheel//?print=1.

29. R. Lawler, "Google X Built a Fully Self-Driving Car from Scratch, Sans Steering Wheel and Pedals," *TechCrunch,* May 27, 2014, http://techcrunch.com/2014/05/27/google-x-introduces-a-fully-self-driving-car-sans-steering-wheel-and-pedals/.

30. L. Gannes, "Google's New Self-Driving Car Ditches the Steering Wheel," *Recode,* May 27, 2014, http://recode.net/2014/05/27/googles-new-self-driving-car-ditches-the-steering-wheel/.

31. R. W. Lucky, "The Drive for Driverless Cars," *IEEE Spectrum,* June 26, 2014, http://spectrum.ieee.org/computing/embedded-systems/the-drive-for-driverless-cars.

32. C. Smith, "'I No Longer Have to Go to See the Doctor': How the Patient Portal is Changing Medical Practice," *Journal of Participatory Medicine* 6 (2014): e6.

33. L. Collar, "Are Physicians Still Relevant?," *Sapphire Equinox*, April 5, 2014, http://sapphireequinox .com/blog/are-physicians-still-relevant/.

34. "Walter de Brouwer: Check Your Emails—and Your Heart—with This 'Emergency Room in Your Hand,'" *Independent*, August 26, 2013, http://www.independent.co.uk/news/business/analysis-and -features/walter-de-brouwer-check-your-emails--and-your-heart--with-this-emergency-room-in-your -hand-8784569.html.

35. A. Verghese, "Prepared Text of Commencement Remarks by Abraham Verghese," *Stanford News*, June 16, 2014, http://med.stanford.edu/news/all-news/2014/06/prepared-text-of-commencement -remarks-by-abraham-verghese.html.

36. S. Strauss, "Clara M. Davis and the Wisdom of Letting Children Choose Their Own Diets," *Canadian Medical Association Journal* 175, no. 10 (2006): 1199–1201.

37. V. Mehta, "Learning from the Wisdom of the Body," *Huffington Post*, July 30, 2011, http://www .huffingtonpost.com/viral-mehta/mind-body-experience-_b_912703.html.

38. W. Cannon, "Walter Bradford Cannon," *Wikipedia*, accessed August 13, 2014, http://en .wikipedia.org/wiki/Walter_Cannon.

39. "Who Owns Your Personal Data? The Incorporated Woman," *The Economist*, June 27, 2014, http://www.economist.com/node/21606113/print.

40. Y.-A. de Montjoye et al., "openPDS: Protecting the Privacy of Metadata Through SafeAnswers," *PLoS One* 9, no. 7 (2014): e98790.

41. L. Hardesty, "Own Your Own Data," *MIT News*, July 9, 2014, http://newsoffice.mit.edu/2014/ own-your-own-data-0709.

42. "The Geek Guide to Insurance," *The Economist*, April 5, 2014, http://www.economist.com/node /21600147/print.

43. U. E. Reinhardt, "The Illogic of Employer-Sponsored Health Insurance," *New York Times*, July 3, 2014, http://www.nytimes.com/2014/07/03/upshot/the-illogic-of-employer-sponsored-health -insurance.html.

44. P. Fronstin, M. J. Sepúlveda, and M. C. Roebuck, "Consumer-Directed Health Plans Reduce the Long-Term Use of Outpatient Physician Visits and Prescription Drugs," *Health Affairs* 32, no. 6 (2013): 1126–1134.

45. A. Lewis and V. Khanna, "The Cure for the Common Corporate Wellness Program," *Harvard Business Review*, January 30, 2014, http://blogs.hbr.org/2014/01/the-cure-for-the-common-corporate -wellness-program/.

46. S. Begley, "Exclusive: 'Workplace Wellness' Fails Bottom Line, Waistlines—RAND," *Reuters*, May 24, 2013, http://www.reuters.com/article/2013/05/24/us-wellness-idUSBRE94N0XX20130524.

47. J. P. Caloyeras et al., "Managing Manifest Diseases, but Not Health Risks, Saved PepsiCo Money Over Seven Years," *Health Affairs* 33, no. 1 (2014): 124–131.

48. R. K. Parikh, "Do Workplace Wellness Programs Work?," *Los Angeles Times*, September 15, 2013, http://articles.latimes.com/2013/sep/15/opinion/la-oe-parikh-employee-wellness-programs-20130912.

49. K. Pho, "Do Corporate Wellness Programs Work?," *USA Today*, September 9, 2013, http://www .usatoday.com/story/opinion/2013/09/09/corporate-wellness-programs-column/2790107/.

50. S. R. Johnson, "Firms Revamping Employee Wellness Programs," *Modern Healthcare*, May 24, 2014, http://www.modernhealthcare.com/article/20140524/MAGAZINE/305249980/?template =printpicart.

51. "Annual Checkups Generally Don't Lengthen Lives, and They Do Carry Some Health Risks," *Washington Post*, June 30, 2014, http://www.washingtonpost.com/national/health-science/annual -checkups-generally-dont-lengthen-lives-and-they-do-carry-some-health-risks/2014/06/30/d51ff5d0 -61cb-11e3-8beb-3f9a9942850f_story.html.

52. S. Duffy, "What If Doctors Could Finally Prescribe Behavior Change?," *Forbes*, April 17, 2014, http://www.forbes.com/sites/sciencebiz/2014/04/17/what-if-doctors-could-finally-prescribe-behavior -change/.

53. M. A. M. Davies, "How to Make Wearables Stick: Use Them to Change Human Behavior," *Venture Beat*, March 2, 2014, http://venturebeat.com/2014/03/02/how-to-make-wearables-stick-use -them-to-change-human-behavior/.

54. L. Wagner, "Wellness Startups Find a Channel to Better Health: Employers," *Venture Beat*, July 31, 2013, http://venturebeat.com/2013/07/31/wellness-startups-find-a-channel-to-better-health-employers/.

55. V. Gidwaney, "How Wearables Will Transform the Health Insurance Game," *HealthWorks Collective*, May 12, 2014, http://healthworkscollective.com/veer-gidwaney/163271/how-wearables-will-transform-health-insurance-game.

56. D. Nield, "In Corporate Wellness Programs, Wearables Take a Step Forward," *CNN Money*, April 15, 2014, http://tech.fortune.cnn.com/2014/04/15/in-corporate-wellness-programs-wearables-take-a-step-forward/.

57. J. Gownder, "Wearables Require a New Kind of Ecosystem," *ZDNet*, January 30, 2014, http://www.zdnet.com/wearables-require-a-new-kind-of-ecosystem-7000025802/.

58. P. Olson, "Get Ready for Wearable Tech to Plug into Health Insurance," *Forbes*, June 19, 2014, http://www.forbes.com/sites/parmyolson/2014/06/19/wearable-tech-health-insurance/.

59. C. O. Werle, B. Wansink, and C. R. Payne, "Is It Fun or Exercise? The Framing of Physical Activity Biases Subsequent Snacking," *Marketing Letters*, May 27, 2014, http://papers.ssrn.com/sol3/papers.cfm?abstract_id=2442383.

60a. E. Topol, *The Creative Destruction of Medicine* (New York, NY: Basic Books, 2012), 126–127.

60b. N. Gohring, "This Company Saved $300k on Insurance by Giving Employees Fitbits," *Cite World*, July 7, 2014: http://www.citeworld.com/article/2450823/internet-of-things/appirio-fitbit-experiment.html.

60c. P. Olson, "Wearable Tech Is Plugging into Health Insurance," *Forbes*, June 19, 2014, http://www.forbes.com/sites/parmyolson/2014/06/19/wearable-tech-health-insurance/.

61. S. Lohr, "Salesforce Takes Its Cloud Model to Health Care," *New York Times*, June 26, 2014, http://bits.blogs.nytimes.com/2014/06/26/salesforce-takes-its-cloud-model-to-health-care/.

62. M. Sullivan, "Salesforce and Philips Partner in Ambitious Health Data Venture," *Venture Beat*, June 26, 2014, http://venturebeat.com/2014/06/26/salesforce-com-and-philips-partner-in-ambitious-health-data-venture/.

63. M. Lev-Ram, "What's the Next Big Thing in Big Data?," *Fortune*, June 2, 2014, http://fortune.com/2014/06/02/fortune-500-big-data/.

64. M. McLuhan, *The Gutenberg Galaxy* (Toronto, Canada: University of Toronto Press, 1962).

65. H. Waters, "New $10 Million X Prize Launched for Tricorder-Style Medical Device," *Nature* 17, no. 7 (2011): 754.

66. A. S. Brown, "Star Trek Comes Back to Earth," *The Bent of Tau Beta Pi*, Fall 2012, http://www.tbp.org/pubs/Features/F12Brown.pdf.

67. "The Dream of the Medical Tricorder," *The Economist*, November 29, 2012, http://www.economist.com/news/technology-quarterly/21567208-medical-technology-hand-held-diagnostic-devices-seen-star-trek-are-inspiring.

68. V. Wadhwa, "Why Our Medicine Will Soon Be Cooler Than Star Trek's," *Venture Beat*, April 7, 2014, http://venturebeat.com/2014/04/07/why-our-medicine-will-soon-be-cooler-than-star-treks/.

69. "Choosing Wisely: Five Things Physicians and Patients Should Question," ABIM Foundation, accessed August 13, 2014, http://www.choosingwisely.org/doctor-patient-lists/.

70. A. Pai, "Survey: One Third of Wearable Device Owners Stopped Using Them Within Six Months," *MobiHealthNews*, April 3, 2014, http://mobihealthnews.com/31697/survey-one-third-of-wearable-device-owners-stopped-using-them-within-six-months/.

71. "Mobile Thought Leadership," FICO, December 2013, http://www.biztositasiszemle.hu/files/201403/fico_mobile_thought_leadership_brief_global_3035ex.pdf.

72a. C. Miller, "Apple Airs New TV Ad "Strength" Focused on Wearables and Fitness Apps (Video)," *9 to 5 Mac*, June 4, 2014, http://9to5mac.com/2014/06/04/apple-airs-new-tv-ad-focused-on-wearables-and-fitness-apps/.

72b. A. D. Marcus, "A Patients' Group Scores a Win in Muscular Dystrophy Drug Research," *Wall Street Journal*, August 4, 2014, http://online.wsj.com/articles/a-patients-group-scores-a-win-in-muscular-dystrophy-drug-research-1407194541#printMode.

72c. E. Steel, "'Ice Bucket Challenge' Has Raised Millions for ALS Association," *New York Times*, August 18, 2014, http://www.nytimes.com/2014/08/18/business/ice-bucket-challenge-has-raised-millions-for-als-association.html.

73. S. Lohr, "New Curbs Sought on the Personal Data Industry," *New York Times,* May 28, 2014, http://www.nytimes.com/2014/05/28/technology/ftc-urges-legislation-to-shed-more-light-on-data-collection.html.

74a. A. Ekert and R. Renner, "The Ultimate Physical Limits of Privacy," *Nature* 507 (2014): 443–447.

74b. S. Gottlieb and C. Klasmeier, "Why Your Phone Isn't as Smart as It Could Be," *Wall Street Journal,* August 7, 2014, http://online.wsj.com/articles/scott-gottlieb-and-coleen-klasmeier-why-your-phone-isnt-as-smart-as-it-could-be-1407369163#printMode.

74c. S. Fellay, "Changing the Rules of Health Care: Mobile Health and Challenges for Regulation," American Enterprise Institute, August 4, 2014, http://www.aei.org/paper/economics/innovation/technology/changing-the-rules-of-health-care-mobile-health-and-challenges-for-regulation/.

75a. R. Hurley, "Can Doctors Reduce Harmful Medical Overuse Worldwide?," *British Medical Journal* 349 (2014): g4289.

75b. E. Dwoskin, "Big Data's High-Priests of Algorithms," *Wall Street Journal,* August 8, 2014, http://online.wsj.com/articles/academic-researchers-find-lucrative-work-as-big-data-scientists-1407543088#printMode.

INDEX

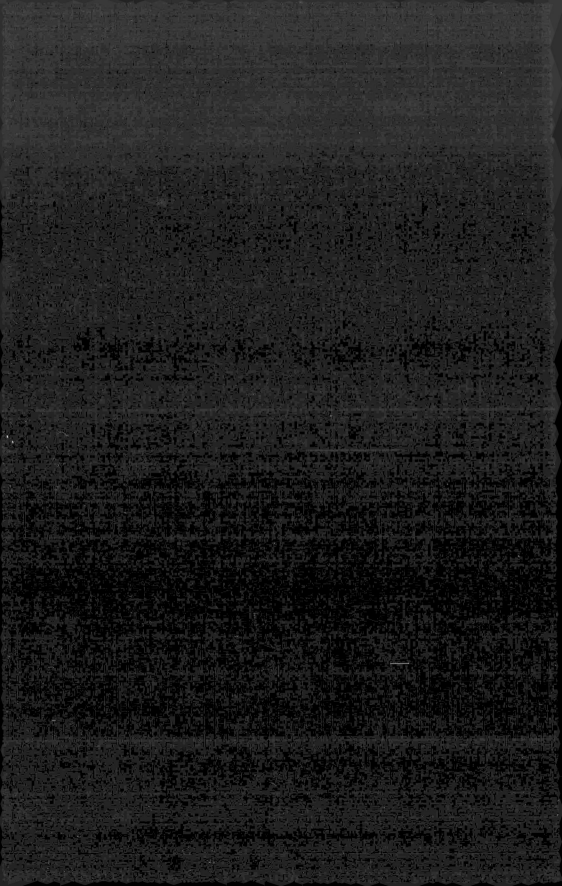